DENTISTRY AND ORAL SCIENCES

CONTEMPORARY USE OF PLANT EXTRACTS IN DENTISTRY

SCIENTIFIC EVIDENCE FOR PHYTOTHERAPY AND ETHNOPHARMACOLOGY

DENTISTRY AND ORAL SCIENCES

Additional books and e-books in this series can be found on Nova's website under the Series tab.

DENTISTRY AND ORAL SCIENCES

CONTEMPORARY USE OF PLANT EXTRACTS IN DENTISTRY

SCIENTIFIC EVIDENCE FOR PHYTOTHERAPY AND ETHNOPHARMACOLOGY

CARLOS ROBERTO EMERENCIANO BUENO
EDITOR

nova
Medicine & Health
New York

Library of Congress Cataloging-in-Publication Data

Names: Emerenciano Bueno, Carlos Roberto, editor.
Title: Contemporary use of plant extracts in dentistry: scientific evidence for phytotherapy and ethnopharmacology / [edited by] Carlos Roberto Emerenciano Bueno.
Identifiers: LCCN 2020010694 (print) | LCCN 2020010695 (ebook) | ISBN 9781536176506 (hardcover) | ISBN 9781536176513 (adobe pdf)
Subjects: LCSH: Materia medica, Dental. | Materia medica, Vegetable. | Ethnopharmacology.
Classification: LCC RK701 .C66 2020 (print) | LCC RK701 (ebook)| DDC 615.1024/6176--dc23
LC record available at https://lccn.loc.gov/2020010694
LC ebook record available at https://lccn.loc.gov/2020010695

Published by Nova Science Publishers, Inc. † New York

It's always challenging to write anything… especially a book. Keeping this in mind, we should thank all the ones who made this possible, whether in a motivational or in a contributory way.

I dedicate this book…
…to my beloved wife and daughter Vanessa & Helena Bueno.
…to my colleagues and co-authors, who made this possible.
…to my eternal supervisor Professor Eloi Dezan Junior.

Carlos Roberto Emerenciano Bueno

Contents

PREFACE

Since ancient times, mankind has used plants as a valuable source of natural products for maintaining human health, to treat or prevent diseases. The common knowledge around plants healing properties, known as folk medicine, has been transmitted over the centuries for generations among human communities. The use of natural products and herbal medicines have been documented in the past, once antibacterial activity of plant extracts has been reported since the late 1800s and some of these traditional medicines are still used, especially in the last decade, with more intensive studies for natural therapies. Active compounds produced during vegetal metabolism are responsible for the antimicrobial and biological properties, interacting with specific chemical receptors in the human body and, due to these components, plants extracts are popular as anti-inflammatory, anti-bacterial or anti-fungal drugs. However, in the absence of scientific studies, the use of aleatory plant extracts may lead to harmful adverse effects. Previously considered empirical, current data on the antimicrobial activity and biocompatibility of numerous plants have been scientifically confirmed. Phytosciences, as ethnopharmacology or phytotherapy are emerging multidisciplinary area, with almost unlimited sources and several aspects to be discussed. Recently, there has been a growing trend to seek natural drugs as part of dental treatment. In dentistry, the association of plant extracts with restorative dentistry, endodontics or periodontics materials have been used to reduce inflammation, as antimicrobial enhancer agent, antiseptics, antifungals, antioxidants, analgesics or even as mouth rinse to prevent or reduce dental plaque. Thus, this book will address the use of plant extract in different fields of dentistry, highlighting its use in cariology, restorative dentistry, endodontics and periodontics, besides other uses of herbal in dentistry. As will be shown and stated, the vast variety of different plants described in literature with medicinal properties makes impracticable to discuss all extracts found in scientific literature. Therefore, this book will contribute with some of these extracts and different methodologies to assess, as an introduction to new research and new researchers. Also, different *in vivo* and *in vitro* tests used to evaluate biological response, such as biocompatibility and antimicrobial activity in dental treatment will be discussed.

Chapter 1 - The use of herbs, herbs extracts and medicinal plants, incorporated in traditional medicine have a long and ancient history in medicine and dental practice around the world for centuries, to prevent, control or recover health against several diseases. Plants are considered the mankind's first medicine, used mainly as antiseptics, analgesics, anti-inflammatory or with antimicrobial purpose. According to the World Health Organization, near 80% of the populations of developing countries still use medicinal plants as a therapeutic resource. Over the years, many plants scientifically demonstrated biological and antimicrobial properties due to the interactions with specific chemical receptors within the body, becoming promising therapeutic agents. Thus, this chapter introduces historic findings of the use of plant extracts in archaic medicine and dentistry, initially used as medicaments for body and, consequently, oral disease.

Chapter 2 - Oral diseases are a major health problem, with periodontal and caries among the most important infectious disease, which influence quality of life. The relationship between oral disease and oral microbiota is well stablished in literature, since more than 750 species are found in oral cavity. Regardless the number of new antibiotics introduced in the market in the last years by pharmacological industry, resistance that pathogenic microorganisms develop against antibiotics has increased. Due to side effects and drug resistance, researches around the globe have been looking for new antimicrobial agents or antimicrobial enhancers, such as those from herbal sources. Medicinal plants and byproducts are constantly indicated and used throughout the world in several areas of medicine and dentistry to induce favorable responses and to treat different diseases. Also, plants naturally produce secondary metabolites that can be used as antimicrobials. There are several ways of producing herbal extracts and retrieve the active compound, as well as different tests to be performed in order to assess the antimicrobial potential. This chapter will briefly discuss the main techniques used and highlight the main properties of some compounds present in plants such as *Myracrodruon urundeuva*, Curcumin, Green tea, Lemon grass, Chamomile, Aloe Vera, Cinnamon, Psidium, Citrus and Capsicum. Due to the huge variety of plants in the literature, it is impracticable to describe all extracts with antibacterial properties. Therefore, this chapter mentions some of the extracts with such properties, which may serve as an introduction to new research and new researchers.

Chapter 3- Inflammation is an inner response of a host to an external agent, encompassing complex mediators and events. The use of anti-inflammatory substances is applicable for the treatment of some conditions. The anti-inflammatory property of phytotherapics turns them into therapeutic option to conventional medicine and stimulates studies for use in humans. Herbals are widely used in popular medicine in many countries. However, the effectiveness of many of them remains poorly accessed. So, experimental researches aiming to investigate their pharmaceutical properties are essential to determine these paths and compatibility. This chapter will embrace experiments assessing the biocompatibility of extracts through cell culture, edema induction, subcutaneous tests and associations made with different extracts aiming to enhance the effectiveness of some compounds already used in daily practice. In addition, several promising plant extracts with scientifically proved results will be described.

Chapter 4 - The use of plant extract for health treatment have been reported over the years. For the treatment of diseases that affect the oral cavity is not different, specifically for dental caries treatment. The

American Academy of Cariology (AAC) defines the cariology as "the science and art of understanding the etiology, mechanisms of the disease known as dental caries including initiation, reversal, progression, diagnosis, prognosis, risk management, prevention, non-surgical and surgical therapies, and oral health-focused outcomes." The use of herbal therapy is proposed in different stages of the mechanism of the dental caries disease, mainly in the diagnosis, prevention and treatment outcomes. This chapter will show the application of herbal therapy in the diagnosis and prevention as well as its application of herbal therapy regarding the treatment of the dental caries disease by restorative dentistry.

Chapter 5 - Studies of the herbal therapies applicability in dentistry field increase prevention and treatment of several diseases. The natural products show anti-inflammatory, antioxidant, and antimicrobial properties. According to the World Health Organization, phytotherapy is the use of herbal substances with therapeutic values, involving minimal or no industrial processing. Some endodontic materials may cause defects on the dentin and/or being an irritant to the tissues, besides of limited antimicrobial effectiveness. The herbal alternatives can prevent adverse effects of synthetic drugs as toxicity and microbial resistance. In addition, herbal products include cost-effectiveness, increase quality of life, nutritional values, easy availability and increased service life. This chapter will present studies of the several herbal alternatives with different potential in endodontic applications: irrigating solutions, intracanal medication, addition in endodontic sealer and for repair materials and other applications.

Chapter 6 - Periodontal diseases continue to be the most commonly occurring oral diseases in modern times. Plaque-induced gingivitis and periodontitis are caused by the penetration of pathogens from the bacterial plaque into the connective tissue, resulting in an inflammatory condition. Gingivitis affects the connective tissue of the gingiva, while periodontitis affects the entire periodontal apparatus. Many adjuvant therapeutic modalities have been tested for the treatment of these conditions. Among them, herbal therapies have been shown anti-inflammatory, antioxidant and antimicrobial properties. These phytotherapic are incorporated into mouth rinses, dentifrices, chewing gums, adhesives, and gels in order to prevent and even treat gingivitis. With regards to periodontitis, gels, chips, and extracts containing herbs have been shown benefits when used as adjuvants to scaling and root planing. In addition, its benefits are also observed in wound healing following periodontal surgery. Hence, this chapter will present aspects of phytotherapy in periodontics.

Chapter 7 - Alternative treatments or coadjutants should be studied and proposed, especially considering the global trend and boosting the world health organization towards natural substances and medicinal plants, regarding to their advantages as a function of its diversity, flexibility, accessibility, availability and wide acceptance. In this context, current researches have evaluated the effectiveness of natural substances, medicinal plants, phytoterapy and homeopathics: (1) as storage media for avulsed teeth or root surface treatment before teeth replantation; (2) as coadjutant to improve osteointegration and reduce peri-implantitis in dental implants; (3) as an alternative for anesthetic agents; (4) within treatment for bone remodeling during orthodontic movement or rapid maxillary expansion; (5) as hemostatic agents; and (6) as dental plaque disclosing agents. This chapter will discuss several studies regarding to all these related topics.

In: Contemporary Use of Plant Extracts … ISBN: 978-1-53617-650-6
Editor: C. R. Emerenciano Bueno

Chapter 1

EMPIRICAL USE OF PLANT EXTRACTS: HERBAL CARE IN MEDICINE AND DENTISTRY

Carlos Roberto Emerenciano Bueno*

Department of Endodontics, São Paulo State University (UNESP),
Araçatuba School of Dentistry, Araçatuba, São Paulo, Brazil

ABSTRACT

The use of herbs, herbs extracts and medicinal plants incorporated in traditional medicine has a long and ancient history going back centuries in medicine and dental practice around the world to prevent, control or recover health against several diseases. Plants are considered mankind's first medicine, which were used mainly as antiseptics, analgesics, anti-inflammatory or with antimicrobial purpose. According to the World Health Organization, near 80% of the populations of developing countries still use medicinal plants as a therapeutic resource. Over the years, many plants scientifically demonstrated biological and antimicrobial properties due to the interactions with specific chemical receptors within the body, becoming promising therapeutic agents. Thus, this chapter introduces historic findings of the use of plant extracts in archaic medicine and

* Corresponding Author's Email: dentistabueno@gmail.com.

dentistry, initially used as medicaments for body and, consequently, oral disease.

An initial historic overview will link, along this book, the millennial empirical use of plants and its extracts to actual researches and findings concerning the use of plants extracts in dentistry.

Keywords: dentistry, ethnopharmacology, medicinal plants, phytotherapy, plant extracts

Historical Use of Natural Products with Medicinal Purpose: History and Evolution

Diseases of the human mouth may be considered as ancient as humankind, even if the knowledge of its importance and the role played in systemic conditions came to evidence centuries later. Quoting the American Poet Pearl S. Buck (1892-1973): "If you want to understand today, you have to search yesterday". Therefore, if we want to understand current investigations of certain plant extracts, we have to look into the past, where our ancestors spent years discovering which plants have healthy effects and which have harmful effects, based only in observation and experience, as the most empirical way.

Herbal products have been used for centuries as a way to recover health and prevent diseases, surrounded by myths, legends and traditions, used as a therapeutic source, mainly by physicians and philosophers. In this context, the human kind depended on nature for ancient basic needs as feeding, shelters, clothing and medicines.

It's impressive to observe the large variety of medicinal plants around the world: about 70,000 plant species have been used with healing objectives (Pan et al. 2014) but it's estimated that less than 1–10% of plant species of the world have been studied chemically and pharmacologically for their potential medicinal value (Verpoorte 2000). The plant parts used in herbal therapy include seeds, berries, roots, leaves, fruits, bark, flowers, or even the whole plants (Jack 1997). Prehistoric excavations sites showed evidence that medicinal herbs were used by humans, as isolated extracts from determined plant, representing the most ancient kind of medication (Kuruppu et al. 2019). A 60,000-year-old burial site in Iraq revealed eight different medicinal plants inside the tombs, suggesting a supernatural significance and medicinal value (Pan et al. 2014).

The earliest herbal records date from a period near 2500 - 3000 BC when the Chinese emperor Shen Nong (or Shennong), considered the father of Chinese pharmaceutics, cataloged near 365 medicinal herbs and poisons (dried parts of medicinal plants), in a document titled *Pen T'sao*, freely translated as "the botanical basis of pharmacy", making this probably the first herbarium in history. Around 1,000 plants and 11,000 prescriptions were described, registered on bamboo slats (Wiart 2006, França et al. 2008). This catalogue led to one of the oldest Chinese herbal text, resulted from a compilation of general nature knowledge, nowadays republished as The Divine Farmer's Materia Medica: "...at that time, Shen Nong encountered 70 herbs in one day, determining which were medicines and which were poisons." (Yang 1998).

Interestingly, the first note of *Aloe* dates back to 2100 BC, found on Sumerian clay tables, created at the time of the King of Akkad, regarding medicinal properties of this plant, also called "plant of immortality", because its use against infections and parasites (Miraldi & Baini 2018). Queens of Egypt considered *Aloe* to be the source of their beauty and pharaohs took it in their afterlife (Petrovska 2012) while African hunters used aloe as a natural deodorant (Wiart 2006).

In ancient Egypt, the primary documents that constitute the medical treatise are the papyri of Hearst (named after Phoebe Hearst), Edwin Smith, and George Ebers. In this last one, a compilation of herbal knowledge and folk medicine was written in hieratic Egyptian dating to 1550 BC, totaling over 842 remedies for illnesses and injuries, historically known as the Ebers Papyrus, one of the oldest, longest and most complete preserved medical documents, currently kept at the library of the University of Leipzig, in Germany. Apparently, the Eber Papyrus functioned as a guide for three kinds of healers: the ones who dealt with internal and external remedies, surgeons who treated wounds and fractures, and sorcerers or exorcists, who act against the demons of disease, containing many incantations meant to turn away disease-causing demons and evidence of a long tradition of empiricism (Magner 1992, Rogers 2011).

Historic records in stone tablets from the Sumerian period left by Assyrians report inflammatory disease treatment with the use of willow leaves, in order to relieve symptoms. This may also be found in the Eber papyrus, with a complete description focusing on classic inflammatory characteristics: “When you examine a man with an irregular wound… and that wound is inflamed… [there is] a concentration of heat; the lips of that wound are reddened and that man is hot in consequence…then you must make cooling substances for him to draw the heat out…leaves of the willow”. In addition, the papyrus suggests alternatives such as onion crushed in honey (Jack 1997). Among the treatments observed in the papyrus, there is a mention to cure dental pain using the following recipe: “...knead a paste and apply on the tooth, with a part of cumin, a part of incense and a part of onion” (Ring 1998).

Opium is used since prehistoric period, known for its sedative properties. Poppy (*Papaver somniferum*) seeds were used by the Sumerians, around 5000 years ago, described as the “joy plant”. Traces of poppy seeds were also found in a Swiss Neolithic village. In addition, opium traces were found in an Egyptian tomb from the 15th century BC and around Thebes, when received the name “Theban opium”. The Ebers Papyrus describes a blend of substances using opium to effectively sedate children (Cohen 1969, Booth 1999, Duarte 2005).

In Mexican culture, ancient civilization as the Aztec and Mayan, developed several uses for medicinal herbs. The use of pepper (*Capsicum* spp.) dates back to more than 7000 years, used by the Colombian Indians, Mayas and Aztecs for treating snake bites, cold, asthma, coughs and to relieve toothaches. Capsaicin (an alkaloid that makes pepper hot) is one of the active ingredients in pepper that are related to the anti-microbial, anti-carcinogenic and analgesic properties in pepper. After the Spanish conquest, the use of local medicinal herbalism ceased because the introduction of new and different products from the Old World (Galarza

1981, Bosland 1996, Andrews 1999, Cortez-Gallardo et al. 2004, Fattori et al. 2016, Saleh et al. 2018).

Homer, the famous Greek author of *Ilia* and *Odyssey* (around 800 BC), described 63 plant species from Minoan, Mycenaean, and Egyptian Assyrian pharmacotherapy, named after mythological characters from these legendary tales: Elecampane (*Inula helenium* L) was named in honor of Elena from the Trojan War and plants from genus *Artemisia* were derived from the Greek word *artemis* (healthy) (Toplak Galle 2005, Petrovska 2012).

According to literature, Muhammad was born in Mecca around the year 570 and introduced the rudiments of oral hygiene into the Arab world, incorporating it into the Muslim religion. The prophet recommended oral hygiene with a chewing stick named *siwak* (or *miswak*), a branch from the *Salvadora persica* tree, which wood contains sodium bicarbonate and tannic acid, among other astringent beneficial compounds. The branch must be immersed in water for 24 hours until the fibers are separated, making a natural "toothbrush", giving the *S. persica* tree (or Arak tree) the common name of "tooth brush tree" (Ring 1998, Wu et al. 2001). The term "chewing stick" may mislead to an erroneous use, since the stick is chewed only briefly to separate its fibers, before use as a toothbrush (Wu et al. 2001).

Theophrastus (371-287 BC), a Greek native of Eresos in Lesbos, was the successor to Aristotle. Later known as "the father of botany" due to classification and description of medicinal plants, Theophrastus expanded botanical science with his books of Plant Etiology (De Causis Plantarium) and Plant History (De Historia Plantarium), describing more than 500 medicinal plants such as cinnamon, iris rhizome, mint, pomegranate, cardamom, monkshood among others (Petrovska 2012).

The roman Gaius Plinius Secundus, also known as "Pliny the Elder" (23 AD-79), a contemporary of Pedanius Dioscorides, was a Roman author, a naturalist and natural philosopher, but also a naval and army commander of the early Roman Empire. He travelled throughout Germany and Spain and wrote about 1000 medicinal plants in his book *Naturalis Historia* (Natural History), which became an editorial model for encyclopedias, incorporating all knowledge of medicinal plants at the time (Toplak Galle 2005, Petrovska 2012).

Historically, Marco Polo's journeys (1254-1324) in tropical Asia, China, and Persia, the discovery of America (1492), and Vasco Da Gama's journeys to India (1498), brought different medicinal plants into Europe, leading to several attempts for cultivation in botanical gardens those herbs from the new and old world (Petrovska 2012).

In North America, skulls unearthed in indigenous cemeteries showed evidence of oral infections, such as pathological bone resorption. These tribes had a wide variety of creams and potions with which they tried to maintain oral hygiene. In addition to the pleasurable effect of smoking, tobacco was also used for a cleansing effect. However, it was used for chewing associated with crushed shells, to achieve a proper consistency, causing dental erosion or tooth fracture. Plant gums, resins, and roots were also popular for oral cleansing and disease prevention. In 1788, a Quaker botanist, William Bastram, toured the southern Cherokee territory and described a variety of *Silphium*, which gum was collected by the indigenous. This amber-colored gum, after drying, had a pleasant fragrance and a slightly bitter taste, used in chewing to clean teeth and flavor the breath. When preventive treatment failed, pastes, roots, and herbs were applied inside the teeth, aiming to reduce pain and cure infection. An almost universal remedy for toothache among the local tribes, later adopted by the colonizers, was the bark of the prickly ash (*Zanthoxylum americanum*), also referred to by Europeans as the "toothache tree". Also, the first Germans to stablish in Pennsylvania learned from local tribes how to cook abele (*Populus alba*) root bark and apply the hot product to sore teeth (Ring 1998).

During the medieval period (Middle Ages), *Mandragora officinarum* was highly valued as a healing plant, used as a narcotic by the ancient Babylonians and Egyptians. In the first century, Aulus Celsus, a Roman encyclopaedist also known for his medical work, boiled this vegetable and used the liquid to treat tooth pain, highlighting its importance. Due to the similarity of its root to the human body, many legends have emerged. A widely copied and read manuscript provides the following instructions for the correct and safe collection of the plant: "Man should not uproot the root, as it would endanger his life. Therefore, the high part of the plant should be tied to a black dog and the animal should be guided by pulling the plant until the mandrake is out of the ground. At this moment, the plant makes a terrible moan and the dog falls dead. To survive, the harvester must have its ears plugged." (Ring 1998).

While the 15th, 16th, 17th and 18th centuries were a prosperous era for phytotherapy, the 19th and early 20th came with a decline in the therapeutic use of drugs derived from plant extracts. By that time, different authors stated that those drugs possessed shortcomings mainly due to destructive action of enzymes. Since active compounds are normally more abundant from well-maintained natural sources, standardized methods for preparation/usage and ideal conditions for cultivation/manipulation of medicinal plants were proposed. The rebirth of phytotherapy relied on advanced scientific information regarding plants compounds (Kovacevic 2000, Nelson & Cox 2005, Sewell & Rafieian-Kopaei 2014).

The immersion and understanding of organic chemistry triggered the modern phytotherapy and the ages between 1800 and 1900 were paramount to the discovery and development of new drugs from natural extracts: in 1803, the German pharmacist Friederich Sertürner retrieved the first active substance from a plant: morphine was isolated from opium, extracted from *Papaver somniferum* (Miraldi & Baini 2018).

Historically, willow tree (*Salix sp.*) has been used with medicinal purpose since 6000 years ago, leading to investigation and creation of the first synthetic drug in 1897: the aspirin, derived from the salicylic acid extracted from willow barks (DerMarderosian & Beutler 2011, Carmona & Pereira 2013). The period from 1901 to 1980 showed antimicrobial agents derived from fungi and bacteria (Booth 1999, de los Santos et al. 2015, Gaynes 2017).

In 1978, the World Health Organization (WHO) recognized the need to appreciate use of medicinal plants and herbal medicines with prophylactic and healing purpose, through the Alma-Ata declaration, since 70-95% of the population of developing countries use traditional medicine in their basic health care and 85% use plants or extracts (Report of the

International Conference on Primary Health Care 1978, Tilburt & Kaptchuk 2008, Rosa 2011, WHO 2011). Over the last 30 years, the number of people using natural medicines has risen constantly (Miraldi & Baini 2018).

However, the dissemination of traditional medicines is widely spread, since it is used as self-medication and home remedies or even as dietary supplements in healthy nourishment. According to the WHO, is difficult to control quality and ensure safety, concerning production of traditional medicine. Thus, scientific evidence needs to improve in order to better assess the use of natural products (WHO 2011).

The term phytotherapy derives from the Greek *phyton* which means "plant" and from *therapeia*, meaning "treatment" and consist of the internal/external use of plants or extracts as a therapeutic approach to treat symptoms and diseases, whether *in natura* or in medicines forms (Marassi & Rossi 2015). Ethnopharmacology is a division of ethnobiology, focused on the study of the complex relationships between plants and animals with human societies and may also be defined as "the exploitation interdisciplinary scientific knowledge of biologically active agents traditionally employed or observed by the men" (Bruhn & Holmstedt 1982). Herbalism or herbal medicine are other common names found in literature, used to refer to the use of plant and its extracts (which contain parts of plants as active ingredients) in traditional or folk medicine (Pan et al. 2014).

The advantages of herbal medicine are related to its compounds. Scientists around the globe investigate medicinal plants to find chemical substance responsible for the therapeutic effect (Williamson 2001). Isolated compounds may present antimicrobial, antioxidant or anti-inflammatory characteristics, but the extract itself may show enhanced activity due to the entire complex, named phytocomplexes, possibly due to synergy, bioavailability or cumulative effects (Schmidt et al. 2008, Gomez Castellanos et al. 2009, Carmona & Pereira 2013, Nazemi Salman et al. 2016, Miraldi & Baini 2018).

In order to analyze the active component, the natural product is extracted from the source, then concentrated, fractionated and purified, generating a single active compound (Koehn & Carter 2005). These compounds are flavonoids, coumarins, iridoid glycosides, phenolic acids, resins, triterpens, phytoesters, choline, carotenoids, tannins, vitamins and essential oils (Bhardwaj & Bhardwaj 2012, Buggapati 2016). However, as previously stated, greater biological effects may be resulted from the combination of different compounds (phytocomplex) and the isolation process may reduce the main effect (Raskin & Ripoll 2004).

On the other hand, this phytocomplexity complicates the standardization of extracts preparation and, consequently, the development of an evidence-based herbal medicine (Cravotto et al. 2010). Yet, there may be variation on the chemical plant composition, since is directly dependent of weather, soil type and available local soil nutrients, which varies from each region. Therefore, urbanized, contaminated, or artificially fertilized areas are not adequate for production of medicinal plants, which should be cultivated in environments that mimic the wild as much as possible, providing a well-balanced medium with biotic and abiotic interactions. This natural metabolic route may be related to the production of secondary metabolites, responsible for the medicinal effects (Carmona & Pereira 2013).

With the advent of modern assessment techniques, current results and ongoing researches show that plant extracts have a promising future in health science, since extracts could offer an effective addition to enhance antimicrobial spectrum of antibiotics or as an alternative to antibiotics or anti-inflammatory drugs, representing a different approach to therapeutic strategies for infection in general. Natural extracts have been investigated in contemporary medicine against cancer (Gorlach et al. 2015, Zheng et al. 2016, Kuruppu et al. 2019). In 1967, Hartwell published the first volume of several manuscripts, concerning the use of plants against cancer, reporting over 3000 species of plants which had been described to have anti-cancer properties (Hartwell 1967). Years later, this research was extended showing over 350 plant species reported to be used against cancer (Graham et al. 2000). Actual reports show that, over 60% of currently used anti-cancer agents are derived from natural sources, such as marine organisms and plant extracts (Cragg & Newman 2005).

The use of plant extracts is also observed in treatment of diabetes mellitus: *Bahuinia* sp., *Syzygium sp.* and *Cissus sicyoides* L. showed hypoglycemic effects (Zanoello et al. 2001, Pepato et al. 2002, Prince et al. 2003, Pepato et al. 2004) and effectiveness against inflammatory skin disease (Dawid-Pać 2013).

Currently in dentistry, plant extracts have been evaluated mainly for biological compatibility (Mohammad et al. 2015, Bueno et al. 2018, dos Santos et al. 2019), antimicrobial activity (Brighenti et al. 2008, Kurian et al. 2016, Cavenago et al. 2017, Bueno et al. 2018, Sangalli et al. 2018) or as a therapeutic adjunctive to enhance properties of certain medication (Cavenago et al. 2017, Valentim et al. 2017).

Lastly, it's also important to state that, beside all investigation of the promising application of plant extracts, the growing use may present issues related to adverse reactions, caused by factors as wrong species of plants used by mistake, plants gathered from unsuitable area for cultivation (especially in areas with uncontrolled use of pesticides), contamination with toxic substances such as heavy metals (mercury or arsenic) or the concomitant use with other drugs (Muzi et al. 2001, Ernst 2002a, Ekor 2014).

Several untested plants are used by the population without any pharmacovigilance, still relying on empirical knowledge passed through generations. Thereby, there is an unknown chance of possible adverse reactions, contraindications and interactions with pharmaceutical or functional food, since the mode of action may be unclear (Ekor 2014).

The illusory idea that herbal medicine and plant extracts are totally safe, devoided of adverse reactions and may be used without any control, leads to increase the cases of life-threatening conditions. According to the World Health Organization (WHO), the use of incorrect species is a threat to consumer safety. To guarantee the quality of traditional medicines, protocols established in the Pharmacopoeias must be followed, as the correct identification of the plant species, analysis of the purity and confirmation of the presence and minimum concentration of the active ingredients (Brandao et al. 2013).

With the increasing use of medicinal plants, the WHO published the Monographs on Selected Medicinal Plants, a list of species with recognized medicinal benefits and the accepted means to correctly use them, with the intent to: provide scientific information on the safety, efficacy, and quality control/quality assurance of widely used medicinal plants, in order to facilitate their appropriate use in Member States; to provide models to assist Member States in developing their own monographs or formularies for these or other herbal medicines; and to facilitate information exchange among Member States (Essential Medicines and Health Products Information Portal 2020).

The content of these monographs was obtained by a systematic review of scientific literature, including: review articles; bibliographies in review articles; many pharmacopoeias-the International, African, British, Chinese, Dutch, European, French, German, Hungarian, Indian, and Japanese; as well as many other reference books. Draft monographs were widely distributed, and some 100 experts in more than 40 countries commented on them. Experts included members of WHO's Expert Advisory Panels on Traditional Medicine, on the International Pharmacopoeia and Pharmaceutical Preparations, and on Drug Evaluation and National Drug Policies; and the drug regulatory authorities of 16 countries (Essential Medicines and Health Products Information Portal 2020).

The volume 1 of the WHO monographs on selected medicinal plants was published in 1999 and contains 28 monographs. In 2004, volume 2 was published with 30 monographs and the volume 3 presented 31 monographs in 2007. The 4th volume containing 28 monographs was published in 2009 and in 2010, additional 30 monographs were published in a 5th volume, entitled Monographs on Medicinal Plants Commonly Used in the Newly Independent States (NIS) (WHO 1999, 2004, 2007, 2009, 2010).

A great number of species substitutions and mislabeling, suggesting that current surveillance methods are not adequate to control the herbal medicine market was pointed by Palhares et al. (2015). In addition, the authors stated that traditional methodologies of species identification are, in general, not appropriate to correctly identify a plant species. Therefore, as a resource of standardization, Palhares et al. (2015) suggested the use of DNA barcode as a first screening step in the quality control of herbal medicine, making the process safer, more reliable, and cheaper, discarding substitutions, without the need for more expensive chemical analyses that are otherwise necessary.

Without a scientific detailed action mechanism and components found in plants used in extracts, toxic compounds may be present, causing cellular toxicity, hepatotoxicity, poisoning (Ernst 2002b, Rietjens et al. 2005, Mei et al. 2010, Byeon et al. 2019) or even a carcinogenic effect (Mei et al. 2010, Poivre et al. 2017), evidencing the need for a toxicity assessment associated with pharmacovigilance and standardized regulatory policies on herbal medicines to promote a safe use (Zhou et al. 2013, Byeon et al. 2019).

At last but not least, Shanley & Luz (2003) brought to attention the impacts of uncontrolled consumption of medicinal plants on forest degradation. This scenario was reported in Africa, where the overharvesting of medicinal plants for exportation along with the increase of urbanization resulted devastation of different species, leaving locals habitants without medicinal remedies (Cunningham 1993). In Brazil, to avoid a similar scenario in Amazonia forest, impacts of land-use and its correct management must be studied, since it may affect primary forest medicinal plants. Plants particularities should also be taken into consideration, such as low-densities occurrence, differences in growing time to reach reproductive age and vulnerability to logging or fire. In this context, the rapid expansion of logging, ranching, mining, and agricultural observed in eastern Amazonia already led to significant changes in forest composition (Veríssimo et al. 1992, Cunningham 2000, Gerwing 2002).

The degradation of forests may lead to loss of potential medicinal plants, besides natural consequences that will influence in occurrence of different species, such as sole erosion and elevation of local temperature. The concern about this degradation led to the search of several efforts to conserve the genetic diversity of medicinal plants through seed banks, tissue culture and creation of forest genetic reserves. Also, a conscientious citizen/population associated with relevant research could provide a viable support to conserve valuable ecosystems and local habitants' medicinal needs (Vieira 1999, Shanley & Luz 2003, Senior et al. 2017).

Conclusion

The ancient empirical use of plant extracts by mankind served as a pillar to current investigations around certain plants. Nowadays, plant extracts have been growing with promising scientific-based results and, considering our biodiversity around the globe, there is still much to discover and learn. The following chapters in this book will evidence several extracts used in different fields of dentistry, such as endodontics, periodontics, restorative dentistry, cariology and dental trauma, among several other applications.

As previously stated, beside promising results, caution with overharvesting and with the use of plant extracts should be taken, especially if extracts are used without safety proof, as biological tests (toxicity, carcinogenicity, genotoxicity, among others). Therefore, continuous investigation and literature update are primordial for dissemination of results.

References

Andrews, J. *Pepper Trail: History and Recipes from around the world.* USA: University of North Texas Press, 1999, 256 p.

Bhardwaj, A; Bhardwaj, SV. Role of Medicinal Herbs in Prevention and Treatment of Dental Diseases. *Ann Ayurvedic Med*, 2012, 1(3), 95-101.

Booth, M. *Opium - a History*. New York, St Martin's Griffin, 1st Edition, 1999.

Bosland, PW. Capsicums: Innovative Uses of an Ancient Crop. In: *Progress in new crops* (Janick J, editor) USA: ASHS Press, 1996, 479-87.

Brandao, M; Cosenza, GP; Pereira, FL; Vasconcelos, AS; Fagg, CW. Changes in the trade in native medicinal plants in Brazilian public markets. *Environ Monit Assess*, 2013, 185, 7013–23.

Brighenti, FL; Luppens, SB; Delbem, AC; Deng, DM; Hoogenkamp, MA; Gaetti-Jardim Junior, E; et al. Effect of Psidium cattleianum leaf extract on Streptococcus mutans viability, protein expression and acid production. *Caries Res*, 2008, 42(2), 148-54.

Bruhn, JG; Holmstedt, B. Ethnopharmacology, objectives, principles and perspectives. In: Beal JL, Reinhard E. (Ed.). *Natural products as medicinal agents*. Stuttgart: Hippocrates Verlag, 1981, 405-30.

Bueno, CRE; Valentim, D; Jardim-Junior, E; et al. Tissue reaction to Aroeira (*Myracrodruon urundeuva*) extracts associated with microorganisms: an *in vivo* study. *Braz. oral res*, 2018, 32, e42.

Buggapati, L. Herbs in Dentistry. *Int J Pharm Sci Invent*, 2016, 5(6), 07-12.

Byeon, JH; Kil, JH; Ahn, YC; Son, CG. Systematic Review of Published Data on Herb Induced Liver Injury. *J Ethnopharmacol*, 2019, 233, 190-96

Carmona, F; Pereira, AMS. Herbal medicines: old and new concepts; truths and misunderstandings. *Rev Bras Farmacogn [Braz J Pharmacogn]*, 2013, 23(2), 370-85.

Cavenago, BC; Carpio-Perochena, AE; Ordinola-Zapata, R; Estrela, C; Garlet, GP; Tanomaru-Filho, M; Weckwerth, PH; Andrade, FB; Duarte, MAH. Effect of Using Different Vehicles on the Physicochemical, Antimicrobial, and Biological Properties of White Mineral Trioxide Aggregate. *J Endod*, 2017, 43(5), 779-86.

Cohen, MM. The history of opium and opiates. *Tex Med*, 1969, 65, 76-85.

Cortez-Gallardo, V; Macedo-Ceja, JP; Hernández-Arroyo, M; Arteaga-Aureoles, G; Espinosa-Galván, D; Rodríguez-Landa, JF. Pharmacognosy: brief history of its origins and their relation with the medical sciences. *Rev Biomed*, 2004, 15(2), 123–36.

Cragg, GM; Newman, DJ. Plants as a source of anti-cancer agents. *J Ethnopharmacol*, 2005, 100(1-2); 72-9.

Cravotto, G; Boffa, L; Genzini, L; Garella, D. Phytotherapeutics: an evaluation of the potential of 1000 plants. *J Clin Pharm Ther*, 2010, 35(1), 11-48.

Cunningham, AB. African medicinal plants: Setting priorities at the interface between conservation and primary health care. Paris: UNESCO. *People and Plants Working Paper 1*, 1993, 39 p.

Cunningham, AB. Applied Ethnobotany: People; Wild Plant Use and Conservation 1st Ed. *Routledge*, 2001, 320 p.

Dawid-Pać, R. Medicinal plants used in treatment of inflammatory skin diseases. *Postepy Dermatol Alergol*, 2013, 30(3), 170-7.

de los Santos, BP; Kanis, LA; Pereira, JR. Herbal Medicines in Dentistry: History, Obtainment Methods, And Properties Of *Copaifera Multijuga Hayne* And *Baccharis Dracunculifolia DC*. *J Res in Dent*, 2015, 3(6), 859-68.

DerMarderosian, A; Beutler, JA. Willow Bark. In: *The Review of Natural Products* (eds A. DerMarderosian, J. A. Beutler). Facts and Comparisons Publishing Group, St. Louis, 2011, 13-43.

dos Santos, AF; Pacheco, JM; Silva, PAO; Bedran- Russo, AK; Rezende, TMB; Pereira, PNR; Ribeiro, APD. Direct and transdentinal biostimulatory effects of grape seed extract rich in proanthocyanidin on pulp cells. *Int Endod J*, 2019, 52, 424-38.

Duarte, DF. Opium and Opioids: A Brief History. *Rev Bras Anestesiol*, 2005, 55(1), 135-46.

Ekor, M. The growing use of herbal medicines: issues relating to adverse reactions and challenges in monitoring safety. *Front Pharmacol*, 2014, 4, 177.

Ernst, E. Heavy metals in traditional Indian remedies. *Eur J Clin Pharmacol*, 2002a, 57(12), 891-6.

Ernst, E. Toxic heavy metals and undeclared drugs in Asian herbal medicines. *Trends Pharmacol Sci*, 2002b, 23(3), 136–9.

Essential Medicines and Health Products Information Portal. *A World Health Organization Resource*. Available at: https://apps.who.int/medicinedocs/en/p/about/ [Accessed in: January 2020].

Fattori, V; Hohmann, MS; Rossaneis, AC. Capsaicin: Current Understanding of Its Mechanisms and Therapy of Pain and Other Pre-Clinical and Clinical Uses. *Molecules*, 2016, 21(7), e844.

França, ISX; et al. Medicina popular: benefícios e malefícios das plantas medicinais [Folk medicine: benefits and harms of medicinal plants]. *Rev Bras Enferm*, 2008, 61(2), 201-8.

Galarza, J. Mexican Codices of the National Library of Paris. Archivo General de la Nacion INAH Seminarios de códices. Mexico City, Mexico. French and Spanish., 1981, 3-130.

Gaynes, R. The Discovery of Penicillin-New Insights After More Than 75 Years of Clinical Use. *Emerg Infect Dis*, 2017, 23(5), 849-853.

Gerwing, JJ. Degradation of forests through logging and fire in the eastern Brazilian Amazon. *For Ecol Manag*, 2002, 157, 131-41.

Gomez Castellanos, JR; Prieto, JM; Heinrich, M. Red lapacho (*Tabebuia impetiginosa*) - a global ethnopharmacological commodity? *J Ethnopharmacol*, 2009, 121, 1-13.

Gorlach, S; Fichna, J; Lewandowska, U. Polyphenols as mitochondria-targeted anticancer drugs. *Cancer Lett*, 2015, 366(2), 141-9.

Graham, JG; Fabricant, MLQDS; Farnsworth, NR. Plants used against cancer - an extension of the work of Jonathan Hartwell. *J Ethnopharmacol*, 2000, 73, 347–77.

Hartwell, JL. Plants used against cancer. A survey. *Lloydia*, 1967, 30, 379-436.

Jack, DB. One hundred years of aspirin. *The Lancet*, 1997, 350(9075), 437-39.

Koehn, FE; Carter, GT. The evolving role of natural products in drug discovery. *Nat Rev Drug Discov*, 2005, 4, 206-20.

Kovacevic, N. *Fundamentals of Pharmacognosy*. Beograd: Personal edition, 2000, 170–1.

Kurian, B; Swapna, DV; Nadig, RR; Ranjini, MA; Rashmi, K; Bolar, SR. Efficacy of calcium hydroxide, mushroom, and *Aloe vera* as an intracanal medicament against *Enterococcus faecalis*: An *in vitro* study. *Endodontol*, 2016, 28, 137-42.

Kuruppu, AI; Paranagama, P; Goonasekara, CL. Medicinal plants commonly used against cancer in traditional medicine formulae in Sri Lanka. *Saudi Pharm J*, 2019, 27(4), 565-573.

Magner, LN. A History of Medicine. CRC Press, 1992, ISBN 9780824786731.

Marassi, CG; Rossi, A. Phytotherapeutic approaches. In: *European Handbook of Dermatological Treatments*, 2015, 2nd edition: 1481-85.

Mei, N; Guo, L; Fu, PP; Fuscoe, JC; Luan, Y; Chen, T. Metabolism, Genotoxicity; and Carcinogenicity of Comfrey. *J Toxicol Environ Health B Crit Rev*, 2010, 13(7-8), 509-26.

Miraldi, E; Baini, G. Medicinal plants and health in human history: from empirical use to modern phytotherapy. *J Siena Academy Sci*, 2018, 10, 7-12.

Mohammad, SG; Raheel, SA; Baroudi, K. Histological Evaluation of *Allium sativum* Oil as a New Medicament for Pulp Treatment of Permanent Teeth. *J Contemp Dent Pract*, 2015, 16(2), 85-90.

Muzi, G; Dell'omo, M; Madeo, G; Abbritti, G; Caroli, S. Arsenic poisoning caused by Indian ethnic remedies. *J Pediatr*, 2001, 139(1), 169.

Nazemi, Salman B; Vahabi, S; Mohebbi, Rad M; Bayat, N. Use of Herbs and Medicinal Plants in Dentistry: A Review. *J Dent Sch*, 2016, 35(2), 133-149.

Nelson, D; Cox, M. *Lehninger Principles of Biochemistry*. 6th ed. New York: W. H. Freeman, 2012, 1328 p.

Palhares, RM; Gonçalves Drummond, M; dos Santos Alves Figueiredo Brasil, B; Pereira Cosenza, G; das Graças Lins Brandão, M; Oliveira G. Medicinal Plants Recommended by the World Health Organization: DNA Barcode Identification Associated with Chemical Analyses Guarantees Their Quality. *PLoS ONE*, 2015, 10(5), e0127866.

Pan, SY; Litscher, G; Gao, SH; Zhou, SF; Yu, ZL; Chen, HQ; et al. Historical perspective of traditional indigenous medical practices: the current renaissance and conservation of herbal resources. *Evid Based Complement Alternat Med*, 2014, 2014, 525340.

Pepato, MT; Baviera, AM; Vendramini, RG; Brunetti, IG. Evaluation of toxicity after one-months treatment with *Bauhinia forficata* decoction in stretozotocin-induced diabetic rats. BMC Complement *Altern Med, 2004*, 4(7), 1-7.

Pepato, MT; Keller, EH; Baviera, AM; Kettelhut, IC; Vendramini, RC; Brunetti, IL. Anti-diabetic activity of *Bauhinia forficata* decoction in stretozotocin-diabetic rats. *J Ethnopharmacol*, 2002, 81(2), 191-7.

Petrovska, BB. Historical review of medicinal plants' usage. *Pharmacogn Rev*, 2012, 6(11), 1-5.

Poivre, M; Nachtergael, A; Bunel, V; Philippe, ON; Duez, P. Genotoxicity and Carcinogenicity of Herbal Products. In: *Toxicology of Herbal Products* (Pelkonen O, Duez P, Vuorela P, Vuorela H, editors), 2017, 179-215.

Prince, PSM; Kamalakkannan, N; Menon, VP. *Syzigium cumini* seed extracts reduce tissue damage in diabetic rat brain. *J Ethnopharmacol*, 2003, 84, 205-9.

Raskin, I; Ripoll, C. Can an apple a day keep the doctor away? *Curr Pharm Des*, 2004, 10, 3419-29.

Report of the International Conference on Primary Health Care, jointly sponsored by the World Health Organization and the United Nations Children's Fund, *Alma-Ata – URSS*, 6 to 12 September, 1978.

Rietjens, IM; Martena, MJ; Boersma, MG; Spiegelenberg, W; Alink, GM. Molecular mechanisms of toxicity of important food-borne phytotoxins. *Mol Nutr Food Res*, 2005, 49(2), 131-58.

Ring, ME. *Dentistry: An Illustrated History*. 1st Ed. Manole publishing company, 1998.

Rogers, K. *Medicine and Healers Through History*. 1st Edition. Britannica Educational Publishing, 2011, ISBN 9781615303670.

Rosa, C; Câmara, SG; Béria, JU. Representations and use intention of phytotherapy in primary health care. *Cienc Saude Col*, 2011, 16, 311-18.

Saleh, BK; Omer, A; Teweldemedhin, B. Medicinal uses and health benefits of chili pepper (*Capsicum* spp.): a review. *MOJ Food Process Technol*, 2018, 6(4), 325–328.

Sangalli, J; Júnior, EGJ; Bueno, CRE; et al. Antimicrobial activity of *Psidium cattleianum* associated with calcium hydroxide against *Enterococcus faecalis* and *Candida albicans*: an *in vitro* study. *Clin Oral Investig*, 2018, 22(6), 2273-79.

Schmidt, B; Ribnicky, D; Poulev, A; Logendra, S; Cefalu, W; Raskin, I. A natural history of botanical therapeutics. *Metabolism*, 2008, 57, S3-S9.

Senior, RB; Hill, JK; del Pliego, PG; Goode, LK; Edwards, DP. A pantropical analysis of the impacts of forest degradation and conversion on local temperature. *Ecol Evol*, 2017, 7(19), 7897-7908.

Sewell, RDE; Rafieian-Kopaei, M. The history and ups and downs of herbal medicine usage. *J HerbMed Pharmacol*, 2014, 3(1), 1-3.

Shanley, P; Luz, L. The Impacts of Forest Degradation on Medicinal Plant Use and Implications for Health Care in Eastern Amazonia. *BioScience*, 2003, 53(6), 573-84.

Tilburt, JC; Kaptchuk, TJJ. Herbal medicine research and global health: An ethical analysis. *Bull World Health Organ*, 2008, 86, 594-9.

Toplak Galle, K. Domestic medicinal plants. *Zagreb: Mozaic book*, 2005, 60-1.

Valentim, D; Bueno, CRE; Marques, VAS; Vasques, AMV; Cury, MTS; Cintra, LTA; Dezan Junior, E. Calcium hydroxide associated with a new vehicle: *Psidium cattleianum* leaf extracts. Tissue response evaluation. *Braz Oral Res*, 2017, 31, 1-8.

Veríssimo, A; Barreto, P; Mattos, M; Tarifa, R; Uhl, C. Logging impacts and prospects for sustainable forest management in an old Amazonian fron- tier: The case of Paragominas. *For Ecol Manag*, 1992, 55, 169-99.

Verpoorte, R. Pharmacognosy in the new millennium: lead finding and biotechnology. *J Pharma Pharmacol*, 2000, 52, 253–262.

Vieira, RF. Conservation of medicinal and aromatic plants in Brazil. In: *Perspectives on New Crops and New Uses*. Janick J (editor). Alexandria (VA) ASHS Press, 1999, 152-59.

WHO (World Health Organization). *Monographs on Medicinal Plants Commonly Used in the Newly Independent States (NIS)*. Geneva 2010, 452 p.

WHO (World Health Organization). *Monographs on selected medicinal plants.*, Volume 1, Geneva 1999, 295 p.

WHO (World Health Organization). *Monographs on selected medicinal plants.*, Volume 2. Geneva 2004, 375 p.

WHO (World Health Organization). *Monographs on selected medicinal plants.*, Volume 3, Geneva 2007, 390p.

WHO (World Health Organization). *Monographs on selected medicinal plants*. Volume 4, Geneva 2009, 456p.

WHO, "the world traditional medicines situation," in *Traditional Medicines: Global Situation, Issues and Challenges*, WHO, Geneva, Switzerland, 2011.

Wiart, C. Ethnopharmacology of medicinal plants: Asia and the Pacific. New Jersey: Humana Press, 2006, 228p.

Williamson, EM. Synergy and other interactions in phytomedicines. *Phytomedicine*, 2001, 8, 401-9.

Wu, CD; Darout, IA; Skaug, N. Chewing sticks: timeless natural toothbrushes for oral cleansing. *J Periodont Res*, 2001, 36, 275-84.

Yang, S. The Divine Farmer's Materia Medica: A Translation of the Shen Nong Ben Cao Jing. Blue Poppy Enterprises, Inc., 1998, 198p.

Zanoello, AM; Melazzo-Mazzanti, C; Kerpel Gindri, J; Andreane Filappi, A; Prestes, D; Cecim, M. Efeito protetor do *Syzygium cumini* contra *Diabetes mellitus* induzido por aloxano em ratos [Protective effect of Syzygium cumini against Alloxane-induced Diabetes mellitus in rats]. *Acta Farmaceutica Bonaerense*, 2001, 21(1), 31-6.

Zheng, YM; Shen, JZ; Wang, Y; Lu, AX; Ho, WS. Anti-oxidant and anti-cancer activities of *Angelica dahurica* extract via induction of apoptosis in colon cancer cells. *Phytomedicine*, 2016, 23(11), 1267-74.

Zhou, J; Ouedraogo, M; Qu, F; Duez, P. Potential genotoxicity of traditional Chinese medicinal plants and phytochemicals: an overview. *Phytother Res*, 2013, 27(12), 1745-55.

In: Contemporary Use of Plant Extracts … ISBN: 978-1-53617-650-6
Editor: C. R. Emerenciano Bueno

Chapter 2

ANTIMICROBIAL PROPERTIES OF PLANT EXTRACTS

Leopoldo Cosme-Silva[1,*], Renan Dal-Fabbro[2], Rayana Duarte Khoury[3], Francine Benetti[4], Juliana Quintino Trizzi[2], Eloi Dezan Junior[2] and Carlos Roberto Emerenciano Bueno[2]

[1]Department of Restorative Dentistry, Faculty of Dentistry, Federal University of Alagoas (UFAL), Maceió, Alagoas, Brazil
[2]Department of Endodontics, Sao Paulo State University (UNESP), Araçatuba School of Dentistry, Araçatuba, São Paulo, Brazil
[3]Department of Restorative Dentistry, Institute of Science and Technology, São Paulo State University (UNESP), São José dos Campos, São Paulo, Brazil
[4]Department of Restorative Dentistry, Federal University of Minas Gerais (UFMG), School of Dentistry, Belo Horizonte, Minas Gerais, Brazil

[*] Corresponding Author's Email: leopoldocosme@gmail.com.

ABSTRACT

Oral diseases are a major health problem, with periodontal and caries among the most important infectious disease, which influence quality of life. The relationship between oral disease and oral microbiota is well stablished in literature, since more than 750 species are found in oral cavity. Regardless the number of new antibiotics introduced in the market in the last years by pharmacological industry, resistance that pathogenic microorganisms develop against antibiotics has increased.

Due to side effects and drug resistance, researches around the globe have been looking for new antimicrobial agents or antimicrobial enhancers, such as those from herbal sources. Medicinal plants and byproducts are constantly indicated and used throughout the world in several areas of medicine and dentistry to induce favorable responses and to treat different diseases. Also, plants naturally produce secondary metabolites that can be used as antimicrobials. There are several ways of producing herbal extracts and retrieve the active compound, as well as different tests to be performed in order to assess the antimicrobial potential. This chapter will briefly discuss the main techniques used and highlight the main properties of some compounds present in plants such as *Myracrodruon urundeuva, Curcumin, Green tea, Lemon grass, Chamomile, Aloe Vera, Cinnamon, Psidium, Citrus* and *Capsicum.* Due to the huge variety of plants in the literature, it is impracticable to describe all extracts with antibacterial properties. Therefore, this chapter mentions some of the extracts with such properties, which may serve as an introduction to new research and new researchers.

Keywords: antibacterial agents, ethnopharmacology, medicinal plants, phytotherapy, plant extracts

1. CONCEPT AND PRODUCTION OF PLANT EXTRACTS

A plant extract is a substance with useful properties that are separated from the tissue of a plant, normally by handling it with a solvent, to be used for a special purpose. Plant-based natural elements can be obtained from any part of the plant (bark, leaves, flowers, roots, fruits, and seeds) (Zhang et al. 2018). This section will cover the concept and production of plant extracts, reflections on microbiology, oral and radicular biofilms, types of studies available to evaluate antimicrobial action, as well as the properties of some components that have been studied and used clinically.

Although herbal extracts come in many designs, they have one frequent feature: extracts represent naturally occurring phytochemicals (plant-produced compounds) that have been extracted from the dormant organic material of the plant that provided them. The main benefit of using extracts over raw herb is that, once extracted from the plant matrix, the phytochemicals circumvent the need for digestion and are far more immediately absorbable (Bimakr et al. 2011, Azmir et al. 2013).

Extracts are typically classified by the solvent employed to make them and/or by their design. Some of the more traditional solvents that are utilized include water, alcohol, glycerin, and vinegar. The intrinsic characteristics of each of these solvents will bring several phytochemicals in an herb. The original extracts were primarily obtained through aqueous extraction or alcoholic fermentation. In the past, the plainness of this procedure, as well as the tools, materials and heating methods, indicated that the extractor was common people rather than a scientist. Nowadays, this activity calls upon the use of precise automatons and adapted materials. It has benefited from improvements in process engineering, phytochemistry and analytics. Furthermore, new technologies to support extraction are being developed (Sasidharan et al. 2011, Zhang et al. 2018).

The process of extracting the compounds should be simple, fast, economic, in agreement with the local regulation, effective and selective when needed (Zhang et al. 2018). Below we list the main used processes:

- Pressing: One of the more typical extraction, pressing may be used complementary or before another process, for instance, to prepare the materials. It causes mechanical perturbation and gives a liquid product.
- Distillation and hydro distillation: By straight heating or steam, this method is mainly used for oils and volatile components. It may cause degradation of the components.
- Solid/Liquid extraction: It consists of the extraction or separation of one active or more from dense materials working on the solubility in a

liquid to reach the soluble part and the insoluble part or fractionation of a homogenous solution. The main typical Solid/Liquid extractions are:

- Maceration: It simply implies you chop up or grind up the plant, put it in a container and cover with your solvent (usually a mixture of alcohol and water, or just straight alcohol) at room temperature. It presents the drawback of long extraction time and low extraction efficiency (Zhang et al. 2018).
- Digestion: It is a sort of maceration with slender warming during the extraction process, given that the temperature does not alter the active ingredients of plant material. The commonly used temperatures ranges between 35° and 40°C, no higher than 50°C. This method is employed with the tougher plant parts or those that contain poorly soluble elements. The parts are introduced in a vessel with the liquid pre-heated to the designated temperatures, and it is maintained for a time that may vary within half an hour and 24 hours, shaking the container periodically (Sasidharan et al. 2011).
- Decoction: This method is used for the extraction of the water-soluble and heat stable elements from plants by boiling it in water for an appropriated time, cooling, filtering and passing enough cold water through the drug to provide the required volume (Bimakr et al. 2011). The decoction cannot be used for the extraction of thermolabile or volatile elements (Zhang et al. 2018).
- Infusion: It is a dilute solution of simply soluble components of the raw drug, carried out by soaking the plants' parts to use in a volume of boiling water, left to stand 15 minutes and then strained through a filter (Azmir et al. 2013).
- Lixiviation: It is the method of separating soluble from insoluble elements by dissolving the former in water or some other solvent, always with cold, fresh and new solvent. The blend of substances is put into a proper vessel, the solvent poured over it, and the entire allowed to stand until a strong

solution is achieved, which is then drawn off from the remainder. This process is reproduced as often as needed until the desired quantity of soluble material has been removed (Azmir et al. 2013).

– Percolation: The solvent is gently passed through the plant, inside a percolator, little by little, filling itself with active ingredients, and is slowly pushed away by a different pure solvent that is added from above. It is an extractive system that is not suggested in the case of plants that tend to expand a lot, which hinders the solvent from flowing precisely (Zhang et al. 2018).

Medicinal plants represent a significant role in human health. Apart from conventional uses, many compounds isolated from them have beneficial medicinal features for treating distinct diseases. Today, oral care products mixed with medicinal plant extracts are earning attention due to their low toxicity and fewer side effects all over the world. These herbal extracts have been employed in dentistry for decreasing inflammation, as antimicrobial plaque agents, as antiseptics, antioxidants, antimicrobials, antivirals and analgesics. They further assist in healing and are efficient in managing microbial biofilm in gingivitis and periodontitis (Sinha & Sinha 2014).

The foremost diseases of the teeth involve biofilm as the main factor. Proper dental care is crucial for reducing tooth decay and periodontal diseases. Prevention of dental caries is challenging, as the incidence of the disease is very high in the general community and it happens in economically deprived people who cannot afford the commercially accessible oral hygiene products (Kumar et al. 2013). In this scenario, in developing countries, the herbal medicines are judged to be safe, efficient and cheaper choices compared to synthetic chemicals (Taheri et al. 2011).

However, it is crucial to be critical and skeptical about herbal medicine. Further research should be performed to assess the effectiveness as possible pharmaceutical sources and/or support their use as medications. At the same time, caution must be taken when promoting herbal medicines because, along with their therapeutic potential, there is a risk for misapplication, therefore further studies are needed to prove use limitations by each herb. Clinicians must be able to assimilate new knowledge, update it, and place it in the arsenal of modern medicine for the general benefit of society.

2. Assessment Techniques and Antimicrobial Properties of Plant Origin Compounds

Initially, the terms antimicrobial and antibacterial must be defined, in order to clarify the text and avoid confusion. The primary difference is the type of microorganism they act upon. Antibacterial acts against bacteria cells, while antimicrobial agents have superior range, covering other microorganisms, such as bacteria, fungi and some viruses.

Antibacterial therapy, a keystone in modern medical practice, provides one of the only pharmacologic treatments that cure oral diseases. Antimicrobial properties are paramount for compounds of natural origin to have high clinical relevance, in this case, some concepts should be appropriated clarified.

The meanings of bacteriostatic and bactericidal seem to be straightforward: "bacteriostatic" indicates that the agent inhibits the growth of bacteria (it keeps them in the stationary stage of growth) and "bactericidal" suggests that it kills bacteria. The bactericidal substance from plants attacks microbes by modifying the cell wall, lipids, enzymes, or protein synthesis inside the cell – sometimes even making a combination of these mechanisms. By disturbing the cell wall composition of existing cells and inhibiting the development of new cells, bactericidal substances induce bacterial cells to die, consequently lowering the quantity found in the individual affected. Bactericidal technologies contribute to irreversible cell death and are often preferred for materials that will be used in healthcare facilities, where total kill is targeted to keep aseptic environments. On another hand, bacteriostatic agents change from bactericidal versions in that they inhibit the growth and multiplications of bacterial cells, rather than directly kill them. Bacteriostatic agents from herbal extracts can perform this by hindering the metabolic mechanisms of the bacterial cell, in most cases targeting the protein synthesis. While doing this does not produce outright cell death, it does completely restrain further growth and DNA replication of the bacterial cells. When bacteriostatic agents are used, the treatment will manage the number of bacterial cells. While the bacteria will not be eliminated, their numbers will not increase. Essentially, bacteriostatic medications efficiently keep bacterial cells from replicating, providing reversible results (Pankey & Sabath 2004, Nemeth et al. 2015).

Also, another property that herbal extracts should provide is the ability to act on oral and radicular biofilms. More than 700 distinct bacterial species have been identified in the oral cavity of humans, in this respect, an extensive spectrum of action is timely (Dewhirst et al. 2010). The bacteria existing in the saliva adhere to the teeth and start the development of a dental biofilm beforehand called dental plaque. The primary adherence of bacteria to dental surfaces is introduced by the development of a conditioning film on the clean dental surfaces essentially consisting of salivary glycoproteins. Bacteria adhesion to the pellicle is the next step of biofilm development. In this step the attachment is reversible and those originally attached bacteria can disconnect from the pellicle smoothly. After, stronger bacterial adherence to the pellicle is set via receptor-pairs among bacterial surface adhesins and glycoprotein receptors in the acquired pellicle. The structure of the developing biofilm is defined by local ecological agents at the site of colonization and modifies considerably at different surfaces, even at the same tooth. Through the biofilm development, bacteria are metabolically active employing mainly endogenous nutrients of saliva. This results in the production of an extracellular matrix that provides the co-adherence of the bacteria on the tooth surface and allows protection of the biofilm bacteria (Do et al. 2013). The structure of the dental biofilm varies not only between different sites in the oral cavity but also between people. Bacteria aggregation into biofilms enables them to change their phenotype, reflecting in greater survival in unfriendly conditions with nutrient lack and enhanced resistance to antimicrobial agents (Larsen & Fiehn 2017).

A dental biofilm is first installed in inactive areas of the teeth where the bacteria are guarded. If left undisturbed, due to inadequate dental hygiene methods, the supragingival biofilm may slowly spread forward the root of the tooth into the periodontal pocket, and a subgingival biofilm is established. This can lead to infection in the dental pulp as a result of profound dental caries, dental trauma, or via extra-radicular root canals from deep periodontal pockets (Larsen & Fiehn 2017). This initiates inflammation in the pulp tissue, named pulpitis. If pulpitis is left untreated, the inflammation develops into an irreversible state and the pulp slowly becomes necrotic. As the disease progresses, the microflora in the root canal shifts more complex, and a biofilm will form on the internal surfaces of the root canals (Jhajharia et al. 2015). When the dental pulp is fully necrotic, the biofilm may extend through the apical foramen of the root to the outer wall of the apical part of the tooth producing inflammation in the periapical tissue. This extraradicular biofilm is an example of the biggest challenges in combating apical periodontitis (Nair 2006). In this scenario, the development of substances that may enhance their removal and disinfection of the area, whether synthetic or natural, has gained wide attention recently.

In conjunction with the development and discovery of new antimicrobial compounds, appropriate methods for assessing their ability to act on these environments should be employed. Many plants have been used due to their antimicrobial qualities and the antimicrobial characteristics, however, an extended biological evaluation is indispensable to guarantee their effectiveness and safety. The antimicrobial susceptibility test (AST) is the primary step towards new drug development and it is employed to delimit the effectiveness of possible antimicrobials from biological extracts against a number of diverse microbial species. The main aim is to define its minimum inhibitory concentration. There are many circumstances that may alter the outcome of susceptibility tests and standardized systems are more likely to be reproducible. Sometimes it's challenging to connect collected results, when working with plant extracts, because numerous variables may affect the results, such as the environmental and climatic conditions under which the plant originated, selection of plant extracts, selection of extraction process, antimicrobial test method and test microorganisms (Hammer et al. 1999).

The AST standard tests can be classified into diffusion and dilution methods. Common diffusion experiments involve agar well/disk diffusion, while dilution designs include broth micro/macro dilution. Agar diffusion methods have been extensively employed to assay herbal extracts for antimicrobial action (Salie et al. 1996), although there are restrictions to the method. Disk diffusion is proper for description but not useful for quantification of bioactivity (Hammer et al. 1999). These diffusion methods usually do not discriminate bactericidal and bacteriostatic consequences and are habitually used for introductory screening.

In the agar diffusion method, paper disks, soaked with filter-sterilized herbal extract at the wanted concentration, are deposited onto the surface of a proper solid agar medium. The media is pre-inoculated with the examined organism and zones of inhibition are later measured from the perimeter of the disks to the border of the inhibition zone (Freixa et al. 1998). The broth microdilution technique has afforded a potentially valuable manner for determining minimum inhibitory concentration (MIC) of huge quantities of test samples. MIC, in microbiology, is the lowest concentration of antimicrobials that will inhibit the apparent growth of microorganisms after overnight incubation. MIC is essential in diagnostic laboratories to prove the resistance of microorganisms to an antimicrobial agent and also to control the activity of a novel antimicrobial agent (Cowan 1999).

Briefly, in the broth dilution technique, a stock solution of the extract is initially obtained with solvent (Grierson & Afolayan 1999). Two-fold serial dilutions are produced from the initial well to achieve a concentration range. An identical quantity of bacteria is added to the wells and incubated at 37°C for 24 h. Following incubation, plates are tested for differences in turbidity as a sign of growth. The first well that seems clear is considered to be the MIC of the plant extract. The fundamental principle of this assay is the equivalent to the broth microdilution assay, but the test is performed in a test tube rather than a microtiter plate. A kit of test tubes with varying concentrations of a plant extract with the equal volume is prepared. Tubes are treated with test microorganisms of usual concentrations. Subsequent incubation, tubes are analyzed for changes in turbidity as an indicator of growth (Klancnik et al. 2010).

The above methods are the simplest and most commonly used. Other pharmacological investigations and additional tests to completely assess the antimicrobial activity of herbal extracts are important to be employed in the subsequent steps (Khan et al. 2019).

3. Antimicrobial Activity of Plant Extracts

Bacterial infections can be considered as one of the most important among the infectious diseases. Thus, new products have been developed, either alone or in combination, to fight multi-resistant bacteria (Moghadamtousi et al. 2014). The use of medicinal plants is a millennial tradition and, given the progress of scientific evidence, the use of natural products in the treatment of various diseases has been encouraged. In general, plant extracts have antibacterial, antioxidant, antifungal and anti-inflammatory activities, among other features (Miraj & Alesaeidi 2016, Masoudi et al. 2017).

3.1. Antimicrobial Components of Extracts

The antimicrobial capacity of the plant extract may be attributable to phenolic compounds as well as secondary metabolites, such as hydroxyl groups of active constituents (Ayala-Zavala et al. 2011, Siddiqui et al. 2015). In response to microbial aggression, plants synthesize these compounds so they can act as antimicrobials against various strains. In general, these compounds interfere with bacterial growth, alter cell membrane permeability, interfering with electron transport and nutrient absorption (Zhang et al. 2006; Padmini et al. 2010). Additional enzyme inhibition is observed, altering microbial adhesins and host receptors, hindering microbial adhesion. Elevated phenols levels may lead to protein precipitation and inhibition of microbial growth. It's also important to keep in mind the complexity composition of extracts, regarding different compounds, named phytocomplex. Thus, antimicrobial activity depends on bioavailability, cumulative effect or synergistic effect of different components (Daglia et al. 2002, Badria & Zidan 2004, Matsumoto et al. 2004, Crivelaro de Menezes et al. 2010).

Among the components that provide the antimicrobial capacity to plant extracts are flavonoids, coumarins, iridoid glycosides, phenolic acids, resins, triterpens, phytoesters, choline, carotenoids, tannins, vitamins and essential oils. Among them, flavonoids and essential oils are worthy of special attention as they can be found in most extracts.

Flavonoids are bioactive compounds from the group of polyphenols that are found in vegetables, fruits, cereals, teas, coffee, cocoa, wine, fruit juice and soy. These compounds have several biological properties as antioxidant, anti-inflammatory (Xu & Lee 2001, Matsuda et al. 2002, Alvesalo et al. 2006, Haenen et al. 2006, Moon et al. 2006). The presence of flavonoids in plants plays a role in phytoalexin accumulation (Harborne & Williams 2000), which acts against bacterial invasion. It is therefore not surprising that flavonoid-rich plants have been used for many years in traditional medicine to treat infectious diseases (Cushnie & Lamb 2005). Flavonoids are divided in subgroups: flavones (widely present in leaves, flowers and fruits as glucosides), flavonols, flavanones, flavanonols, flavanols or catechins, anthocyanins (pigments responsible for colours in plants, flowers and fruits) and chalcones (phloridzin, arbutin, phloretin and chalconaringenin). Flavonols are flavonoids with a ketone group. The most studied flavonols are kaempferol, quercetin, myricetin and fisetin. Onions, kale, lettuce, tomatoes, apples, grapes and berries are rich sources of flavonols. Flavanones, such as hesperitin, naringenin and eriodictyol are another important class which is generally present in all citrus fruits such as oranges, lemons and grapes. Cyanidin, delphinidin, malvidin, pelargonidin and peonidin are the most commonly studied anthocyanins (Panceh et al. 2016).

Kaempferol is a flavonoid that exhibits good antibacterial activity (Beschia et al. 1984) and has been reported to exhibit specific antimicrobial activity against *Staphylococcus aureus, Escherichia coli, Enterococcus faecalis, Pseudomonas aeruginosa, Proteus mirabilis, Bacillus subtilis* (Agarie et al. 2009). In addition, kaempferol may also act synergistically with antibiotics (rifampicin, vancomycin, methicillin, erythromycin and clindamycin) against antibiotic resistant bacteria (Lim et al. 2007, Otsuka et al. 2008), suggesting that kaempferol could be used in combination with these drugs in cases of resistance.

Associations were also studied by Mokhtar et al. (2017). Quercetin and caffeic acid showed antimicrobial activity against *S. aureus* and combination of kaempferol with quercetin for *P. aeruginosa*. Different modes of interaction as synergism, additive, and indifferent were observed but no antagonism was obtained.

Essential oils have several biological properties such as larvicidal, antioxidant, analgesic/anti-inflammatory, fungicidal and antitumor (Chaftar et al. 2016). They can be synthesized in various plant organs, such as buds, flowers, leaves, stems, twigs, seeds, fruits, roots, wood or bark, and are stored in secretory cells, cavities, epidermal cells or trichomes (Adorjan & Buchbauer 2010). The antimicrobial activity of essential oils is closely linked to their chemical composition, which is influenced by several factors including (but not limited to) plant provenance, part of plant used, stage of plant development, climatic conditions and growth (temperature, soil, fertilizers, etc.), as well as the conditions for distillation and storage (Adorjan & Buchbauer 2010, Chaftar et al. 2016).

In the gram negative bacterial cell, lipid constituents of cell membrane are paramount for its normal functioning and play a role in a variety of processes in the bacterial cell. Toxic effects of these components on membrane structure and function have been generally used to explain the antimicrobial action of several essential oils and components (Sikkema et al. 1994).

Studies on the antimicrobial activity of essential oils and their mechanism of action have been highlighted in recent decades. Essence oils are known to cross the cell membrane wall and are related to the disruption of polysaccharides, fatty acid and phospholipids in the membrane wall (Adorjan & Buchbauer 2010; Chaftar et al. 2016). In addition, essential oils have been shown to impair membrane structure and function by binding to proteins and deforming cell wall structure, leading to cell distortion and death (Khan et al. 2014).

4. Plant Extracts with Antibacterial Properties

4.1. Myracrodruon Urundeuva

Myracrodruon urundeuva is popularly known as "aroeira" and is often found on the slopes of the hills (Lorenzi & Matos 2002). Due to its medicinal properties, aroeira has been used as a wound healer, exerting anti-inflammatory and also anti-tumor activity (Albuquerque et al. 2007; Duarte et al. 2009). In addition, the extract of this plant has antimicrobial potential, which was evidenced from the discovery of molecules obtained from *Myracrodruon urundeuva* extracts that have antibacterial as well as antifungal properties (Alves et al. 2009, Figueredo et al. 2014).

Chemical analysis of *Myracrodruon urundeuva* extracts showed that the essential oils extracted from the plant are rich in monoterpenes, the main one being represented by 3-carene (Figueredo et al. 2013). The literature shows that 3-carene substance was responsible for causing plasmolysis leading to leakage of protoplasmic content such as intracellular proteins and potassium ions (Doughari et al. 2012). The cell membrane is known to be responsible for maintaining cell balance (Yao et al. 2012). In addition, 3-Carene may inhibit intracellular tricarboxylic acid cycle activity and glycolysis-associated enzymes and disrupt ATP synthesis and decomposition, leading to bacterial metabolic dysfunction (Shu et al. 2019). Thus, it is assumed that a substance that is capable of altering the bacterial cell membrane is also considered an antimicrobial substance.

Research shows that *Myracrodruon urundeuva* extract was able to reduce the viability of the *Streptococcus mutans* biofilm, suggesting a possible anticariogenic action (Pires et al. 2019). Bueno et al. (2018) demonstrated that *Myracrodruon urundeuva* extract was effective against inactivated microorganisms, such as *Porphyromonas gingivalis, Fusobacterium nucleatum, Porphyromonas endodontalis* and *Enterococcus faecalis*, suggesting the inhibiting power of toxic compounds commonly present in inactivated microorganisms. In addition, when *Myracrodruon urundeuva* extract was associated with established antibiotics, an antibacterial action against Gram positive bacterial strains was noted (Figueredo et al. 2014).

Efficacy against *S. mutans* was evidenced by Crivelaro de Menezes et al. (2010), analyzing caries development in rats. Authors observed that the extracts had a significant effect on *S. mutans* in rats' oral biofilm, decreasing *S. mutans* accumulation and enamel demineralization.

4.2. *Curcumina* (Curcuma longa)

Curcumin is a natural, orange-yellow, phytochemical compound obtained from Curcuma longa rhizomes (Shlar et al. 2017). In recent years, there is growing scientific evidence showing that curcumin has anti-inflammatory, antitumor, antiangiogenic and also antimicrobial activity. The antimicrobial properties of curcumin were first described in 1949 by Schraufstätter & Bernt (1949). Curcumin has the ability to modulate multiple cell signaling pathways and affect many different molecular targets. This pleiotropic capacity has been demonstrated in several studies conducted in the last 50 years (Gupta et al. 2012; Zhou et al. 2011).

Regarding the mechanism of action of curcumin, Rai et al. (2008) proposes that curcumin may prevent bacterial cell proliferation by inhibiting the assembly dynamics of a bacterial protofilament, which polymerizes to form a ring that is essential for bacterial cell division. In vitro studies show that curcumin may exert antibacterial activity in a range of periodontopathic bacteria such as Porphyromonas gingivalis, Prevotella intermedia, Fusobacterium nucleatum and Treponema denticola indicating that this nutrient may be a potent agent to prevent periodontitis (Izui et al.

2016). Corroborating previous in vitro studies, curcumin was able to decrease microbial load when applied locally to chronic periodontal disease (Anitha et al. 2015). In addition to oral bacteria, curcumin was also effective against other bacteria. This information has been proven through promising data on the inhibitory effect of curcumin on Helicobacter pylori, decreasing gastritis symptoms and inducing bacterial eradication (Sarkar et al. 2016).

Regarding the mechanism of action of curcumin, Rai et al. (2008) proposes that curcumin may prevent bacterial cell proliferation by inhibiting the assembly dynamics of a bacterial protofilament, which polymerizes to form a ring that is essential for bacterial cell division. In vitro studies show that curcumin may exert antibacterial activity in a range of periodontopathic bacteria such as *Porphyromonas gingivalis, Prevotella intermedia, Fusobacterium nucleatum* and *Treponema denticola* indicating that this nutrient may be a potent agent to prevent periodontitis (Izui et al. 2016). Corroborating previous *in vitro* studies, curcumin was able to decrease microbial load when applied locally to chronic periodontal disease (Anitha et al. 2015). In addition to oral bacteria, curcumin was also effective against other bacteria. This information has been proven through promising data on the inhibitory effect of curcumin on *Helicobacter pylori*, decreasing gastritis symptoms and inducing bacterial eradication (Sarkar et al. 2016).

4.3. *Camellia sinensis*

Green tea is produced from the *Camellia sinensis* plant, being the most consumed liquid in the world, except for water. The therapeutic potential of tea was described by Sharangi (2009), which includes antioxidant effect, anticancer, antimutagenic and ability to control blood pressure, in addition to antimicrobial effect. The antimicrobial capacity of green tea may be related to the ability of the plant's active compounds to bind bacterial adhesions by disrupting bacterial surface receptors (Padmini et al. 2010). In addition, active compounds attack the cell wall/membrane causing release of intracellular constituents such as ribose and sodium glutamate as well as altering protein and nucleic acid synthesis leading to inhibition of bacterial growth. Finally, active compounds can denature membrane proteins, resulting in potassium ions leakage, inhibition of cell respiration and bacterial cell lysis (Padmini et al. 2010, Zhang et al. 2006).

The antimicrobial action of green tea has been shown to be effective against several oral bacteria. Tea's active compounds have been shown to restrict the development and colonization of harmful bacteria such as *Porphyromonas gingivalis, Prevotella intermedia* and *Prevotella nigrescens*, producing therapeutic effects on periodontal health; prevent *Streptococcus mutants* from adhering to tooth surfaces by demonstrating anti-caries action (Khurshid et al. 2016). In addition, green tea active compounds may be useful when combined with other antimicrobial agents: tetracycline against *Staphylococcus aureus* and *Staphylococcus epidermidis*; penicillin against *Staphylococcus epidermidis*; with penicillin, oxacillin, ampicillin/sulbactam, and imipenem against methicillin-resistant *Staphylococcus aureus* and with chloramphenicol, ciprofloxacin, and cefotaxime against isolates of *Escherichia coli* (Reygaert 2014).

4.4. *Cymbopogon*

Cymbopogon citratus (Lemon grass) is commonly used as a medicine, especially in tropical regions for the treatment of infectious diseases and various other diseases and disorders due to its antimicrobial and pharmacological properties (Jeong et al. 2009). Essential oils may be primarily responsible for the pharmacological action of lemon grass. These oils are complex and volatile, characterized by a strong odor and synthesized by aromatic plants during the production of secondary metabolites, which act to protect the plant against microorganisms. The chemical composition of the essential oil of *Cymbopogon citratus* may vary according to the geographical origin of the plant, but it is basically composed of hydrocarbon terpenes, alcohols, ketones, esters and mainly aldehydes and the essential oil consists mainly of citral (Shah et al. 2011).

Cymbopogon citratus essential oil has shown antibacterial effect against *Bacillus subtilis*, *Escherichia coli*, *Staphylococus aureus*, *Salmonella paratyphi* and *Shigella* flexneri (Shah et al. 2011). *Cymbopogon citratus* essential oil was also effective in the control of *Streptococcus mutans* biofilm, highlighting the promising potential of this natural substance for the development of anti-cariogenic products (Almeida et al. 2013). In addition to the antimicrobial action, it has been proven that this essential oil can also alter the adhesion of cariogenic microorganisms in tooth enamel (Oliveira et al. 2017).

Cymbopogon nardus, also extracted from a type of lemongrass, was another tested specie. The main chemical components of this essential oil are antiseptics, geraniol, and citronellol, hence its extensive use in household disinfectants and soaps

Guandalini Cunha et al. (2020) assessed the cytotoxicity and antimicrobial effects of citronella oil (*Cymbopogon nardus*) and commercial mouthwashes on *Staphylococus aureus* and *Candida albicans* biofilms (in formation–adhesion phase and 24h-biofilm formation) in prosthetic materials. Both concentrations of the citronella-based mouthwash presented superior antibiofilm effects compared to commercial alcohol-free solutions against *S. aureus* and *C. albicans*. At high concentrations, all solutions tested demonstrated toxic effects on epithelial cells. However, after serial dilution, considering the concentrations of the active principles of commercial mouthwashes, citronella had the lowest cytotoxic effect and shows a viable alternative for future mouthwash formulation.

4.5. *Matricaria chamomilla*

Chamomile (*Matricaria chamomilla L.*) is a medicinal plant belonging to the *Asteraceae* family native to Europe and Asia. It contains flavonoids, coumarins and essential oils that give chamomile extract antiseptic, sedative and protective effect against mucosal ulcers. The main components of the essential oil extracted from chamomile flowers are α-bisabolol and azulenes terpenoids, including derivatives of chamazulene and acetylene (Miraj & Alesaeidi 2016).

Chamomile aqueous and alcoholic extract is used to treat skin infections caused by pathogenic bacteria, oral lesions, respiratory system infection and digestive disorders. Munir et al. (2014) evaluated chamomile extract against strains of *Staphylococcus aureus*, and *Salmonella typhi*. In the study, gram-positive bacteria such as *Staphylococcus aureus* were more vulnerable than gram-negative bacteria such as *Escherichia coli* in relation to chamomile antimicrobial activity (Munir et al. 2014).

The antibacterial capacity of chamomile extract has also been investigated against *Enterococcus faecalis,* which is a bacterium of great interest in dentistry, especially in endodontics, as it is a microorganism commonly found in endodontic treatment failure. In a study conducted by Shakya et al. (2019), *Enterococcus faecalis* was cultivated in human teeth and the antimicrobial action of chamomile was evaluated. The study showed that *Enterococcus faecalis* was susceptible to chamomile at different time intervals when compared to two others commonly used endodontic antibacterial agents: chlorhexidine and calcium hydroxide.

4.6. *Aloe barbadensis Miller* and *Aloe aborescens*

Aloe Vera is a predominantly warm-weathered cactus-like plant that belongs to the *Liliaceae* family, which has about 360 species, but only two species are cultivated commercially: *Aloe barbadensis Miller* and *Aloe aborescens* (Nair et al. 2016). The pharmacological action of aloe vera extract is well known due to its antifungal, anti-inflammatory, antioxidant, anti-tumor as well as antibacterial properties (Nair et al. 2016). Aloe vera is made up of aloeferon that acts on wound healing and contains acemannan, which is a mucopolysaccharide that has antifungal, antimicrobial action and activates the immune system for antibody production. In addition, it is composed of another substance also responsible for antibacterial action: anthraquinone (Barreto et al. 2005).

The antibacterial action of aloe vera extract is related to bacterial cell wall disruption (Rahmani et al. 2015). The best antibacterial activity of aloe vera was found to be related to acetone extract when compared to aqueous and ethanol extracts (Nair et al. 2016). The antimicrobial activity of Aloe vera juice was also evaluated. In the study, the authors found that plant juice was more effective mainly against Gram-positive bacteria (Alemdar & Agaoglu 2009). Other studies have confirmed that aloe vera juice has been considered bacteriostatic against *Staphylococcus aureus*, *Streptococcus pyogenes* and *Salmonella paratyphi* (Agarry et al. 2005, Reynolds & Dweck 1999).

4.7. *Cinnamomum*

Cinnamon is a native plant of Sri Lanka that can be obtained from the bark of *Cinnamomum* trees and belongs to the *Lauraceae* family. Not only the bark, but the leaves can also be used in medicine due to its antifungal, antioxidant, antidiabetic, anti-inflammatory, nematicide, insecticidal, anticancer and antibacterial effects. With respect to antibacterial action, cinnamon has a wide variety of secondary metabolites that exhibit antibacterial properties (Vasconcelos et al. 2018). Basically, the antibacterial action of cinnamon has been attributed to the presence of essential oils such as eugenol. This antimicrobial action occurs by changes in the cell membrane of bacteria, inhibition of bacterial cell division and inhibition of motility and biofilm formation (Vasconcelos et al. 2018).

In a study conducted by Gupta et al. (2013), it was shown that *Cinnamomum* was effective against the planktonic form and biofilm of *Enterococcus faecalis* (Gupta et al. 2013). Abbaszadegan et al. (2016) also demonstrated that *Cinnamomum* essential oil is an efficient antibacterial agent against *E. faecalis* in both planktonic and biofilm forms, being cytocompatible with L929 fibroblasts (Abbaszadegan et al. 2016). Thus, this substance proves its potential to be used as an antimicrobial agent in root canal treatment (Abbaszadegan et al. 2016). Cinnamon extract was added in a mouthwash and its action was evaluated in patients with gingivitis dental plaque (Gupta & Jain 2015). The results of this randomized clinical trial demonstrated that cinnamon may be an effective agent because of its ability to reduce plaque levels and gingivitis, highlighting its antibacterial power.

4.8. *Psidium catleianum* and *Psidium Guava*

*Psidium spp (*Myrtaceae family*)* are species of plants native from Brazil, also found in Uruguay and the Caribbean islands (Patel 2012). The fruits are popularly known in Brazil as *araçá, yellow-araçá, red-araçá, rosa-araçá, araçá-de-comer, araçá-da-praia, araçá-de-coroa, araçá-do-campo, common guava or yellow guava (Mitra et al. 2012).*

The extract from *araçá fruits (Psidium cattleianum)* has bioactivity such as antiproliferative action, antidiabetic and also antimicrobial properties. This bioactivity may be related to the content of vitamin C and antioxidants present in the fruit acetone extract. Also, the reported bioactivity of *Psidium cattleianum* can be attributed to the high content of phenolic compounds *(up to 768mg 100g^{-1} fresh fruit pulp)*, which are secondary metabolites with high antioxidant capacity (Medina et al. 2011, Verma et al. 2013).

In 2008, Brighenti et al. (2008) tested the effect of *Psidium cattleianum* leaf extract in *Streptococcus mutans* and evidenced its antimicrobial activity, showing that leaf extract kills *S. mutans* grown in biofilms when applied at high concentrations and inhibits *S. mutans* acid production in low concentrations. This efficacy against *S. mutans* was also confirmed by Crivelaro de Menezes et al. (2010), when performing a study assessing caries development in rats. Authors observed that the extracts had a significant effect on *S. mutans* in rats' oral biofilm, decreasing *S. mutans* accumulation and enamel demineralization.

dos Santos et al. (2017) evidenced 13 bioactive phenolic compounds in methanolic extracts of *Psidium guajava*, especially elagic acid, gallic acid, rutin and catechin, which contributes to a greater use of this fruit with pharmaceutical/medicinal purposes, as a rich source of polyphenols. Besra

& Kumar (2018) found that the most active part of *Psidium guajava* against *Streptococcus mutans* and *Lactobacilus acidophilus* was extract from the leaves and methanol fraction was more successful in the extraction of phytochemicals from plant samples than aqueous solvent, as methanol extracts show higher antimicrobial activity than aqueous extracts against both the test pathogens.

The *araçá* contains flavonoids and anthocyanidins which are well-known antimicrobial agents. The effect of these compounds is related to their reaction with the microbial cell membrane that inactivates essential enzymes, or the formation of complexes with metal ions, limiting their accessibility to microbial metabolism. The extract of *araçá* fruits exhibited antibacterial activity *(in vitro)* against *Salmonella enteritidis,* which is known to be an enteric pathogen of food origin, often described in the literature related to the occurrence of intoxication in humans (Medina et al. 2011). The extract was able to inhibit the growth of planktonic and biofilm forms of anaerobic bacteria such as *Streptococcus mutans, Porphyromonas gingivalis, Prevotella intermedia* and facultative bacteria such as *Aggregatibacter actinomycetemcomitans (*Salineiro et al. 2009, Sangalli et al. 2009). In addition, Sangalli et al. (2018) showed that the association of *araça* extract with calcium hydroxide-based drugs, commonly used in endodontics, was more effective against *Enterococcus faecalis* and *Candida albicans* when compared to isolated calcium hydroxide pastes.

Interestingly, *Psidium cattleianum* extracts reduced survival rates of breast cancer cells (MCF-7) and colon cancer cells (Caco-2), by a mechanism other than toxicity since these extracts did not affect fibroblast cells (3T3) (Medina et al. 2011).

Considering the *Psidium* genus, the antimicrobial potential was also observed in *Psidium densicomum*, against *Enterecoccus faecalis,* an important pathogen associated with endodontic infection that can show resistance to a wide range of antimicrobial agents, showing results significantly better than that observed when using chlorhexidine (Castilho et al. 2013).

4.9. *Citrus sp*

Citrus plant (*Rutaceae* Family) is native to tropical Asia but it is also found in all tropical and subtropical country, known for an abundance of bioactive components, nutraceuticals and functional compounds in the flavedo and albedo of the peels. The peels of citrus fruits are rich in the polymethoxylated flavones, tageretin, nobiletin and sinensetin. Citrus flavonoids exert interesting pharmacological effects as antioxidant, anti-inflammatory, blood lipid-lowering and cholesterol-lowering agents.

The major active biological constituents in Citrus herbs/fruits are flavonoids (neohesperidosides, rutinosides), especially with bioactive compounds like naringin, hesperidin and alkaloids, mainly synephrine, with beneficial medical effects on human health (Pellati et al. 2002, Ramful et al. 2010, Escobedo-Avellaneda et al. 2014). Phenolic compounds like flavonoids are known to exhibit antioxidant, antiatherogenic, anti-inflammatory, anti-carcinogenic, antiviral, antimicrobial and antiallergenic activities (Escobedo-Avellaneda et al. 2014). The soluble fiber, or pectin, which is effective for heart health, is also an anticancer agent. Interestingly, the anticancer potential of Citrus is most effective when the whole fruit is eaten, possibly due to a synergistically components effect to amplify one another's (Suryawanshi 2011).

4.9.1. Citrus aurantium

Citrus aurantium, commonly known as bitter orange, is a valuable source of medicinally important compounds besides minerals, vitamins and antioxidants. It’s used in traditional medicine for healing several diseases. The leaves, fruit, barks, flower and root are used for stomach ache, vomiting, blood pressure, cough, cold, bronchitis, dysentery, diarrhea and fever, among other popular applications. *C. aurantium* peel contains flavonoids, coumarins, triterpenes, vitamin C, carotene and pectin (Suryawanshi 2011, Karthikeyan & Karthikeyan 2014).

A review of *Citrus aurantium* medicinal properties also emphasized that important biologically active compounds of the fruits are phenethylamine alkaloids octopamine, tyramine, N-methyltyramine, hordenine and synephrine, a primary synthesis compound with pharmacological activities (vasoconstriction, elevation of blood pressure and relaxation of bronchial muscle) (Suryawanshi 2011).

Essential oil from *C.aurantium* was tested for antibacterial activity in by agar diffusion method and showed active against *S. aureus, S. pyogenes, P. aeruginosa* (Ross et al. 1980, Karthikeyan & Karthikeyan 2014).

It's also important to state that Bitter orange contains synephrine and octopamine, chemicals components that may induce hypertension. This was observed as a possible association of acute lateral-wall myocardial infarction and a supplement with bitter orange (Nykamp et al. 2004).

4.9.2. Citrus sinensis

Popularly known as common Orange, is a widely global grown fruit crop, with global production reported to be near 120 million tons (Shakthi Deve et al. 2014).

Extracts from Orange peels showed potent antibacterial activity against *Enteric* and *Klebsiella pneumonia* pathogens (Akdemir Evrendilek 2015, Mehmood et al. 2015), besides anti-inflammatory effects of saponins (Just et al. 1998). Terpenoids found in ethanolic extracts are speculated to be involved in membrane disruption by the lipophilic compounds (Alams et al. 2005). Another secondary metabolite compound also found in ethanolic extract is alkaloid, which shows toxicity against cells of foreign organisms (Shetty et al. 2016). Components as tannin form irreversible complexes with proline rich protein resulting in the inhibition of cell protein synthesis (Shimada 2006).

Regarding antimicrobial effects against oral bacteria, peel extracts from *C. sinensis* was tested *in vitro* in aqueous and ethanolic extracts (cold and hot) against *Streptococcus mutans* and *Lactobacillus acidophilus*. Using agar well diffusion method, it was possible to observe that dental caries pathogens were inhibited most by hot ethanolic extract followed by cold ethanolic extract. Aqueous extracts were effective at very high concentrations (Shetty et al. 2016).

4.9.3. Other Citrus spp

Citrus auratium var. *bergamia also known as bergamot, showed* antimicrobial properties of flavonoid-rich ethanolic fractions derived from its peel against Gram-negative bacteria (*Escherichia coli*, *Pseudomonas putida*, *Salmonella enterica*) and Gram-positive bacteria (*Listeria innocua*, *Bacillus subtilis*, *Staphylococcus aureus*, *Lactococcus lactis*) *(Fisher & Philips 2006, Mandalari et al. 2007).*

Citrus reticulata var. *Kinnow* showed antibacterial activity by the extracts of methanol, ethanol, acetone and petroleum ether against *Staphylococcus aureus, Escherichia coli, Pseudomonas aeruginosa,* and *Klebsiella pneumoniae*. In addition, acetone extract demonstrated superior antibacterial properties, inhibiting all four pathogenic bacterial strains (Yashaswini & Arvind 2018).

Citrus unshiu is a seedless and easy-peeling citrus species, also known as unshu mikan and showed antimicrobial activity against pathogenic bacteria such as *Bacillus cereus*, *Staphylococcus aureus*, and *Listeria monocytogenes*, when used the acid-hydrolyzed peel extract (Min et al. 2014).

4.10. Capsicum spp

Pepper (genus *Capsicum*) is one of the oldest utilized crops, member of the *Solanaceae* family and consists of approximately 31 species. Capsaicin, an alkaloid that makes pepper hot, along with its minor capsaicinoids (norcapsaicin, nordihydrocapsaicin, nornordihydrocapsaicin, homocapsaicin and homodihydrocapsaicin) are the active ingredients in pepper that are related to the anti-microbial properties (Bosland 1996, Saleh et al. 2018).

Interesting results were observed by Mokhtar et al. (2017), studying the antimicrobial activity of pepper polyphenols and capsaicinoids (coumarin, caffeic acid, narangin, kaempferol, rutin, quercetin, capsaicin, and dihydrocapsaicin) against pathogen bacteria. The phenolic compounds had the most important activity with the highest inhibition zones obtained with caffeic acid, quercetin, and kaempferol. The clinical strains *Staphylococcus aureus* were more sensitive to quercetin whereas kaempferol was more active against the strains *S. aureus, S. typhimurium* and *P. aeruginosa*. The interaction between these three polyphenols was studied against *S. aureus* and *P. aeruginosa*. Different modes of interaction as synergism, additive, and indifferent were noticed but no antagonism was obtained. The best combination was quercetin and caffeic acid for *S. aureus* and kaempferol with quercetin for *P. aeruginosa*.

5. Other Plant Extracts with Antimicrobial Properties

There is a huge variety of plant extracts with antimicrobial properties. Perumal Samy et al. (1998) tested 34 Indian medicinal plants from 18 different families, searching for antibacterial properties against *Escherichia coli*, *Klebsiella aerogenes*, *Proteus Tulgaris*, and *Pseudomonas aerogenes*. The authors found 16 plants with significant antibacterial activity, such as *Cassia fistula*, *Terminalia arjuna* and *Vitex negundo* among others. In addition, the authors observed that, the aqueous extract generally exhibited a superior degree of antibacterial activity.

Another extensive research was conducted by Panda et al. (2017). The authors tested *in vitro* different parts of 35 medicinal plants belonging to 21 families, used by local tribal of the Similipal Biosphere Reserve (India) to treat infections. From each plant, three extracts were prepared with different solvents (water, ethanol, and acetone) and tested for antimicrobial (*E. coli, S. aureus, C. albicans*); anthelmintic (*C. elegans*); and antiviral (*enterovirus 71*) bioactivity. Strong antibacterial effects were observed by plants such as *Alangium salviifolium, Antidesma bunius, Bauhinia racemosa, Careya arborea, Caseria graveolens, Cleistanthus patulus*, *Colebrookea oppositifolia, Crotalaria pallida, Croton roxburghii, Holarrhena pubescens*, *Hypericum gaitii, Macaranga peltata, Protium serratum, Rubus ellipticus,* and *Suregada multiflora.* On the other hand, strong antifungal effects were observed by *Alstonia scholaris, Butea monosperma, C. arborea, C. pallida, Diospyros malbarica, Gmelina arborea, H. pubescens, M. peltata, P. serratum, Pterospermum acerifolium, R. ellipticus,* and *S. multiflora.*

Plants such as *A. salviifolium, A. bunius, Aporosa octandra, Barringtonia acutangula, C. graveolens, C. pallida, C. patulus, G. arborea, H. pubescens, H. gaitii, Lannea coromandelica, M. peltata, Melastoma malabathricum, Millettia extensa, Nyctanthes arbor-tristis, P. serratum, P. acerifolium, R. ellipticus, S. multiflora, Symplocos cochinchinensis, Ventilago maderaspatana,* and *Wrightia arborea* inhibit survival of *C. elegans* and could be a potential source for anthelmintic activity. Additionally, plants such as *A. bunius, C. graveolens, C. patulus, C. oppositifolia, H. gaitii, M. extensa, P. serratum, R. ellipticus,* and *V. maderaspatana* showed anti-enteroviral activity. Most of the plants, whose traditional use as anti-infective agents by the tribals was well supported, show *in vitro* inhibitory activity against an enterovirus, bacteria (*E. coil, S. aureus*), a fungus (*C. albicans*), or a nematode (*C. elegans*) (Panda et al. 2017).

Final Considerations

The development of bacterial resistance as well as undesirable side effects of the antibiotics has triggered the search of new antibacterial agents. The antimicrobial potency of plants is believed to be due to synergistic and biologically active phytocomplex components such as tannins, saponins, phenolic compounds, essential oils and flavonoids. Although previous articles have already evidenced the effects of many herbal extracts, new research with updated methodologies and analyzes as well as randomized clinical trials are of paramount importance to establish a solid and safe usage protocol. Also, the dentistry/medical community must be updated to be able to use new therapeutic sources in the daily clinical routine. The antibacterial activity observed in the several studies in this chapter may explain the folk therapy/traditional medicine that have been using plant extracts to successful treat different diseases for generations.

Due to the huge variety of plants in the literature, it is impracticable to describe all extracts with antibacterial properties. Therefore, this chapter mentioned some of the extracts with such properties, which may serve as an introduction to new research and open mind of new researchers.

REFERENCES

Abbaszadegan A, Dadolahi S, Gholami A, Moein MR, Hamedani S, Ghasemi Y, Abbott PV. Antimicrobial and cytotoxic activity of *cinnamomum zeylanicum*, calcium hydroxide, and triple antibiotic paste as root canal dressing materials. *J Contemp Dent Pract* 2016;17:105–13.

Adorjan B, Buchbauer G. Biological properties of essential oils: an updated review. *Flavour Fragr J* 2010;25:407–26.

Agarie S, Kawaguchi A, Kodera A, Sunagawa H, Kojima H, Nose A, Nakahara T. Potential of the common ice plant, Mesembryanthemum crystallinum as a new high-functional food as evaluated by polyol accumulation. *Plant Prod Sci* 2009;12:37–46.

Agarry O, Olaleye M, Bello-Michael C. Comparative antimicrobial activities of aloe vera gel and leaf. *African J Biotechnol* 2005;4:1413–1414.

Akdemir Evrendilek G. Empirical prediction and validation of anti-bacterial inhibitory effects of various plant essential oils on common pathogenic bacteria. *Int J Food Microbiol* 2015;202:35–41.

Alams K, Skaug N, Ahmad I. An *in vitro* antimicrobial comparison of miswak extract with commercially available non-alcohol mouth rinses. *Int J Dent Hyg* 2005;3:18–24.

Albuquerque UP, Medeiros PM, Almeida ALS, Monteiro JM, de Freitas Lins Neto EM, de Melo JG, dos Santos JP. Medicinal plants of the caatinga (semi-arid) vegetation of NE Brazil: A quantitative approach. *J Ethnopharmacol* 2007;114:325–354.

Alemdar S, Agaoglu S. Investigation of in vitro antimicrobial activity of Aloe vera juice. *J Anim Vet Adv* 2009;8:99–102.

Almeida RBA, Akisue G, Cardoso LML, Junqueira JC, Jorge AOC. Antimicrobial activity of the essential oil of *Cymbopogon citratus* (DC) Stapf. on *Staphylococcus* spp., *Streptococcus mutans* and *Candida* spp. *Rev Bras Plantas Med.* 2013;15:474–482.

Alves PM, Queiroz LMG, Pereira JV, Pereira MDSV. *In vitro* antimicrobial, antiadherent and antifungal activity of Brazilian medicinal plants on oral biofilm microorganisms and strains of the genus *Candida*. *Rev Soc Bras Med Trop* 2009;42:222–224.

Alvesalo J, Vuorela H, Tammela P, Leinonen M, Saikku P, Vuorela P. Inhibitory effect of dietary phenolic compounds on Chlamydia pneumoniae in cell cultures. *Biochem Pharmacol* 2006;71:735–741.

Anitha V, Rajesh P, Shanmugam M, Priya B, Prabhu S, Shivakumar V. Comparative evaluation of natural curcumin and synthetic chlorhexidine in the management of chronic periodontitis as a local drug delivery: A clinical and microbiological study. *Indian J Dent Res* 2015;26:53–56.

Ayala-Zavala JF, Vega-Vega V, Rosas-Domínguez C, Palafox-Carlos H, Villa-Rodriguez JA, Siddiqui MW, Dávila-Aviñaa JE, González-Aguilar GA. Agro-industrial potential of exotic fruit byproducts as a source of food additives. *Food Res Int* 2011;44:1866–74.

Azmir J, Zaidul I, Rahman M, Sharif K, Mohamed A, Sahena F, Omar AKM. Techniques for extraction of bioactive compounds from plant materials: A review. *J Food Eng* 2013;117,426–436.

Badria FA, Zidan OA. Natural products for dental caries prevention. *J Med Food* 2004;7:381–4.

Barreto L, Feitosa SC, De Araújo J, Chagas K, Costa K. Acción antimicrobiana in vitro de dentífricos conteniendo fitoterápicos. *Av Odontoestomatol* 2005;21:195–201.

Beschia M, Leonte A, Oencea I. Phenolic compounds with biological activity. *Bull Univ Galati Faso* 1984;6:23–7.

Besra M, Kumar V. In vitro investigation of antimicrobial activities of ethnomedicinal plants against dental caries pathogens. *3 Biotech* 2018;8(5):257.

Bimakr M, Rahman RA, Taip FS, Ganjloo A, Salleh LM. Selamat J, Zaidul ISM. Comparison of different extraction methods for the extraction of major bioactive flavonoid compounds from spearmint (*Mentha spicata L.*) leaves. *Food and Biop Proc* 2011;89,67–72.

Bosland PW. Capsicums: Innovative Uses of an Ancient Crop. In: Janick J editor. *Progress in new crops*. USA: ASHS Press 1996:479–87.

Brighenti FL, Luppens SB, Delbem AC, Deng DM et al. Effect of *Psidium cattleianum* leaf extract on streptococcus mutans viability, protein expression and acid production. *Caries res* 2008;42(2):148–54.

Bueno CRE, Valentim D, Jardim Junior ÉG, Mancuso DN, Sivieri-Araujo G, Jacinto RC, Cintra LTA, Dezan-Junior E. Tissue reaction to Aroeira (*Myracrodruon urundeuva*) extracts associated with microorganisms: an in vivo study. *Braz Oral Res* 2018;32:e42.

Castilho AL, Saraceni CHC, Díaz IEC, et al. New trends in dentistry: plant extracts against *Enterococcus faecalis*. The efficacy compared to chlorhexidine. *Braz oral res* 2013;27(2): 109–15.

Chaftar N, Girardot M, Labanowski J, Ghrairi T, Hani K, Frère J, Imbert C. Comparative evaluation of the antimicrobial activity of 19 essential oils. *Adv Exp Med Biol* 2016;901:1–15.

Cowan, MM. Plant products as antimicrobial agents. *Clin Microb Rev* 1999;12,564–582.

Crivelato de Menezes TE, Botazzo Delbem AC, Lourenção Brighenti F, et al. Protective efficacy of *Psidium cattleianum* and *Myracrodruon urundeuva* aqueous extracts against caries development in rats. *Pharm Biol* 2010;48(3):300–5.

Cushnie TPT, Lamb AJ. Antimicrobial activity of flavonoids. *Int J Antimicrob Agents* 2005;26:343–56.

Daglia M, Tarsi R, Papetti A, Grisoli P, Dacarro C, Pruzzo C, Gazzani G. Antiadhesive effect of green and roasted coffee on *Streptococcus mutans* adhesive properties on saliva-coated hydroxyapatite beads. *J Agric Food Chem* 2002;50: 1225–9.

Dewhirst FE, Chen T, Izard J, Paster BJ, Tanner AC, Yu WH, Wade WG. The human oral microbiome. *J Bacteriol* 2010;192,5002–5017.

Do T, Devine D, Marsh PD. Oral biofilms: molecular analysis, challenges, and future prospects in dental diagnostics. *Clin Cosmet Investig Dent* 2013;5,11–19.

Dos Santos WNL, Sauthier MCS, dos Santos AMP, et al. Simultaneous determination of 13 phenolic bioactive compounds in guava (*Psidium guajava* L.) by HPLC-PAD with evaluation using PCA and Neural Network Analysis (NNA). *Microchem J* 2017;133:583–92.

Doughari JH, Ndakidemi PA, Human IS, Benade S. Antioxidant, antimicrobial and antiverotoxic potentials of extracts of Curtisia dentata. *J Ethnopharmacol* 2012;141:1041–50.

Duarte MR, Schroder LM, Toledo MG, M. Y, Machado AA, Modolo AK. Anatomia foliar comparada de espécies de aroeira: Myracrodruon urundeuva ALLEMÃO E Schinus terebinthifolius RADDI. *Visão Acadêmica* 2009;10:18–28.

Escobedo-Avellaneda Z, Gutiérrez-Uribe J, Valdez-Fragoso A, Torres JA, Welti-Chanes J. Phytochemicals and antioxidant activity of juice, flavedo, albedo and comminuted orange. *J Funct Foods* 2014; 6: 470–81.

Figueredo FG, Ferreira EO, Lucena BFF, Torres CMG, Lucetti DL, Lucetti ECP, Silva JM, Santos FA, Medeiros CR, Oliveira GM, Colares AV, Costa JG, Coutinho HD, Menezes IR, Silva JC, Kerntopf MR, Figueiredo PR, Matias EF. Modulation of the antibiotic activity by extracts from amburana cearensis A. C. Smith and anadenanthera macrocarpa (Benth.) Brenan. *Biomed Res Int* 2013;2013:1–5.

Figueredo FG, Lucena BFF, Tintino SR, Matias EFF, Leite NF, Andrade JC, Nogueira LF, Morais EC, Costa JG, Coutinho HD, Rodrigues FF. Chemical composition and evaluation of modulatory of the antibiotic activity from extract and essential oil of Myracrodruon urundeuva. *Pharm Biol* 2014;52:560–5.

Fisher K, Philips CA. The effect of lemon, orange and bergamot essential oils and their components on the survival of *Campylobacter jejuni*, *Escherichia coli* O157, *Listeria monocytogenes*, *Bacillus cereus* and

Staphylococcus aureus in vitro and in food systems. *J Appl Microbiol* 2006;101(6):1232–40.

Freixa B, Vila R, Vargas L, Lozano N, Adzet T, Cañigueral S. Screening for antifungal activity of nineteen Latin American plants. *Phyto Res* 1998;12,427–430.

Grierson DS, Afolayan AJ. Antibacterial activity of some indigenous plants used for the treatment of wounds in the Eastern Cape, South Africa. *J Ethnopharmacol* 1999;66,103–106.

Guandalini Cunha B, Duque C, Sampaio Caiaffa K, Massunari L, Araguê Catanoze I, dos Santos DM, de Oliveira SHP, Guiotti AM, Cytotoxicity and antimicrobial effects of citronella oil (*Cymbopogon nardus*) and commercial mouthwashes on *S. aureus* and *C. albicans* biofilms in prosthetic materials. *Arch Oral Biol* 2020;109:104577.

Gupta A, Duhan J, Tewari S, Sangwan P, Yadav A, Singh G, Juneja R, Saini H. Comparative evaluation of antimicrobial efficacy of Syzygium aromaticum, Ocimum sanctum and Cinnamomum zeylanicum plant extracts against Enterococcus faecalis: A preliminary study. *Int Endod J* 2013;46:775–83.

Gupta D, Jain A. Effect of Cinnamon Extract and Chlorhexidine Gluconate (0.2%) on the Clinical Level of Dental Plaque and Gingival Health: A 4-Week, Triple-Blind Randomized Controlled Trial. *J Int Acad Periodontol.* 2015;17:91–8.

Gupta SC, Patchva S, Koh W, Aggarwal BB. Discovery of curcumin, a component of golden spice, and its miraculous biological activities. *Clin Exp Pharmacol Physiol* 2012;39:283–99.

Haenen GRMM, Arts MJTJ, Bast A, Coleman MD. Structure and activity in assessing antioxidant activity in vitro and in vivo A critical appraisal illustrated with the flavonoids. *Environ Toxicol Pharmacol* 2006;21:191–8.

Hammer KA, Carson CF, Riley TV. Antimicrobial activity of essential oils and other plant extracts. *J Appl Microbiol* 1999;86,985–990.

Harborne JB, Williams CA. Advances in flavonoid research since 1992. *Phytochemistry* 2000;55:481–504.

Izui S, Sekinc S, Maeda K, Kuboniwa M, Takada A, Amano A, Nagata H. Antibacterial Activity of Curcumin Against Periodontopathic Bacteria. *J Periodontol* 2016;87:83–90.

Jeong MR, Park PB, Kim DH, Jang YS, Jeong HS, Choi SH. Essential Oil Prepared from Cymbopogon citrates Exerted an Antimicrobial Activity Against Plant Pathogenic and Medical Microorganisms. *Mycobiology* 2009;37:48.

Jhajharia K, Parolia A, Shetty KV, Mehta LK. Biofilm in endodontics: A review. *J Int Soc Prev Community Dent* 2015;5, 1–12.

Just MJ, Recio MC, Giner RM, Cueller MJ, Manez S, Bilia AR, et al. Anti-inflammatory activity of unusual lupine saponins from Bupleurum fruticescens. *Planta Med* 1998;64:404–7.

Karthikeyan V, Karthikeyan J. *Citrus aurantium* (Bitter Orange): A Review of its Traditional Uses, Phytochemistry and Pharmacology. *International Journal of Drug Discovery and Herbal Research* 2014;4(4): 766–772.

Khan MSA, Ahmad I, Cameotra SS. Carum copticum and Thymus vulgaris oils inhibit virulence in Trichophyton rubrum and Aspergillus spp. *Braz J Microbiol* 2014;45:523–31.

Khan ZA, Siddiqui MF, Park S. Current and Emerging Methods of Antibiotic Susceptibility Testing. *Diagnostics (Basel)* 2019;9(2):E49.

Khurshid Z, Zafar MS, Zohaib S, Najeeb S, Naseem M. Green Tea (*Camellia Sinensis*): Chemistry and Oral Health. *Open Dent J* 2016;10:166–73.

Klancnik A, Piskernik S, Jersek B, Mozina SS. Evaluation of diffusion and dilution methods to determine the antibacterial activity of plant extracts. *J Microbiol Methods* 2010;81,121–126.

Kumar G, Jalaluddin M, Rout P, Mohanty R, Dileep CL. Emerging trends of herbal care in dentistry. *J Clin Diagn Res* 2013;7,1827–1829.

Larsen T, Fiehn NE. Dental biofilm infections - an update. APMIS 2017;125,376–384.

Lim YH, Kim IH, Seo JJ. In vitro activity of kaempferol isolated from the Impatiens balsamina alone and in combination with erythromycin or clindamycin against Propionibacterium acnes. *J Microbiol* 2007;45:473–7.

Lorenzi H, Matos FJA. Plantas medicinais do Brasil: nativas e exóticas. São Paulo: Instituto Plantarum de Estudos Da Flora [Medicinal plants from Brazil: native and exotic. Sao Paulo: Plantarum Institute of Flora Studies] 2002:512p.

Mandalari G, Bennett RN, Bisignano G, et al. Antimicrobial activity of flavonoids extracted from bergamot (*Citrus bergamia Risso*) peel, a byproduct of the essential oil industry. *J Appl Microbiol* 2007; 103(6): 2056–64.

Masoudi M, Rafieian Kopaei M, Miraj S. A comparison of the efficacy of metronidazole vaginal gel and Myrtus (*Myrtus communis*) extract combination and metronidazole vaginal gel alone in the treatment of recurrent bacterial vaginosis. *Avicenna J Phytomedicine* 2017;7:129–36.

Matsuda H, Ninomiya K, Shimoda H, Yoshikawa M. Hepatoprotective principles from the flowers of Tilia argentea (linden): structure requirements of tiliroside and mechanisms of action. *Bioorg Med Chem* 2002;10:707–12.

Matsumoto M, Tsuji M, Okuda J, Sasaki H, Nakano K, Osawa K, Shimura S, Ooshima T. Inhibitory effects of cacao bean husk extract on plaque formation *in vitro* and *in vivo*. *Eur J Oral Sci* 2004;112: 249–52.

Medina AL, Haas LIR, Chaves FC, Salvador M, Zambiazi RC, Da Silva WP, Nora L, Rombaldi CV. Araçá (*Psidium cattleianum Sabine*) fruit extracts with antioxidant and antimicrobial activities and antiproliferative effect on human cancer cells. *Food Chem* 2011;128, 916–922.

Mehmood B, Dar KK, Ali S, Awan UA, Nayyer AQ, Ghous T, et al. Short communication: in vitro assessment of antioxidant, antibacterial and phytochemical analysis of peel of *Citrus sinensis*. *Pak J Pharm Sci* 2015;28:231–9.

Min KY, Kim HJ, Lee KA, Kim KT, Paik HD. Antimicrobial activity of acid- hydrolyzed *Citrus unshiu* peel extract in milk. *J Dairy Sci* 2014;97(4): 1955–60.

Miraj S, Alesacidi S. A systematic review study of therapeutic effects of Matricaria recuitta chamomile (chamomile). *Electron Physician* 2016;8:3024–31.

Mitra SK, Irenaeus TKS, Gurung MR, Pathak PK. Taxonomy and importance of Myrtaceae. *Acta Horticulturae* 2012;959, 23–34.

Moghadamtousi SZ, Kadir HA, Hassandarvish P, Tajik H, Abubakar S, Zandi K. A review on antibacterial, antiviral, and antifungal activity of curcumin. *Biomed Res Int* 2014;2014:186864.

Mokhtar M, Ginestra G, Youcefi F, Filocamo A, Bisignano C, Riazi A. Antimicrobial Activity of Selected Polyphenols and Capsaicinoids Identified in Pepper (*Capsicum annuum L.*) and Their Possible Mode of Interaction. *Curr Microbiol* 2017; 74(11):1253–60.

Moon YJ, Wang X, Morris ME. Dietary flavonoids: Effects on xenobiotic and carcinogen metabolism. *Toxicol Vitr* 2006;20:187–210.

Munir N, Iqbal AS, Altaf I, Bashir R, Sharif N, Saleem F, Naz S. Evaluation of antioxidant and antimicrobial potential of two endangered plant species Atropa belladonna and Matricaria chamomilla. *African J Tradit Complement Altern Med* 2014;11:111–7.

Nair GR, Naidu GS, Jain S, Nagi R, Makkad RS, Jha A. Clinical Effectiveness of Aloe Vera in the Management of Oral Mucosal Diseases- A Systematic Review. *J Clin Diagn* Res 2016;10:1–7.

Nair PN. On the causes of persistent apical periodontitis: a review. *Int Endod J* 2006;39,249–281.

Nemeth J, Oesch G, Kuster SP. Bacteriostatic versus bactericidal antibiotics for patients with serious bacterial infections: systematic review and meta-analysis. *J Antimicrob Chemother* 2015;70,382–395.

Nykamp DL, Fackih MN, Compton AL. Possible association of acute lateral-wall myocardial infarction and bitter orange supplement. *Ann Pharmacother* 2004, 38: 812–16.

Oliveira MAC de, Borges AC, Brighenti FL, Salvador MJ, Gontijo AVL, Koga-Ito CY. Cymbopogon citratus essential oil: effect on polymicrobial caries-related biofilm with low cytotoxicity. *Braz Oral Res* 2017;31:89.

Otsuka N, Liu M-H, Shiota S, Ogawa W, Kuroda T, Hatano T, Tsuchiya T. Anti-methicillin resistant Staphylococcus aureus (MRSA) compounds isolated from Laurus nobilis. *Biol Pharm Bull* 2008;31:1794–7.

Padmini E, Valarmathi A, Ushaarani M. Comparative analysis of chemical composition and antibacterial activities of and Menthaaspicata Camelliaasinensis. *Asian J Exp Biol Sci* 2010;1:772–81.

Panche AN, Diwan AD, Chandra SR. Flavonoids: an overview. *J Nutr Sci* 2016; 29(5):e47.

Panda SK, Padhi L, Leyssen P, Liu M, Neyts J, Luyten W. Antimicrobial, Anthelmintic, and Antiviral Activity of Plants Traditionally Used for Treating Infectious Disease in the Similipal Biosphere Reserve, Odisha, India. *Front Pharmacol* 2017; 23;8:658.

Pankey GA, Sabath LD. Clinical relevance of bacteriostatic versus bactericidal mechanisms of action in the treatment of Gram-positive bacterial infections. *Clin Infect Dis* 2004;38,864–870.

Patel S. Exotic tropical plant *Psidium cattleianum*: a review on prospects and threats. *Reviews in Environmental Science and Bio/Technology* 2012;11,243–248.

Pellati F, Benvenuti S, Melegari M, Firenzuoli F. Determination of adrenergic agonists from extracts and herbal products of *Citrus aurantium* L. var. *Amara* by LC. *J Pharm Biomed Anal* 2002; 29(6): 1113–19.

Perumal Samy R, Ignacimuthu S, Sen A. Screening of 34 Indian medicinal plants for antibacterial properties. *J Ethnopharmacol* 1998;62(2):173–82.

Pires JG, Braga AS, de Andrade FB, Saldanha LL, Dokkedal AL, de Oliveira RC, Magalhães AC. Effect of hydroalcoholic extract of myracrodruon urundeuva All. and Qualea grandiflora Mart. leaves on the viability and activity of microcosm biofilm and on enamel demineralization. *J Appl Oral Sci* 2019;27:e20180514.

Rahmani AH, Aldebasi YH, Srikar S, Khan AA, Aly SM. Aloe vera : Potential candidate in health management via modulation of biological activities. *Pharmacogn Rev* 2015;9:120–6.

Rai D, Singh JK, Roy N, Panda D. Curcumin inhibits FtsZ assembly: an attractive mechanism for its antibacterial activity. *Biochem J* 2008;410:147–55.

Ramful D, Bahrun T, Bourdon E, Tarnus E, Aruoma OI. Bioactive phenolics and antioxidant propensity of flavedo extracts of Mauritian citrus fruits: potential prophylactic ingredients for functional foods application. *Toxicology* 2010;278(1):75–87.

Reygaert WC. The antimicrobial possibilities of green tea. *Front Microbiol* 2014;5.

Reynolds T, Dweck AC. Aloe vera leaf gel: A review update. *J Ethnopharmacol* 1999;68(1–3):3–37.

Ross SA, El-keltawi NE, Megalla SE. Antimicrobial activity of some egyptian aromatic plants. *Fitoterapia* 1980;51: 201–5.

Saleh BK, Omer A, Teweldemedhin B. Medicinal uses and health benefits of chili pepper (*Capsicum* spp.): a review. *MOJ Food Process Technol* 2018;6(4):325–328.

Salie F, Eagles PF, Leng HM. Preliminary antimicrobial screening of four South African Asteraceae species. *J Ethnopharmacol* 1996;52, 27–33.

Salineiro FCS, Bianco KG, Gaetti Jardim-Júnior E. Evaluation of antimicrobial activity of plant extracts from the Brazilian savannah on Streptococcus mutans. *J Appl Oral Sci* 2009; 485 abstract 307.

Sangalli J, Dezan-Junior E, Gaetti-Jardim E Jr. Antimicrobial activity of six plant extracts from the Brazilian savanna on microbial biofilms. *Braz Oral Res* 2009; 23(Supplement 1):294 Abstract PNe073.

Sangalli J, Júnior EGJ, Bueno CRE, Jacinto RC, Sivieri-Araujo G, Gomes-Filho JE, Cintra LTA, Dezan-Junior E. Antimicrobial activity of Psidium cattleianum associated with calcium hydroxide against Enterococcus faecalis and Candida albicans: an in vitro study. *Clin Oral Investig* 2018;22(6):2273–79.

Sarkar A, De R, Mukhopadhyay AK. Curcumin as a potential therapeutic candidate for Helicobacter pylori associated diseases. *World J Gastroenterol* 2016;22:2736–48.

Schraufstätter E, Bernt H. Antibacterial action of curcumin and related compounds. *Nature* 1949;164:456–7.

Sasidharan S, Chen Y, Saravanan D, Sundram KM, Yoga L. Extraction, isolation and characterization of bioactive compounds from plants' extracts. *Afr J Tradit Complement Altern Med* 2011;8,1–10.

Shah G, Shri R, Panchal V, Sharma N, Singh B, Mann AS. Scientific basis for the therapeutic use of Cymbopogon citratus, stapf (Lemon grass). *J Adv Pharm Technol Res* 2011;2:3–8.

Shakthi Deve A, Sathish Kumar T, Kumaresan K, Rapheal VS. Extraction process optimization of polyphenols from Indian *Citrus sinensis* as novel antiglycative agents in the management of diabetes mellitus. *J Diabetes Metab Disord* 2014;13:11.

Shakya VK, Luqman S, Tikku AP, Chandra A, Singh DK. A relative assessment of essential oil of Chrysopogon zizanioides and Matricaria chamomilla along with calcium hydroxide and chlorhexidine gel against Enterococcus faecalis in ex vivo root canal models. *J Conserv Dent* 2019;22:34–9.

Sharangi AB. Medicinal and therapeutic potentialities of tea (Camellia sinensis L.) - A review. *Food Res Int* 2009;42:529–35.

Shetty SB, Mahin-Syed-Ismail P, Varghese S et al. Antimicrobial effects of *Citrus sinensis* peel extracts against dental caries bacteria: An *in vitro* study. *J Clin Exp Dent* 2016;8(1):e71–7.

Shimada T. Salivary proteins as a defense against dietary tannins. *J Chem Ecol* 2006;32:1149–63.

Shlar I, Droby S, Rodov V. Modes of antibacterial action of curcumin under dark and light conditions: A toxicoproteomics approach. *J Proteomics* 2017;160:8–20.

Shu H, Chen H, Wang X, Hu Y, Yun Y, Zhong Q, Chen W, Chen W. Antimicrobial Activity and Proposed Action Mechanism of 3-Carene against Brochothrix thermosphacta and Pseudomonas fluorescens. *Molecules* 2019;24:3246.

Siddiqui MW, Ayala-Zavala JF, Dhua RS. Genotypic variation in tomatoes affecting processing and antioxidant attributes. *Crit Rev Food Sci Nutr* 2015;55:1819–35.

Sikkema J, De Bont JA, Poolman B. Interactions of cyclic hydrocarbons with biological membranes. *J Biol Chem* 1994; 269(11):8022–28.

Sinha DJ, Sinha AA. Natural medicaments in dentistry. *Ayu* 2014;35:113–8.

Suryawanshi JAS. An overview of *Citrus aurantium* used in treatment of various diseases. *Afr J Plant Sci* 2011; 5(7): 390–5.

Taheri JB, Azimi S, Rafieian N, Zanjani HA. Herbs in dentistry. *Int Dent J* 2011;61:287–96.

Vasconcelos NG, Croda J, Simionatto S. Antibacterial mechanisms of cinnamon and its constituents: A review. *Microb Pathog* 2018;120:198–203.

Verma AK, Rajkumar V, Banerjee R, Biswas S, Das AK. Guava (Psidium guajava L.) Powder as an Antioxidant Dietary Fibre in Sheep Meat Nuggets.Asian-Australas. *J Anim Sci* 2013;26:886–95.

Xu HX, Lee SF. Activity of plant flavonoids against antibiotic-resistant bacteria. *Phytother Res* 2001;15:39–43.

Yao X, Zhu X, Pan S, Fang Y, Jiang F, Phillips GO, Xu X. Antimicrobial activity of nobiletin and tangeretin against Pseudomonas. *Food Chem* 2012;132:1883–90.

Yashaswini P, Arvind. Antimicrobial Properties of Orange (*Citrus reticulata* var. *Kinnow*) Peel Extracts against Pathogenic Bacteria. *Int J Curr Microbiol App Sci* 2018; 7(3): 737–46.

Zhang QW, Lin LG, Ye WC. Techniques for extraction and isolation of natural products: a comprehensive review. *Chin Med* 2018;13,20.

Zhang YM, White SW, Rock CO. Inhibiting bacterial fatty acid synthesis. *J Biol Chem* 2006;281:17541–4.

Zhou H, Beevers CS, Huang S. The Targets of Curcumin. *Curr Drug Targets.* 2011;12:332–47.

In: Contemporary Use of Plant Extracts … ISBN: 978-1-53617-650-6
Editor: C. R. Emerenciano Bueno

Chapter 3

BIOCOMPATIBILITY OF PLANT EXTRACTS

Marina Tolomei Sandoval Cury[1,*], Gabriel Pereira Nunes[1], Ana Maria Veiga Vasques[1], Juliano Milanezi de Almeida[2], Henrique Rinaldi Matheus[2], Alexandre Henrique dos Reis-Prado[3], Eloi Dezan Junior[1] and Carlos Roberto Emerenciano Bueno[1]

[1]Department of Endodontics, São Paulo State University (UNESP), Araçatuba School of Dentistry, Aracatuba, São Paulo, Brazil
[2]Department of Surgery and Integrated Clinic, Division of Periodontics, São Paulo State University (UNESP), Araçatuba School of Dentistry, Aracatuba, Sao Paulo, Brazil
[3]Department of Restorative Dentistry, Federal University of Minas Gerais (UFMG), School of Dentistry, Belo Horizonte, Minas Gerais, Brazil

* Corresponding Author's Email: ma.tolomei@gmail.com.

ABSTRACT

Inflammation is an inner response of a host to an external agent, encompassing complex mediators and events. The use of anti-inflammatory substances is applicable for the treatment of some conditions. The anti-inflammatory property of phytotherapics turns them into therapeutic option to conventional medicine and stimulates studies for use in humans. Herbals are widely used in popular medicine in many countries. However, the effectiveness of many of them remains poorly accessed.

So, experimental researches aiming to investigate their pharmaceutical properties are essential to determine these paths and compatibility. This chapter will embrace experiments assessing the biocompatibility of extracts through cell culture, edema induction, subcutaneous tests and associations made with different extracts aiming to enhance the effectiveness of some compounds already used in daily practice. In addition, several promising plant extracts with scientifically proved results will be described.

Keywords: biocompatibility, ethnopharmacology, inflammation, phytotherapy, plant extracts

1. INFLAMMATION

Inflammation is the inner response of the hosts' blood vessels to an external agent, mainly characterized by fluids and defense cells reaching the interstice (Lope et al. 1987), and clinically observed through redness, heat, swelling, pain, and loss of function (Dassoler et al. 2004). Innumerous reasons can trigger an inflammatory process, however, the cascade of events is basically the same. The inflammatory agent induces the activation of phospholipase A2, which will release arachidonic acid and other substances. According to Dassoler et al. (2004), cytokines, histamine, serotonin, leukotrienes, and prostaglandins increase vascular permeability in order for all leukocytes to reach the inflamed tissues. Any interruption in this cascade results on reduced release of such mediators and yields to normal hemodynamic behavior (Lope et al. 1987).

Even this mechanism being efficient, the complexity of the events and mediators related to the inflammatory response are capable to induce, sustain and to aggravate many lesions (Sosa et al. 2002). Non-steroidal anti-inflammatories (NSAIDs) are the most used drugs by the population and not rarely related to adverse gastric reactions, collapse of kidneys' activity, reduction of the efficacy of diuretics and inhibition of the angiotensin-converting enzyme (Gaddi et al. 2004).

The anti-inflammatory properties of the herbal extracts may consist of a plausible alternative to NSAIDs. The main idea for the use of phytotherapics is not to replace conventional medicine, but to increase the therapeutic options with equivalent medicines, also branded, of lower costs and more accurate spectrum (Lapa et al. 2003).

2. BIOCOMPATIBILITY

This chapter will describe the conceptual aspects of biocompatibility, emphasizing the natural extracts used in dentistry and the methods to evaluate biocompatibility and to monitor these organic species.

In accordance with the 1986 conference of the European Society for Biomaterials, biocompatibility is defined as the capacity of any substance to exhibit an appropriate response by a host, with no damage to body tissues (Duncan & Izzo 2005). The use of a substance on a living tissue creates an area of contact, which may display biological and structural stability. The interface between substance and tissue is dynamic and depends on the biocompatibility of the tested material. This positive interaction depends on the type, form, size, physical property, composition and location of the material, and also factors related to the host. Nowadays, the assessment of biocompatibility also comprises the replaced and adjacent tissues.

Not only the absence of reported pain nor periapical alterations observed in x-ray images are signs to determine biocompatibility. The success of materials used in health science is related with three essential factors:

1. Properties of the material;
2. Design of the device;
3. Biocompatibility of their compounds.

The biocompatibility of biological materials may be evaluated through analysis of composition, cell culture tests, animal and human experimentation. These methodologies are regulated and standardized by government bodies, such as *International Standards Organization* (ISO), *Federation Dentaire Internationale* (FDI) and *American Dental Association* (ADA). These organizations affirm that isolated testing is not enough to assure secure use. All biocompatibility tests might follow some requirements: to be performed in a manner to mimic the real use of the material; the conditions shall befit the time of permanence of this material in contact with the tissue; and the reactions of the material may be considered for the understanding of the biological response.

3. Biocompatibility Tests

The acceptance and security of any product shall be based in experiments proving, among other positive properties, their biocompatibility. Biological assays for evaluation of biocompatibility can encompass *in vitro* and *in vivo* designs. These tests are essential to identify not only substances with positive effects over tissues, but also the ones that present adverse reactions and might not be used in any condition. Different methodologies have been proposed to identify the substances that can be indicated for further studies in humans.

For example, the placement of samples in the subcutaneous connective tissue of rodents is considered suitable for evaluating the biocompatibility of endodontic materials (Bueno et al. 2016, 2017, 2018, 2019, Benetti et al. 2019), however, it is known that the tissues' response may not be essentially the same observed in pulpal and periapical tissues. The normative disclosed by the ADA (1972, 1982, Stanley 1992) and International Organization for Standardization (1997) considers the methodology of subcutaneous implantation valid for preliminary phases of histocompatibility evaluation.

3.1. Cell Cultures

First studies with cell cultures obtained from animals are dated from the beginning of 20th century (Carrel 1912, Harrison 1970). Tests with cell cultures aim to evaluate the behavior these cells isolated from systemic variations, observing if the material possess the potential to damage or not these cells. These tests can be considered relatively quick and with considerable ease standardization (Cintra et al. 2017).

For this type of experiment, the extract is placed in intimate contact with the cultivated biological material, or this contact is interposed by some kind of barrier (e.g., filter of membrane). The results are commonly related with the determination of growth, cell function and integrity of cells' genetics. The main limitation of *in vitro* testing is the difficulty to connect its results to the complexity of an organism.

Cells cultures are obtained from normal tissues, primary cultures or cells lineage stablished by enzymatic, mechanical of chemical degradation (Freshney 1994). For cell culture tests, three methods may be used:

- **Organ culture:** the features of the tissue are partially maintained. The three-dimensional architecture is favored by the culture in plaques or gel matrix, providing a gas-liquid interface.
- **Tissue culture:** the cellular proliferation occurs when a sample of the tissue in placed in a growth medium.
- **Cell culture:** cellular suspensions are mechanically, chemically and enzymatically obtained.

The MTT test, used to determine the viability of cells is based on the quantitative evaluation of living cells after exposure to the treatment and incubation in the vital dye MTT [3-(4,5-Dimethylthiazol-2-yl)-2, 5diphenyltetrazolium bromide] (Cintra et al. 2017). MTT is a blue formazan salt produced from active mitochondrial proteins of living cells, and hence, directly proportional to the number of viable cells in the culture.

After performance of "initial" tests such cell culture, the running of "secondary" tests are imperative.

3.2. Subcutaneous Tests

The use of subcutaneous implants started with Torneck (1966). His pioneering research analyzed the reaction of rats' subcutaneous tissue in direct contact with implanted polyethylene tubes.

Performed in rats, accesses the response of the subcutaneous connective tissue against the insertion of polyethylene tubes filled with the materials to be tested in their interior. After initial protocol for anesthesia, trichotomy, and antisepsis of the dorsum of the animals, a single incision is performed. Then, tissues are divulsed in both sides of the medial line and polyethylene tubes are insert, filled with the material to be tested. At the end of the surgical procedure, four sites (two on each side of the incision) are obtained and the skin is sutured. After the analysis periods, euthanasia is performed and the specimens are submitted to histological processing for histological and immunohistochemical analyses (Bueno et al. 2016, 2017, 2018, 2019, Benetti et al. 2019).

The microscopy analysis allows the observation of the responses within the connective tissues in contact with the material. The parameters evaluated are phenomena related to the inflammatory infiltrate, repair and features of the remains of the material. In addition, it is possible to identify other tissue damages, such as abscess and vascular alterations (e.g., swelling and hyperemia) and also to analyze presence of macrophages and multinucleated giant cells, evaluating angiogenesis, fibroblastic proliferation, fibrosis and even presence of mineralization. These evaluations are usually based on distribution by inflammatory scores (qualitative) or cell count (quantitative).

3.3. Tests in Tibia

Bony defects are challenging in different fields of Medicine and Dentistry. According to Najjar & Kahn (1977), the tibia and the mandible present very similar processes of repair and remodeling. Thus, many tests are performed in experimental models of rats' and rabbits' tibiae (Öztürk et al. 2008). The surgical procedure follows the standard cautions of anaesthesia, trichotomy and antisepsis of the surgical site. In this model, a 1,5mm incision is performed in the medial side of the legs until reaching the tibial metaphysis. Soft tissues are dislocated and a monocortical defect is made in the largest later-mesial extension of the bone, using a 2 mm, 3 mm or 3,5 mm trephine under constant irrigation with sterile physiological saline solution. The final step of the surgical intervention is the suture of the tissues.

For efficacy evaluation, the substances are administered to the animals through gastric gavage. Usually, the systemic treatment initiates on the same day of the surgery and is continued until the day prior euthanasia, when the specimens are collected and submitted to specific processing for the analyzes to be performed. The histological analysis is used to evaluate the aspects related with bone repair, such as the presence of granulation tissue, bone formation, arrangement of immature trabeculae, maturation of the bone until the late stages of remodeling, and quantitative analysis of the area of the defect and the adjacent cancellous canal.

In addition, one of the models most used and appropriate to confirm the osteoinductive potential, is the creation of critical size defects, characterized by the incapacity of the organism to spontaneously close the bone wound (Honma et al. 2008). This model allows to evaluate, with significant reliability, the capacity of any substance or material to induce complete repair of the critical defect. With this purpose, the calvaria of rats represents an environment appropriate to provide relevant information for different areas in dentistry (Develioglu et al. 2009). For that, the interparietal and interoccipital sutures are selected for guidance on the creation of the critical side defects of pre-stablish diameter. Then, the defects are filled with the phytotherapics to be tested.

The specimens are submitted for conventional processing to obtain histological sections. These sections are commonly analyzed under light microscopy for evaluation of the quality of the newly formed bone and the types of cells enrolled with the repair process. Well conducted and detailed histological and immunohistochemical evaluations can provide relevant information regarding the mechanisms of bone repair. Also, histometric measurements of the distance between the borders of the original defects and quantification of the area of newly formed bone within the defect can provide an overview of the osteoinductive capacity of the tested material.

3.4. Alveolus

Alveolar repair comprises a series of tissues' processes occurring in the interior of the extraction socket. However, among other conditions, alveolitis severely delays the alveolar repair process (Poi et al. 2000). The positive effects of phytotherapics over socket healing have already been reported in the literature (Uribe-Fentanes et al. 2018).

The pre-clinical experiment to access this condition is conducted as follows: after sedation, the rats are placed in dorsal decubitus and the right superior incisor is extracted in accordance with the protocol of Okamoto & Russo (1973). After extraction, complete ischemia of the socket is obtained by the placement of a paper cone embedded in 1:1000 adrenalin for 15 minutes. After removal of the cone, the animals remain under observation for additional 15 minutes, in order to confirm the absence of the formation of a blood clot. Forty-eight hours later, the animals are examined to verify the presence of alveolitis, identified by the clinical signs of foul-smelling, edema, hyperemia and abscess (Shafer et al. 1987). In this experiment (Shafer et al. 1987), the test group received 5 ml of the phytotherapic added to 45 ml of water *ad libitum*. The changes of solutions were performed daily. Following euthanasia, the specimens were collected and submitted to conventional histological processing.

Another alveolus protocol for testing materials, is the placement of a polyethylene tube containing the test material into the alveolus. Then, a suture is performed and after experimental periods, animals are euthanized. The jaw is separated, cleaned, demineralized and, after histologic and staining protocols, specimens are assessed for inflammatory/repair response (Bueno et al. 2017).

This type of test enables to observe alveolar repair through the presence or absence of bone trabeculae, osteoblastic and osteoclastic activity, signs of resorption, vascularization, inflammatory infiltrate of polymorphonuclear cells, pus, and necrosis. Moreover, healing can also be observed in the analysis of the phases involved with clot formation.

3.5. Pulp Tissues

Pulpal inflammation is a reflex of any aggressive agent to the pulp tissue, characterized by the infiltrate of inflammatory cells and eventual necrosis and abscess. It is known that phytotherapics display anti-inflammatory effects over the pulp (Nossa et al. 2013). The induction of pulpal inflammation in pre-clinical models is obtained by the access to the pulp of the first mandibular molars using a spherical bur ½ attached to high-speed handpieces. The depth of the perforation is equivalent to the diameter of the bur. After preparation of the cavities, the animals are submitted to the treatments to be tested. In endodontics, phytotherapics may be administered intraperitoneally, to assess the pulp tissue response to a systemic administration of the extracts or even the periapical area (bone resorption/formation). Following euthanasia in pre-established periods, the specimens are histologically processed.

This pulpal assessment enables the visualization of the inflammatory condition within the pulp though the assignment of scores from normal tissue (intact layer of odontoblasts and nervous tissue, and absence of inflammatory infiltrate, hyperemia or edema represents 0% of inflammation of the field of view) to severely inflamed pulp (predominance of inflammatory cells, neutrophils, lymphocytes, capillary stuffiness, hemorrhage, and eventual dystrophic calcification represents 67 to 100% of inflammation of the field of view). Additionally, the histopathological analysis provides information regarding the architecture of the affected tissues, intensity of the inflammatory response and the type of leukocytes in predominance (Chidiac et al. 2002, Holt et al. 2005, Castilho et al. 2008). Immunohistochemical and molecular biology techniques (PCR and RT-PCR) are applied to access the expression of proteins and specific genes related to the immune system (Holt et al. 2005, Kawagishi et al. 2006).

3.6. Edemogenic

The immediate inflammatory response observed until 48 hours after inoculation of a flogonenous agent to the interior of body tissues can be analyzed by a test known as "edemogenic". This test consists on the use of a non-toxic dye with an edematous systemic effect when linked to plasmatic albumin (Rutberg 1977). Edemogenic test has been frequently used to evaluate the intensity of the acute inflammatory response through the analysis of the optical density of the dye on a fragment of the inflamed tissue, under spectrophotometry (Gehlen et al. 2004).

The experimental step of this test (Valentim et al. 2017, Bueno et al. 2017, Bueno et al. 2018) initiates by sedation and endovenous injection of 1% at the proportion of 0.2 ml of solution for each 100 g of body weight. Thirty minutes later, the animals are divided into each group. Then, 0.1 ml of each substance to be tested (or herbal extract) is injected with a hypodermic needle in the back of the rats. For the majority of the tests, 5 animals are euthanized by anesthetic overdose at 3 and 6 hours after administration. The specimens are collected from the region of the edema and standardized with a mold. After fixation during 72h at 45ºC and filtration with gauze, the analysis of absorbance is performed in a spectrophotometer (Valentim et al. 2017, Bueno et al. 2017, Bueno et al. 2018).

3.7. Bedsores

Bedsores are cutaneous ulcers observed in hospitalized and/or diabetic patients. The persistence of these ulcers may be mainly explained by the persistence of inflammation and infections caused by local biofilms (Chen & Wen 2011). The antimicrobial feature and the capacity to improve healing observed in phytotherapics can also be observed in animal models of induction of cutaneous ulcers.

In animal test, after sedation, the back of rats is trichotomized and two punchs of 1.5 mm diameter are performed, leaving the dermal wounds exposed. Then, the microorganisms to be inoculated are adjusted to UFC/ml for each strain (e.g., *Staphylococcus aureus*) and pipetted inside the wounds. The ulcer is collected at day zero to serve as the control. After surgery, dipyrone is solved in physiological saline solution ae the dose of 50 mg/kg and orally administered twice a day during the first 48 hours.

Animals' behavioral reactions to pain are recorded. Usually, animals are divided into the experimental groups and analyzed at 2, 7 and 14 days after treatments. Each animal is treated by topical application (i.e., spray containing the phytotherapic) in the morning and in the evening (Shukla et al. 1999), or according to the stablished protocol. Following the periods of analysis, the animals are euthanized, and images recorded with a digital camera for posterior analysis of the wound healing, using an indicated imaging software (Robson et al. 2000).

After recording the images, the 1,5 mm wounds are usually collected and submitted to fixation in buffered 4% formaldehyde solution for histological analysis (inflammatory infiltrate, angiogenesis and fibroplasia) and frozen in specific buffered for counting of myeloperoxidase and dosage of neutrophils and hydroxyproline.

As stated in previous chapter, it is impracticable to cite and describe all herbal extracts with proved biocompatibility reported in literature, since it's estimated that near 70,000 plant species have been used for medicinal purpose and 3000 species were described with anti-cancer properties. Only in India, there are approximately 1,250 medicinal plants (Graham et al. 2000, Amruthesh 2007, Pan et al. 2014).

Therefore, the following sections will mention and describe several plants, which extracts were scientifically tested showing promising results, as am introduction to new possible researches.

4. Biocompatibility of Herbal Extracts

4.1. Arnica

Contrera et al. (1985) reported negative effects when evaluating the action of *Lichnophora ericoide* (Serra Dourada arnica) and *Solidago microglossa* (false arnica) on skin wound healing of rats. The authors observed delayed healing at 10 days and increased local inflammation.

On the other hand, positive results have been found with other species. *Lychnophora pinaster* Mart. and *Symphytum officinale* L. are Arnica species, known at the world medicine by the treatment of skin infections. When administered orally, both species can be toxic due to the presence of sesquiterpenoids lactones, pyrrolizidine alkaloids and saponins (Stickel & Seitz 2000). However, the toxicity risks are minimal when used topically, because the absorption through the skin is 20 to 50 times lower (Carvalho 2004, Staiger 2007). The sesquiterpene lactones are known for their anti-inflammatory activity mediated by inhibition of transcription factor Nuclear Factor-Kappa B (Lyss et al. 1998). This anti-inflammatory activity is attributed to the existence of flavonoids that prevent the activation of inflammatory processes by the presence of free radicals in high concentrations in inflamed tissues (Salvemini et al. 1996). Allantoin, choline and rosmarinic acid are responsible for anti-inflammatory effects and wound healing, proliferation of fibroblasts, chondroblasts and osteoblasts during tissue remodeling, reduced capillary permeability and increased perfusion through vasodilation (Andres et al. 1989, Niedner 1989).

A study in rat used a model of acute inflammation through animal paw edema, stimulating the release of proinflammatory cytokines, serotonin, histamine, kinins, and prostaglandins (Winter et al. 1962), to evaluate extract ointment (Burch & DeHaas 1990, Ferreira et al. 1993). The formulations containing ethanolic extract of *Lynchnophora pinaster* and *Symphytum officiale* were evaluated. After 3 hours of the application of the formulations, it was observed that the application of ointments containing 5 and 10% *Lychnophora pinaster* had lower paw edema, showing the anti-inflammatory activity of the extract; in addition, formulations containing 2 and 5% *Lychnophora pinaster* were more active than Cataflam®. Formulations containing 10 and 16% of *Symphytum officiale* also reduced the edema, and showed similar anti-inflammatory activity than Cataflam®.

Martins et al. (2009) analyzed the cytotoxicity of the extract of Brazilian arnica (*Solidago microglossa*) and Paulist arnica (*Porophyllum ruderale*) in excipient for use in ulcers. These species allowed cell viability after 24 hours, being cytocompatible with human oral mucosa fibroblasts.

4.2. Pomegranate

Punica granatum is a medicinal plant, widely used, with evidence in the ethnopharmacology literature, using its pericarp (external part of the fruit) for treating inflammation in the mouth and throat. Also, based on a popular tradition, its juice has been used to treat cataract (Lorenzi & Matos 2008).

The infusion of *P. granatum* peel is popularly indicated to treat acute inflammation. Its leaf, flower and peel are also used for the treatment of infectious diseases, including genital, urinary and respiratory tract infections (Costa 2001).

Gomes (2017) realized an *in vitro* analysis of the cytocompatibility of pomegranate extract associated with a hydrogel matrix through 3-(4,5-dimethylthiazol-2-yl)-2,5-diphenyltetrazolium bromide (MTT) assay in mouse macrophages. The hydrogel acts as a network of interconnected pores, allowing nutrient retention and an adequate environment for cell proliferation and growth. The pomegranate extract associated with the hydrogen matrix at 100, 50 and 25 mg/mL dilutions did not show cytotoxicity, but the concentration of 12.5 mg/mL was cytotoxic.

Pomegranate extract without association of hydrogel matrix in any of the samples tested was considered cytotoxic.

4.3. Aloe Vera

Aloe vera (*Aloe barbadensis*) is a succulent plant considered to belong in the *Liliaceae* family. This plant has many pharmacological benefits and it has been used for a long time as a medicine for several medical conditions. For example, analgesic, anti-inflammatory, immunoregulation, antioxidant, antineoplastic and healing properties are described. Additionally, no adverse reactions have been reported (Ndhlala et al. 2009, Hashemi et al. 2015, Ali & Wahbi 2017, Wahedi et al. 2017).

Its leaves contain high amounts of polysaccharides, such as acemannan. This immunomodulator has been shown to be a stimulator for cell proliferation, cell differentiation, mineralization and dentin formation (Jittapiromsak et al. 2010). The leaf has a gel, also known as parenchyma, retaining all its nutrients. Juice or gel products are used for medical and cosmetic purposes, including overall health. Some authors have demonstrated that Aloe vera gel may be an appropriate storage for the transportation of an avulsed tooth, because it was capable of maintaining the viability of periodontal ligament cells (Tudose et al. 2009, Badakhsh et al. 2014).

Seventy-five nutrients were identified in Aloe vera gel. The most important compounds are lignin, saponins, fatty acids and some hormones. Firstly, lignin is a cellulose-based substance without known specific medicinal properties, but it allows Aloe vera to penetrate into the human skin when topically applied. Secondly, saponins are glycosides which composing approximately 3% of A. vera gel. It is like soap and contains antiseptic properties. Finally, Aloe vera has fatty acids, as salicylic acid, and some hormones, such as auxins and gibberellins, which present anti-inflammatory function. These anti-inflammatories compounds work more often by stimulating immune system and collagen growth, or by blocking the pathways of irritant agents (Mangaiyarkarasi et al. 2015).

Chithra et al. (1998) treated full thickness dermal wounds extending to subcutaneous tissue in rats either by topical application or oral administration of Aloe vera. The medicine was orally and topically applied. The authors evaluated the presence of glycosaminoglycans (GAGs) in the granulation tissue. Significant qualitative and quantitative changes occurred in GAG content. The results showed an increased content of uronic acid in the Aloe vera treated wounds compared to untreated controls, representing an improved GAG statistic. The maximum amount of urea was presented in granulation tissue on the fourth day, being the highest level measured of GAG during the first week of healing. While the measurement of collagen content in the wound starts to increase, the amount of uronic acid decreases. GAGs are the first components of the extracellular matrix to be synthesized during wound healing, forming a scaffold for the deposition collagen and elastin (Dunphy & Udupa 1955).

Hyaluronic acid produces the major part of GAGs in the wound granulation tissue. Also, the levels of hyaluronic acid and dermatan sulfate were significantly higher in both the topically treated and orally treated groups compared to the untreated groups. Hyaluronic acid plays an important role in the initial process of wound healing, being able to extend its regulatory effects by two possible mechanisms. First, it forms a pericellular layer attached to the cell surface (Underhill & Toole 1979, Knudson & Toole 1985, Shelton 1991), creating a limit of anionic electrochemical activity around fibroblasts which may result in the attraction or localization of cationic growth factors and provides fibroblasts greater accessibility to growth factors. Lastly, the second mechanism may be a result of the cell surface binding of fibroblasts to hyaluronic acid, promoting tyrosine phosphorylation and phospholipid degradation, which provides important intracellular signals for cell function (Turley 1989). Moreover, the interaction of hyaluronic acid with keratinocytes also has an important role in the process of epithelialization (Okasala et al. 1995). The increase of hyaluronic acid in wounds treated with Aloe vera can result in a more stable scar formation due to a more fluid and malleable matrix provided by this acid, facilitating cell mobility and greater early remodelling.

The increase of dermatan sulfate in treated wounds by Aloe vera also plays an important role in rapid wound healing. This component makes the process of healing more resistant because of its contribution to the organization and strength of the *in vivo* fibrillar network (Scott 1988). Aloe vera has a significant influence on PGs and GAGs levels in a wound. Reduced tissue loss and rapid healing can be shown into cold burns and electrical injuries treated with Aloe vera (Heggars et al. 1993, Miller & Koltai 1995). This property of Aloe vera can be partially attributed to the polysaccharides from its gel. Studies have demonstrated that mannose-6-phosphate has healing properties and decreases inflammation (Davis et al. 1994).

Interleukin-1 beta (IL-1β) and tumor necrosis factor-alpha (TNF-α) are the main proinflammatory cytokines, playing an important role in the induction of acute inflammation. Aloe vera can reduce IL-1β and TNF-α levels in cases of peptic ulcers and promotes a cytoprotective effect on the mucosa by stimulating endogenous prostaglandin production (Eamlamnam et al. 2006). Additionally, Aloe vera is able to induce angiogenesis *in vivo*, decreasing vasoconstriction and improving capillary perfusion to provide better wound healing (Moon et al. 1999, Eamlamnam et al. 200).

4.4. Orange Tree

Citrus sinensis (L.) Osbeck (Rutaceae), popularly known as sweet orange, is largely cultivated for commercial purposes (fruits, juices, essential oils). The extract from its leaves or peel is used in the traditional medicine to treat various diseases (Siddique et al. 2012). A wide range of health benefits have been attributed to *Citrus*, such as anticancer, antimicrobial, antioxidant and anti-inflammatory properties (Benavente-Garcia et al. 1995), deeply associated with its flavonoids content (Tripoli et al. 2007).

Pepe et al. (2017) investigated the antioxidant and anti-inflammatory effects of bioavailable flavonoids from a *Citrus Sinensis* extract, involving a huge group of phenolic compounds that affect the production and elimination of reactive oxygen species and the mechanisms of injuries mediated by oxygen free radicals. The bioavailable fraction (8.3% of the total flavonoid fraction) was compared to the original extract, showing higher antioxidant and anti-inflammatory potential at the same concentration. Also, the antioxidant activity was also remarkable at the lowest concentration (10 μg/mL), with a similar effect to the concentrated extract, revealing a positive influence in this *in vitro* test. In an experimental study of colitis induced by trinitrobenzenesulfonic acid in rats, Khan et al. (2016) demonstrated that the juices of *C. sinensis* (orange juice) and *C. paradisi* (grapefruit juice), especially C. paradisi, could be used to treat inflammatory bowel disease.

Garcia et al. (2017) evaluated cytotoxic activity against macrophages of extracts with hexane (100%), dichloromethane/ethanol (1: 1) solvents derived from dried leaves of *Citrus sinensis*. The minimum cytotoxic concentrations for hexane and dichloromethane/ethanol were 125.6 (CC50 1⁄4 35.75 lg/mL) and 125 lg/mL (CC50 1⁄4 86.17 lg/mL), respectively, showing cytotoxic effect at the same level as the standard medicine. The essential oil used for sweet orange peel exhibits cytotoxic activity of 5.51 μg/mL (CC50) against HeLa cells (Liu et al. 2012). Based on hydrogen peroxide elimination, *C. sinensis* juices from a local supermarket presented values of 1.2 ± 0.3 × 103 s-1 and 0.4 ± 0.1 × 103 s-1, being an effective antioxidant activity (Karyakina et al. 2009).

Phytocystatins are cystatins derived from plants, and they are involved in plant development and in response to biotic and abiotic stresses, inhibiting cell activity (Kondo et al. 1991, Margis et al. 1998). Recently, a gene sequence encoding a new phytocystatin called CsinCPI-2 from *Citrus sinensis* was cloned (Leguizamón et al. 2019). Leguizamón et al. (2019) demonstrated that this protein has an anti-inflammatory potential and a pro-osteogenic effect, as evidenced by *in vitro* experiment with macrophages and *in vivo* experiment with rats executed by these authors. Additionally, the pro-osteogenic effect of CsinCPI-2 was observed *in vitro* analysis with human dental pulp cells.

4.5. Green Tea and Turmeric

Green tea comes from the leaves of *Camellia sinensis.* Clinical and laboratory studies suggest that dietary polyphenols from green tea have antioxidant, anticariogenic, anti-inflammatory, thermogenic, probiotic, and antimicrobial properties (Medina-Remón et al. 2017, Mukherjee et al. 2006). Its extract has anti-inflammatory effects, repressing expression of NF-κB and the production of pro-inflammatory cytokines (Nichols & Katiyar 2010). Recently, it has been proposed that its polyphenols content, as catechins, provide a protector effect in green tea (Alipour et al. 2018). Hagiu et al. (2019) endorse that green tea is a powerful anti-inflammatory agent, and depending on the dose it evokes cellular migration during wounds healing. This event is attributed to its polyphenols components, mainly catechins from its leaves.

Catechins from green tea and turmeric have showed anti-inflammatory property during an *in vitro* analysis with human epithelial cells (Jobin et al. 1999, Wheeler et al. 2004, Biswas et al. 2005). Epicatechin-3-gallate is a catechin from green tea. It influences in the anti-inflammatory cellular activity, suppressing and inhibiting production and action of several pro-inflammatory mediators, such as nitric oxide, reactive oxygen species/ reactive nitrogen species and cyclooxygenase-2 COX-2 (Zhong et al. 2012).

Saffron, also known as Curcuma longa, is an Indian spice derived from the rhizomes of the plant. Turmeric is composed of three curcuminoids: curcumin (diferuloylmethane), desmethoxycurcumin and bisdesmethoxycurcumin. Some volatile oils (tumerone, atlantone, and zingiberone), sugars, proteins, and resins can also be included. The inflammatory response is modulated by down-regulating cyclooxygenase-2 activity (COX-2), lipoxygenase and enzymes induced by nitric oxide synthase (Goel et al. 2008). Inhibition of COX-2 and iNOS is likely to be accomplished by curcumin suppression and nuclear factor-kappa B activation (NF-KB), which is involved in the regulation of inflammation and cell proliferation (Surh et al. 2001).

A pilot study examined the effect of curcumin in fifteen patients with pancreatitis, accessing the effects on the pattern of pain and erythrocyte malondialdehyde, an indicator of lipid peroxidation. A significant reduction in the erythrocyte malondialdehyde levels has been detected within the group which curcumin was administered (Durgaprasad et al. 2005).

Starzonek et al. (2019) used green tea and tumeric extract with a high teor of polyphenols (20%) to reduce the inflammatory reaction in the blood and liver tissue. Polyphenol-rich dietary supplements showed a potential to decrease inflammatory responses, but these supplements did not provoke anti-inflammatory effect in horses and ponies. Curcumin is one of three curcuminoids, being the principal compound of saffron, a spice derived from Curcuma longa (Jurenka 2009).

In an experiment performed on mice with acute liver failure, Diao et al. (2019) observed that a pretreatment with green tea extract prevents oedema and necrosis in hepatocytes. The hepatoprotective effects of low, medium and high dose of green tea were associated with the elimination of free radicals and the improvement of superoxide dismutase, catalase and glutathione peroxidase activities in the liver. In addition, green tea decreases apoptosis in the liver.

4.6. Gervão and Cambará

Plants of the genus *Bouchea* are commonly known as "gervão". The leaves of *Bouchea fluminensis* are composed of iridoid and steroid glycosides in the form of crude triterpene mixture presenting anti-inflammatory potential. A purified fraction contains ursolic, oleanolic and micromeric acids (Costa et al. 2003). The anti-inflammatory activity of oleanolic and ursolic acid inhibiting the edema induced by carrageenin or serotonin involves distinct mechanisms, such as inhibition of lipoxygenase and cyclo-oxygenase, inhibition of elastase and inhibition of complementary system. On the latter, process happens possibly through the inhibition on C3-convertase of the classical complementary pathway.

Gochnatia polymorpha is popularly known as cambará in Brazil. Its leaves contain sesquiterpenes and lactones derivate. In a study realized by Moreira et al. (2000), various fractions were obtained from the leaves of *G. polymorpha*. The fraction at a dose of 150 mg/kg, in carrageenin-induced rat paw edema test, provoked significant anti-inflammatory activity. Furthermore, the amino acid 4-hydroxy-N-methyl-proline showed a considerable edema inhibition at a dose of 200 mg/kg (Moreira et al. 2000).

4.7. Sambacaita

In Brazil, *Hyptis pectinata* is popularly known as "sambacaita" or "canudinho". The essential oils extracted from the leaves contains 95.8% of monoterpenes. The extract of *Hyptis pectinata* administered orally at the dose of 600 mg/kg has been tested in rats. The carrageenin-induced rat paw edema test and subplantar injection of arachidonic acid have been performed to observe its antiedematogenic effects. A significant antiedematogenic activity (34.1% inhibition) was exhibited. The findings demonstrated that the aqueous extract of *Hyptis pectinata* acts on both the cyclooxygenase and lipoxygenase pathways (Bispo et al. 2001).

4.8. Sucupira

Pterodon pubescens is known as sucupira in Brazil. An autoimmune model of rheumatoid arthritis using the hydroalcoholic extract of *P. pubescens* seeds has been studied for the prevention and treatment of arthritis (Sabino et al. 1999). Preventive treatment significantly reduced the inflammation level and the incidence of collagen-induced arthritis. Thus, this study provided a scientific basis for the use of *P. pubescens* infusions in the treatment of rheumatoid arthritis (Sabino et al. 1999).

4.9. White Mallow

Sida cordifolia is commonly called "malva branca" (white mallow) in Brazil. A model of carrageenin-induced edema and edema induced by arachidonic acid were used in rats to investigate the anti-inflammatory activity of aqueous extract *S. cordifolia* leaves (Franzotti et al. 2000). There was a reduction of 7.55% in edema at the dose of 800 mg/kg, while the dose of 400 mg/kg of the extract *S. cordifolia* inhibited edema by 28.31%. On the other hand, the dose of 200 mg/kg was ineffective in decreasing edema. This model involves three different phases: (1) histamine and serotonin release, (2) release of kinins, and (3) release of prostaglandins. The model edema induced by arachidonic acid is very sensitive to inhibitors of the lipoxygenase pathway and is resistant to selective cyclooxygenase inhibitors. The present findings demonstrated that the dose 200 mg/kg was ineffective in antiedematogenic potential. Then, the aqueous extract of *S. cordifolia* seems not to interfere with the lipooxygenase pathway but rather with the cyclooxygenase pathway (prostaglandin biosynthesis) (Franzotti et al. 2000).

4.10. Propolis

Propolis has a complex chemical composition. According to *in vitro* (Al-Shaher et al. 2004) and *in vivo* (Silva et al. 2004) studies, it has been considered a substance with low-irritant potential. The most important pharmacological active agents of propolis are flavonoids, phenols and aromatic compounds. Many biological properties of propolis are attributed to flavonoids (Cogulu et al. 2006). Bioflavonoids stimulate enzymes that reinforce the walls of the blood vessels in the periodontium. This function of flavonoids is related to its capacity of inhibiting the synthesis of prostaglandins and providing tissue disinfection.

As an anti-inflammatory agent, propolis inhibits production of prostaglandins, activates the thymus gland and it facilitates the immune system by promoting phagocytic activity (Madarova 1980). Moreover, this substance stimulates cellular immunity, improves healing effects on epithelial tissues (Park et al. 2000) and it aids the synthesis of collagen due to the presence of iron and zinc in its composition (Scheller et al. 1978, Marcucci 1995).

Caffeic acid and phenethyl ester is also responsible for the anti-inflammatory activity of propolis. Ethanolic extract of propolis has good properties for Endodontics, such as promoting bone regeneration and inducing hard tissue bridging in pulpotomies or pulp capping (Ferreira et al. 2007, Parolia et al. 2010).

Martin & Pileggi (2004) conducted an investigation of propolis as new storage media for maintaining viable periodontal ligament (PDL) cells on avulsed teeth. Its performance was compared with Hank's balanced salt solution, milk or saline. Another study suggested its use for hypersensitivity dentin by observing dentinal tubules after the application of propolis on the dental prosthesis (Almas et al. 2001). Propolis has also been tested as a tissue repair agent in wound healing following surgical procedures (Magro Filho & Carvalho 1990, Magro Filho & Carvalho 1994).

Ethanolic extract of propolis produced better anti-inflammatory and analgesic effects in mouse models by inhibiting nitric oxide production (Paulino et al. 2006) than diclofenac (Tan-No et al. 2006). It has also reduced polymorphonuclear leukocyte chemotaxis (Naito et al. 2007). Al Sahaher et al. (2004) realized an *in vitro* study of the effects of propolis on dental pulp cells and periodontal ligament fibroblasts dissolved in DMSO or ethyl alcohol as a first step to be an alternative remedy. Periodontal ligament fibroblasts treated with 1, 2 or 4 mg/mL propolis in both solvents resulted in 75% to 44% of PDL cell viability after 20 h without any toxicity. Nevertheless, the presence of 2 or 4 mg/mL of propolis resulted in 50% of viable cells after 20 h, regardless of the solvent used. Finally, the concentration of 1 mg/mL de propolis were not found to be toxic on dental pulp cells.

Lopes-Rocha et al. (2012) performed a topical administration of propolis on oral wounds. Propolis induced the proliferation of keratinocytes, accelerating the epithelialization, starting at day 3 and ending on day 7 postoperatively, which was significantly faster than other groups.

In an attempt to improve the properties of mineral trioxide aggregate (MTA), Cavenago et al. (2015) manipulated white MTA with aqueous extract and/or propylene glycol from *Arctium lappa L.*, *Casearia sylvestris Sw.* and propolis. According to histological and histomorphometric evaluations of implants in subcutaneous and alveolar bone tissues, no significant difference was found among the experimental groups when compared to the group of MTA manipulated with distilled water, with similar expression of TNF-α and IL-10 cytokines among all groups.

4.11. *Articum Lappa L.*

Arctium lappa Linne is commonly known as burdock. Many active ingredients have been isolated from distinct botanical parts of the plant (root, leaf and seed). *Arctium lappa L.* is used in the traditional medicine as a phytotherapic substance due to its anti-inflammatory (Zhao et al. 2009), anti-allergic activity (Knipping et al. 2008).

The main mechanisms of its anti-inflammatory action are related to inhibition of induced nitric oxide synthase (iNOS) and nitric oxide (NO) production; suppression of proinflammatory cytokines; inhibition of nuclear factor kappa B (NF-kB); activation of antioxidant enzymes and elimination of free radicals (Chan et al. 2011).

4.12. *Casearia Sylvestris SW*

Casearia sylvestris (*Flacourtiaceae* family) is a plant commonly known as "guaçatonga" (Teske & Trentini 2001). Its principal compounds are essential oil (terpenes, triterpenes), saponins, fatty acids, tannins, resins and flavonoids. Anti-inflammatory activity of this herbal medicine has been confirmed in rat paw edema, granulomatous tissue test, vascular permeability, writhing test, gastric ulcer stress-induced and evaluation of gastric secretion (Esteves et al. 2005, De Almeida et al. 2013). In addition, this phytotherapic medicine provides an antioxidant action (Albano et al. 2013).

The propylene glycol extract of *Casearia sylvestris* associated with calcium hydroxide does not interfere in the pH and pH and Calcium Ion Release of calcium hydroxide paste (Duarte et al. 2009).

As stated in section 4.10, *Casearia sylvestris* was also tested in association with endodontic repair cement with mineral trioxide aggregate (MTA), showing similar response to MTA mixed with distilled water (Cavenago et al. 2015).

4.13. *Psidium*

Psidium cattleianum belongs to the family *Myrtaceae* and is usually known as "wild guava" or "guava" (Pott & Pott 1994). *Psidium ssp.* are used as anti-inflammatory agents and for hemostasis (Lozoya et al. 1994, Jaiarj et al. 1999). Moreover, the plants that belong to this family reduce the metastasis of cancer cells (Im et al. 2012) and biocompatibility tests of this species were performed by Ruviére et al. (2008).

The biocompatibility of the aqueous and hydroalcoholic extracts of *Psidium sp* was accessed by edemogenic and morphological analysis in subcutaneous tissues (Novais 2008). The tested extracts were biologically accepted by the organisms, since the overall results of the edema triggered by the hydroalcoholic solution remained high at 7 days, maybe due to the alcohol in its composition, but decreased after its metabolization by the organism. With regard to the morphological analysis of the subcutaneous tissues, the delayed tissue response in all groups presented a positive progression in function of time, indicating that the extract did not hinder the natural progression of the repair.

Valentim et al. (2017) obtained the extract of guava in both vehicles (i.e., water and alcohol). After obtention, the combination of 1 ml of the aqueous or alcoholic extracts, and propylene glycol were manufactured in the proportion of 1 g of calcium hydroxide [$Ca(OH)_2$]. These combinations were edemogenic and subcutaneously tested. The alcoholic extract *plus* $Ca(OH)_2$ presented increased edema at 3h when compared with the other groups. However, at 6h, alcoholic extract *plus* $Ca(OH)_2$ displayed a higher incidence of edema when compared with the other groups. The repair process improved over time when compared with the initial periods. In addition, no significant difference was observed among the combinations, indicating that aqueous and alcoholic extracts of the leaves of *Psidium cattleianum* used as vehicles for $Ca(OH)_2$ exhibit similar tissues' response when compared with groups propylene glycol and control.

Psidium guajava belongs to the family *Myrtaceae* and is popularly known as guava. In Brazil's northwestern, its leaves are used for the treatment of dysentery, digestive issues, inflammation, gingivitis and throat infections (De Albuquerque et al. 2007). Its leaves and barks in composed by tannins, flavonoids, saponins and alkaloids (Tona et al. 2000).

4.14. *Libidibia Ferrea*, *Parapiptadenia Rigida* and *Caesalpinia Ferrea*

Libidibia ferrea and *Parapiptadenia rigida (Fabaceae* family), were analyzed by de Araújo et al. (2014), evidencing the analgesic, antimicrobial and anti-inflammatory activity of aqueous and acetone-water extract, via a leukocyte migration model. Authors stated that those properties were due to appropriate extraction, preserving gallic acid and catechin. *Parapiptadenia rigida* is popularly known as Angico Vermelho. Its bark is used for the treatment of inflammations, gastrointestinal disturbs, tumors and chronic diseases (Souza et al. 2004), possibly due to the positive effects of compounds such as tannins, derivates of catechins and proanthocyanidins (Schmidt et al. 2011).

Caesalpinia ferrea also belongs to the *Fabaceae* family. It contains the following phenolic compounds: tannins, catechins and hydrolysable tannins, such as gallic and ellagic acids (Frasson et al. 2003). The tea from the stem bark has been popularly used in the treatment of diabetes in

Brazil. Vasconcelos et al. (2011) showed the hypoglycemic effect of the stem bark aqueous extract of *C. ferrea* in diabetic rats.

4.15. Horsetail

Equisetum pyramidale L., Equisetaceae, also known as horsetail, is used in folk medicine and commercialized as a remineralizing, anti-inflammatory and diuretic herb (Pott & Pott, 2000). *Equisetum pyramidale L., Equisetaceae* is resilient and has chemotaxonomic markers such as caffeic acid's esters, flavonoids, and styrylate. However, its chemical composition is dependent on the stage of development of the plant (Veit et al. 1995).

Studies evaluating the ethanolic extract of *E. pyramidale* reported a potential positive effect on the second-intension healing process of wounds created in Wistar rats (Oliskovicz et al. 2006, Matias 2010). Camignan et al. (2019) investigated the influence of an ethanolic *E. pyramidale* hydrogel over the healing of cutaneous lesions in an animal model. The size of the wound decreased from 3 to 7 days, possibly because of the phytochemical anti-inflammatories present on the hydrogel. It was also observed increased collagenization and angiogenesis in test groups, with predominance of neutrophils on the third day.

4.16. Grape Seeds

Grapes (*Vitis vinifera)* are cultivated all around the world, and rich in flavonoids, polyphenols, anthocyanins, proanthocyanins, procyanidins and trans-resveratrol (Roy et al. 2005). The extract derived from grape seeds is a natural food supplement with potent modulatory capacity over oxygen-reactive species (Bagchi et al. 1997). Recent studies divulged that grape seeds' extract exhibits antioxidant properties, eliminates free radicals and can be anti-diabetic, cardioprotective, liver protector, anti-carcinogenic, antimicrobial and anti-viral (Kaur et al. 2006, Ye et al. 1999).

Different concentrations of this extract have been related with innumerous positive effects for the treatment of cancer. High concentrations (25 to 100 μg/ml) were cytotoxic or anti-proliferative to cells of bladder, colorectal and mammary cancers. On the other hand, 2.5 μg/ml inhibits the incidence of micronucleus and release of oxygen-reactive species by lymphocytes cultures, confirming the antioxidant property of grape seeds' extract has a protective effect over oxidative stress (Stankovic et al. 2008, Perde-Schrepler et al. 2013, Raina et al. 2013, Dinicola et al. 2014).

The cytotoxicity of grape seed extract over the evolution of oral epidermoid carcinoma (KB cells lineage) was described through MTT assays and Tripan blue by Aghbali et al. (2013). The cells treat with hydroalcoholic extract displayed significant reduction in its viability when compared with control group. Also, its toxicity over KB cells seems to be dose and time dependent, since the more significant cytotoxicity was achieved with the highest concentration and longer treatment with grape seed extract.

dos Santos et al. (2019) accessed the biostimulator effect of different concentrations of proanthocyanins obtained from grape seed extract over a culture of pulp cells. Distinct behaviors were observed among the concentrations, with reduction in their metabolism not higher than 10% when compared with the negative control, independent if applied directly on pulp cells or in the presence of a dentinal barrier. In addition, was observed increased metabolism and collagen synthesis when used in direct contact with pulp cells, indicating that this extract may play a biostimulator and protective role over this tissue.

Yahara et al. (2005) investigated the effects of a proanthocyanin-based extract derived from grape seed administered together with daily diet, on the proportion of 3 mg of extract for each 100 g of the regular feed, over the mineralization of the tibial diaphysis of rats with low circulation levels of calcium. All parameters used to evaluate the bone, except for the periosteal perimeter, were significantly higher in groups supplemented with the extract. These results suggest that the addition proanthocyanins to the diet may be beneficial for the treatment of conditions related with reduced skeletal levels of calcium.

4.17. *Memora Nodosa* (Silva Manso) Miers (*Bignoniaceae*)

Memora nodosa (Silva Manso) Miers (*Bignoniaceae*) is a plant native from Brazillian cerrado. Its leaves and stem are popularly used for wound healing and treatments of ulcers, while its roots, for the treatment of abdominal pain and scabies, mainly due to the rich composition of saponins, flavonoids and essential oils of its leaves and saponins and flavonoids in the roots. An experiment using mice and Wistar rats (Tresvenzol et al. 2013) evaluated the acute toxicity and cicatricial property of ethanolic extracts obtained from the leaves and roots of *Memora nodosa*. The results presented by Tresvenzol et al. (2013) showed that 2000 mg/kg^{-1} of extract did not lead to alterations in the organs of the rats. On the other hand, the mice tested with 5000 mg/kg^{-1} of ethanolic extract presented hydropic degeneration and moderate amount of polymorphonuclear infiltrate in their livers, with no alterations in the spleen and kidneys.

With regards to wound closure, was observed decreased size of the wound over time, more evident between the seventh and the fourteenth day of treatment, explained by the presence of allantoin isolated from the ethanolic extract of *Memora nodosa.* Allantoin stimulated cellular proliferation, leading to a faster epithelialization. No significant differences were observed between test and control regarding fibrin, hyperemia, hemorrhage and inflammatory infiltrate at 4 and 7 days of treatment.

4.18. Chamomile

Chamomile tea is prepared with dried leaves of *Matricaria recutita* (McKay & Blumberg 2006) and suggested to present anti-inflammatory and analgesic properties due to inhibition of cyclooxygenase (COX) (Ortiz et al. 2016). An experiment observed that a lyophilized extract of chamomile suppressed the inflammation and the leucocyte infiltrated induced by the simultaneous inoculation of carragheenin and prostaglandin E1 in rats (Shipochliev et al. 1981).

Also, in a rodent model, Kobayashi et al. (2003) fed the rats with a diet containing 1.2% of ethyl acetate extracted from dry flowers of *M. recutita*. The regression of the induced lesions was dose dependent. Moreover, ethyl acetate in ethanol or non-ethanol vehicles and a hot water infusion of chamomile flowers presented inhibitory influence over the lesions similar to the ones observed with 10 mg/kg of oxatomide.

Another study (Al-Hindawi et al. 1989) reported that the ingestion of alcoholic chamomile extract (1.6 g of fresh herb/kg of body weight) by Wistar rats reduced in 41.1% the edema of their paws when compared with the group receiving carragheenin only.

Tubaro et al. (1984) performed topic application of an ethanolic extract of chamomile in the internal portion of the ears of mice and this treatment reduced the induced edema. The mice tested with 0.25 mg of this extract showed an 8.5% reduction in the edema, while the ones tested with 0.75 mg reached an average of 23.4% of reduction. In addition, 0.75 mg displayed a similar reduction with the treatment with 0.45 mg of benzydamine (26.6%), a non-steroidal anti-inflammatory used as reference.

Della Loggia et al. (1990) found that the topical application of extracts obtained from fresh chamomile at the proportion of 51.8 mg/100 g of bisabolol, 29.6 mg/100 g of matricin or 5.3 mg/100 mg of apigenin (i.e., equivalent to 750 μg of dried chamomile) was as effective as the drug of reference (0.60 mg of benzydamine) for prevention of inflammation in mice with induced edema.

4.19. *Mikania – Asteraceae*

Guaco (*Mikania - Asteraceae*) is popularly used in Brazil, where are found 171 of the 415 species already cataloged. The main properties described for guaco are antimicrobial, anti-inflammatory and analgesic.

Mourão et al. (1999) investigated the acute toxicity and the anti-inflammatory property of the juice of *K. brasiliens* through intraperitoneal injection of 0.25 – 5 g/kg of *K. brasiliens* (aqueous solution) in mice and in Wistar rats induced to intentional edema with carragheenin. The extract was capable to inhibit some aspects and mediators related to inflammation, such as histamine, serotonin, brachinine and prostaglandins, with the optimal activity at the concentration of 0.25 mg/kg.

The decoction of dried leaves and stem of *M. laevigata* and *M. involucrate* were found to suppress the formation of edema following injection with carragheenin and pleurisy in rats (Suyenaga et al. 2002).

4.20. Perungalli

Plumeria acuminata belongs to the family *Apocynaceae* and is popularly known as "perungalli" in southern India. Its methanolic extract was studied by Gupta et al. (2006) through the test of acute toxicity and anti-inflammatory assessment in Wistar rats intentionally induced to inflammation in their hind legs. The acute toxicity assay showed no death of the animal during 72 h following the administration of the doses 500, 750, 1000, 1250, 1500 and 2000 mg/kg^{-1} body weight (b.w.). Also, independent on the dose, no signs of convulsion, ataxia, diarrhea or increased diuresis were observed. The median lethal dose (LD50) was determined to be higher than the highest dose tested. The inhibitory activity of *Plumeria acuminate* extract, with the doses of 250 e 500 mg/kg-1 b.w, was observed after 4 h. Also, the inflammation induced by serotonin and histamine was very similar to the group tested with indomethacin. These results indicate that the extract plays its role in later stages of inflammation, possibly over arachidonic acid's metabolites.

4.21. Cranberry

Vaccinium macrocarpon has been recognized by its medicinal properties due to its polyphenol unique composition. The bioactive components predominant in cranberries are the flavonols, flavon-3-ols, anthocyanins, tannins (e.g., ellagitannins and proanthocyanidins), and phenolic acid derivates (Côté et al. 2010). These phytochemicals are frequently associated with organoleptic (sensorial) features of the fruit, also displaying innumerous biological and physiological properties in animals (Kren & Martinkove 2001).

In order to investigate the effects of cranberry on the expression of pro-inflammatory cytokines, Bodet et al. (2006) exposed macrophages to a non-dialyzable lyophilized material with a high concentration of cranberry juice or lyophilized high concentrated cranberry juice only. This experiment didn't detect cytotoxicity after exposure of macrophages to any of the substances and cell viability was higher than 94% in non-treated controls.

A biocompatibility test of concentrated cranberry juice was conducted by Rajeshwari et al. (2017) through colorimetric MTT test over periodontal fibroblasts isolated from healthy teeth extracted for orthodontic purposes. The results of this test are measured by the intensity of the coloration resultant from the solubilization of formazan crystals, which is directly proportional to the number of viable cells. The concentrated cranberry juice (500 mg/ml) expressed more than 90% viability when compared with chlorhexidine gluconate (0.2%).

4.22. Coconut

Cocos nucifera is used in folk medicine for the treatment of headaches, diarrhea, fever and stomach disorders. Coconut water is a pure and sterile biologic fluid of cytoplasmatic origin, found in the interior of coconuts, rich in sugars, essential amino acids, vitamins, proteins and electrolytes (Yong et al. 2009). On the other hand, is already known that its acidic pH is harmful to cellular metabolism (Moreira-Neto et al. 2009, Souza et al. 2011).

Aqueous extracts obtained from the bark of *C. nucifera* are used for the treatment of arthritis and other inflammatory diseases in Brazilian's northwestern (Esquenazi et al. 2002). An experiment performed with an animal model of inflammation (formalin test and subcutaneous airbag model) showed that this extract (both 50 or 100 mg/kg) significantly reduced the period that the animals licking their paws injected with formalin and decreased the inflammation induced by subcutaneous injection of carragheenin, confirmed by the reduction on cellular migration, overflow of proteins, and expression of tumor necrosis factor -α (Silva et al. 2013).

Extracts of the fibers found in coconut bark were also tested in carragheenin, histamine and serotonin (150 mg/kg) induced edema (Rinaldi et al. 2009). This extract significantly reduced the histamine and the edema of the rats' paws induced by serotonin, pointing to a positive effect on this situation.

A study performed by Padumadasa et al. (2015) indicated that the inflorescence of *Cocos nucifera L* is mainly composed of proanthocyanidins (Diouf et al. 2009). Padumadasa et al. (2016) affirm that proanthocyanidins display anti-inflammatory and antioxidant activities. Moreover, Padumadasa et al. (2016) showed its potent cytotoxic activity over the HeLa lineage of cells.

Innumerous experiments investigated that toxicity of *C. nucifera*. One of them verified positive effects etila's acetate extract obtained from *C. nucifera* fibers over physiological parameters and topic inflammation of animal models (Silva et al. 2009). With regards to the physiological parameters and macroscopic features of lymphoid organs, neither mortality nor symptoms of toxicity were observed in the animals.

Another experiment evaluated the toxicity of a methanol extract of *C. nucifera*'s water (Al-Adhroey et al. 2011). Five female and five male mice received a single oral dose (5000 mg/kg) of this extract. All animals were observed to identify signs of toxicity and mortality 1, 3 and 4 h after administration, and then, twice a day for 14 days. No signs of toxicity or mortality were observed, and the animals gained weight during the observational period.

Zakaria et al. (2006) investigated the biocompatibility of fresh coconut juice and of the aqueous extract of coconut. Both substances presented anti-inflammatory activity, significantly higher with fresh juice. Both extracts at the concentration of 100% completely reduced the edema 300 minutes after administration. Between 4 and 8 h was observed antipyretic activity. Furthermore, both extracts at the concentration of 50% led to hypothermia during the first 3 h. At the third day, group fresh juice showed progression of the repair process to formation of granulation tissue. At day six, the granulation tissue was mature, presenting monocytes and fibers formation that increased over time. On the other hand, group coconut extract showed fibrous cover, indicating fastened repair process.

Evidence suggests that a diet rich in phenolic compounds may significantly improve human health due to their antioxidant property (Naczk et al. 2004). Studies with virgin coconut oil reported that the phenolic concentration was almost seven times higher than in commercial coconut oil, explained by the possible degradation of some biologically active compounds during commercial refinement (Seneviratne et al. 2008). The 1,1-difenil-2-picril-hidrazil test indicated that virgin coconut oil possesses higher antioxidant capacity when compared with the refined product.

During the analysis of antioxidant properties of *C. nucifera's* water extract, it was demonstrated that ethanolic, dried distillate and aqueous extracts have significant antioxidant activity (4.1828; 3.31; 20.83; 1.0179 mg/mL, respectively) (Singla et al. 2011).

Micronutrients, such as inorganic ions and proteins present in coconut water, play vital roles in order to hosts' immune system. Some evidence suggested that coconut oil (6 ml/100g of body weight) administered to animals intoxicated with carbon tetrachloride recovered the activity of antioxidant enzymes (superoxide dismutase and catalase levels) and decreased lipidic peroxidation (Loki & Rajamohan 2003). Coconut water is also rich in L-arginine (30 mg/dL), which can possibly to reduce the formation of free radicals (Boger et al. 1995) and to exhibit antioxidant activity (Salil & Rajamohan 2001). Moreover, coconut water presents ascorbic acid (15 mg/100 ml), responsible for lipidic peroxidation in rats (Das et al. 2001).

4.23. Pepper (*Capsicum* spp)

Capsaicin (an alkaloid that makes pepper hot) and its minor capsaicinoids (norcapsaicin, nordihydrocapsaicin, nornordihydrocapsaicin, homocapsaicin and homodihydrocapsaicin) are the active ingredients in pepper that are related to the anti-microbial, anti-carcinogenic and analgesic properties in pepper. Capsaicin is typically an analgesic drug used to treat neuropathic pain such as diabetic neuropathy and postherpetic neuralgia, as well as osteoarthritis, rheumatoid arthritis and symptomatic treatment of psoriasis (Haroutounian & Finnerup 2018).

The use of capsaicin as an analgesic agent is usually in concentrations ranging from 0.025 to 0.075% as creams, gels and ointments formulations (Graham et al. 2017). Steinke et al. (2017) showed that a single application lasting up to 60 minutes in patients with neuropathic pain produces effective pain relief for up to 12 weeks.

Romero et al. (2019) evidenced the analgesic action of a topic 8% capsain cream in patients with myofascial pain syndrome. This analgesia persisted for almost two months after a single application, without significant adverse effects.

CONCLUSION

Due to some extracts to trigger toxic reactions to the organisms, biocompatibility tests are essential to confirm if rather a substance can be used or not in human medicine. A promising future with the use of herbal extracts can be envisioned since they display high biocompatibility and a huge amount of phytotherapics with positive effects over tissues. It is possible to find in literature a wide amount of species with high biocompatibility, and bibliographic researches must be constant in order to amplify their use in dentistry.

References

ADA. American Dental Association. Council on Dental Materials and Device of the American Dental Association. *J Amer Dent Assoc*, 1972, 84, 375-95.

ADA. American National Standards/American Dental Association. Document n°41 for recommended standard practices for biological evaluation of dental materials. New York, ANSI/ADA, 1982.

Aghbali, A; Hosseini, SV; Delazar, A; Gharavi, NK; Shahneh, FZ; Orangi, M; Bandehagh, A; Baradaran, B. Induction of apoptosis by grape seed extract (*Vitis vinifera*) in oral squamous cell carcinoma. *Bosn J Basic Med Sci*, 2013, 13(3), 186-91.

Al Shaher, A; Wallace, J; Agarwal, S; Bretz, WA; Baugh, D. Effect of propolis on human fibroblasts from the pulp and periodontal ligament. *J Endod*, 2004, 30(5), 359-61.

Al-Adhroey, AH; Nor, ZM; Al-Mekhlafi, HM; Amran, AA; Mahmud, R. Evaluation of the use of *Cocos nucifera* as antimalarial remedy in Malaysian folk medicine. *J Ethnopharmacol*, 2011, 134(3), 988–91.

Al-Hindawi, MK; Al-Deen, IH; Nabi, MH; Ismail, MA. Anti-inflammatory activity of some Iraqi plants using intact rats. *J Ethnopharmacol*, 1989, 26(2), 163 –8.

Al-Shaher, A; Wallace, J; Agarwal, S; Bretz, W; Baugh, D. Effect of propolis on human fibroblasts from the pulp and periodontal ligament. *J Endod*, 2004, 30(5), 359-61.

Albano, MN; da Silveira, MR; Danielski, LG; Florentino, D; Petronilho, F; Piovezan, AP. Anti-inflammatory and antioxidant properties of hydroalcoholic crude extract from *Casearia sylvestris Sw.* (Salicaceae). *J Ethnopharmacol*, 2013, 147(3), 612-7.

Ali, S; Wahbi, W. The efficacy of Aloe vera in management of oral lichen planus: a systematic review and meta-analysis. *Oral Dis*, 2017, 23(7), 913-8.

Alipour, M; Malihi, R; Hosseini, SA; et al. The effects of catechins on related risk factors with Type 2 diabetes: a review. *Prog Nutr*, 2018, 20(1), 12-20.

Almas, K; Mahmoud, A; Dahlan, A. A comparative study of propolis and saline application on human dentin. A SEM study. *Indian J Dent Res*, 2001, 12(1), 21-7.

Amruthesh, S. Dentistry and Ayurveda–III (basics-ama, immunity, ojas, rasas, etiopathogenesis and prevention). *Indian J Dent Res*, 2007, 18(3), 112-9.

Andres, P; Brenneisen, R; Clerc, JT. Relating antiphlogistic efficacy of dermatics containing extracts of Symphytum officinale to chemical profiles. *Planta Medica*, 1989, 55, 66-7.

Badakhsh, S; Eskandarian, T; Esmaeilpour, T. The use of *Aloe vera* extract as a novel storage media for the avulsed tooth. *Iran J Med Sci*, 2014, 39(4), 327–32.

Bagchi, D; Garg, A; Krohn, RL; Bagchi, M; Tran, MX; Stohs, SJ. Oxygen free radical scavenging abilities of vitamins C and E, and a grape seed proanthocyanidin extract *in vitro*. *Res Commun Mol Pathol Pharmacol*, 1997, 95(2), 179–89.

Benavente-Garcia, O; Castillo, J; Sabater, F; Del Rio, JA. Characterization of a *S*-adenosyl-L-methionine: Eriodictyol 4′-*O*-methyltransferase from Citrus aurantium. Developmental changes in the levels of 4′-*O*-methoxyflavonoids and *S*-adenosyl-L-methionine: Eriodictyol 4′-*O*-methyltransferase activity. *Plant Physiol Biochem*, 1995, 33, 263–71.

Benetti, F; de Azevedo Queiroz, ÍO; Oliveira, PHC; Conti, LC; Azuma, MM; Oliveira, SHP; Cintra, LTA. Cytotoxicity and biocompatibility of a new bioceramic endodontic sealer containing calcium hydroxide. *Braz Oral Res*, 2019, 33(0), 42-51.

Bispo, MD; Mourão, RHV; Franzotti, EM; Bomfim, KBR; Arrigoni Blank, MDF; Moreno, MPN; Marchioro, M; Antoniolli, AR. Antinociceptive and antiedematogenic effects of the aqueous extract of *Hyptis pectinata* leaves in experimental animals. *J Ethnopharmacol*, 2001, 76(1), 81-6.

Biswas, SK; McClure, D; Jimenez, LA; Megson, IL; Rahman, I. Curcumi induces glutathione biosynthesis and inhibits NF-kappaB activation and interleukin-8 release in alveolar epithelial cells: mechanism of free radical scavenging activity. *Antioxid Redox Sign*, 2005, 7(1–2), 32-41.

Bodet, C; Chandad, F; Grenier, D. Antiinflammatory activity of a high-molecular-weight cranberry fraction on macrophages stimulated by lipopolysaccharides from periodontopathogens. *J Dent Res*, 2006, 85(3), 235- 239.

Boger, RH; Bode-Boger, SM; Mugge, A; Kienke, S; Brandes, R; Dwenger, A; Frolich, JC. Supplementation of hypercholesterolaemic rabbits with L-arginine reduces the vascular release of superoxide anions and restores NO production. *Atherosclerosis*, 1995, 117(2), 273–84.

Bueno, CRE; Lopes, GA; Valentim, D; Marques, VAS; Vasques, AMV; Cury, MTS; Sivieri-Araujo, G; Jacinto, RC; Cintra, LTA; Dezan-Junior, E. Mixing failures of endodontic sealers: an *in vivo* biocompatibility study. *Braz Dent Sci*, 2017, 20(4), 85-92.

Bueno, CRE; Valentim, D; Jardim Junior, EG; Mancuso, DN; Sivieri-Araujo, G; Jacinto, RC; Cintra, LTA; Dezan-Junior, E. Tissue reaction to Aroeira (*Myracrodruon urundeuva*) extracts associated with microorganisms: an *in vivo* study. *Braz Oral Res*, 2018, 32, 1-9.

Bueno, CRE; Valentim, D; Marques, VAS; et al. Biocompatibility and biomineralization assessment of bioceramic-, epoxy-, and calcium hydroxide-based sealers. *Braz Oral Res*, 2016, 30(1), 81.

Bueno, CRE; Vasques, AMV; Cury, MTS; et al. Biocompatibility and biomineralization assessment of mineral trioxide aggregate flow. *Clin Oral Investig*, 2019, 23(1), 169-177.

Burch, RM; DeHaas, C. A bradykinin antagonist inhibits carrageenan edema in rats. Arch *Pharmacol*, 1990, 342(2), 189-93.

Carmignan, F; Matias, R; Carollo, CA; Dourado, DM; Fermiano, MH; Silva, BAK; Bastos, PRHO. Efficacy of application of Equisetum pyramidale Goldm. hydrogel for tissue restoration of induced skin lesions in Wistar rats. *Braz J Biol*, 2019, Epub May 09, 1-11.

Carrel, A. On the permanent life of tissues outside of the organism. *J Exp Med*, 1912, 15, 516-28.

Carvalho, JCT. Fitoterápicos anti-inflamatórios: Aspectos químicos, farmacológicos e aplicações terapêuticas [Anti-Inflammatory Herbal Medicines: Chemical, Pharmacological Aspects and Therapeutic Applications]. Ribeirão Preto, SP: Tecmed, 2004, 480p.

Castilho, C; Couto, LB; Souza-Gabriel, AE; Perez, DEC; Nunes, FD; Cruz-Filho, AM. Avaliação da atividade anti-inflamatória de AINES em tecido pulpar de ratos [Anti-inflammatory evaluation of NSAIDs in rat's pulps] *Robrac*, 2008, 17(43), 32-8.

Cavenago, BC; Garlet, GP; Duarte, MAH. O efeito do uso de fitoterápicos e da própolis nas propriedades físico-químicas, antimicrobiana e biocompatibilidade do MTA. Tese (Doutorado) – Faculdade de Odontologia de Bauru. Universidade de São Paulo. [The effect of the use of phytotherapics and propolis in physicochemical properties, antimocrobial and biocompatibility of MTA] Thesis - University of São Paulo, 2015, 183p.

Chan, YS; Cheng, LN; Wu, JH; Chan, E; Kwan, YW; Lee, SM; Leung, GP; Yu, PH; Chan, SW. A review of the pharmacological effects of *Arctium lappa* (burdock). *Inflammopharmacology*, 2011, 19(5), 245-54.

Chen, L; Wen, YM. The role of bacterial biofilm in persistent infections and control strategies. *Int J Oral Sci*, 2011, 3(2), 66-73.

Chidiac, JJ; Rifai, K; Hawwa, NN; Massaad, CA; Jurjus, AR; Labbur, SJ; Saadã, NE. Nociceptive behavior induced by dental application of irritants to rat incisors: a new model for tooth inflammatory pain. *Eur J Pain*, 2002, 65(1), 55-67.

Chithra, P; Sajithlal, G; Chandrakasan, G. Influence of Aloe vera on the glycosaminoglycans in the matrix of healing dermal wounds in rats. *J Ethnopharmacol*, 1998, 59(3), 179-86.

Cintra, LTA; Benetti, F; Queiroz, IOA; Ferreira, LL; Massunari, L; Bueno, CRE; Oliveira, SHPO; Gomes-Filho, JE. Evaluation of the cytotoxicity and biocompatibility of new resin epoxy-based endodontic sealer containing calcium hydroxide. *J Endod*, 2017, 43, 2088-2092.

Cogulu, D; Uzel, A; Sorkun, K. Efficacy of propolis as an intracanal medicament against *Enterococcus faecalis*. *Gen Dent*, 2006, 54(5), 319- 22.

Contrera, A; Bernardi, AC; Pozetti, GL; Lopes, RA; Contrera, MGD. Ação da tintura-mãe de *Lichnophora ericoides*, *Aristolochia esperanzae* e *Solidago microglossa*, em feridas cutâneas de ratos [Action of the mother tincture of *Lichnophora ericoides*, *Aristolochia esperanzae* and *Solidago microglossa*, on rat skin wounds]. *Rev Esc Farm Odont*, 1985, 11, 157-60.

Costa, AF. Farmacognosia: farmacognosia experimental. 3rd Edition. Lisboa; *Calouste Gulbenkian Foundation*, 2001, 992p.

Costa, VB; Coube, CS; Marinho, BG; Matheus, ME; Leitão, SG; Fernandes, PD. Antiinflammatory and analgesic activity of *Bouchea fluminensis*. *Fitoterapia*, 2003, 74(4), 364-71.

Côté, J; Caillet, S; Doyon, G; Sylvain, JF; Lacroix, M. Bioactive compounds in cranberries and their biological properties. *Crit Rev Food Sci Nutr*, 2010, 50(7), 666–79.

Das, KK; Das, SN; Dasgupta, S. The influence of ascorbic acid on nickel-induced hepatic lipid peroxidation in rats. *J Basic Clin Physiol Pharmacol*, 2001, 12(3), 187–95.

Dassoler, M; Schwanz, M; Busseto, F; Moreira, EA; Gutierrez, L. Perfil fitoquímico e ensaio farmacológico de *Averrhoa carambola* L. (*Oxalidaceae*) [Phytochemical profile and pharmacological assay of Averrhoa carambola L (*Oxalidaceae*)]. *Jornal Brasileiro de Fitomedicina*, 2004, 2, 4-8.

Davis, RH; Donato, JJD; Hartman, GM; Haas, RC. Anti-inflammatory and wound healing activity of a growth substance in *Aloe* vera. *J A Podiatr Med Assoc*, 1994, 84(2), 77–81.

de Albuquerque, UP; Muniz de Medeiros, P; de Almeida, AL; Monteiro, JM; Machado de Freitas Lins Neto, E; Gomes de Melo, J; dos Santos, JP. Medicinal plants of the caatinga (semi-arid) vegetation of NE Brazil: a quantitative approach. *J Ethnopharmacol*, 2007, 114(3), 325–54.

de Almeida, AB; Sánchez-Hidalgo, M; Martín, AR; Luiz-Ferreira, A; Trigo JR; Vilegas, W; dos santos, LC; Souza-Brito, AR; de la Lastra, CA. Anti-inflammatory intestinal activity of *Arctium lappa L.* (Asteraceae) in TNBS colitis model. *J Ethnopharmacol*, 2013, 146(1), 300-10.

De Araújo, AA; Soares, LAL; Assunção Ferreira, MR; de Souza Neto, MA; da Silva, GR; de Araújo, RF; Jr. Guerra, GC; de Melo, MC.

Quantification of polyphenols and evaluation of antimicrobial, analgesic and anti-inflammatory activities of aqueous and acetone–water extracts of *Libidibia ferrea*, *Parapiptadenia rigida* and *Psidium guajava*. *J Ethnopharmacol*, 2014, 156, 88–96.

Della Loggia, R; Carle, R; Sosa, S; Tubaro, A. Evaluation of the antiinflammatory activity of chamomile [*Chamomilla recutita*] preparations. *Planta Med*, 1990, 56, 657–58.

Develioglu, H; Saraydin, SU; Kartal, U. The bone-healing effect of a xenograft in a rat calvarial defect model. *Dent Mater J*, 2009, 28(4), 396-400.

Diao, JX; Ou, JY; Dai, H; Li, HY; Huang, W; Xie, T; Wang, M; Yang, YG. Antioxidant and Antiapoptotic Polyphenols from Green Tea Extract Ameliorate CCl_4-Induced Acute Liver Injury in Mice. *Chin J Integr Med*, 2019, 1-9.

Dinicola, S; Pasqualato, A; Cucina, A; Coluccia, P; Ferranti, F; Canipari, R; Catizone, A; Proietti, S; D'Anselmi, F; Ricci, G; Palombo, A; Bizzarri, M. Grape seed extract suppresses MDA-MB231 breast cancer cell migration and invasion. *Eur J Nutr*, 2014, 53(2), 421–31.

Diouf, PN; Stevanovic, T; Cloutier, A. Study on chemical composition, antioxidant and anti-inflammatory activities of hot water extract from *Picea marianai* bark and its proanthocyanidin-rich fractions. *Food Chem*, 2009, 113(4), 897–902.

dos Santos, AF; Pacheco, JM; Silva, PAO; Bedran-Russo, AK; Rezende, TMB; Pereira, PNR; Ribeiro, APD. Direct and transdentinal biostimulatory effects of grape seed extract rich in proanthocyanidin on pulp cells. *Int Endod J*, 2019, 52(4), 424–38.

Duarte, MA; Midena, RZ; Zeferino, MA; Vivan, RR; Weckwerth, PH; Dos Santos, F; et al. Evaluation of pH and calcium ion release of calcium hydroxide pastes containing different substances. *J Endod*, 2009, 35(9), 1274-7.

Duncan, R; Izzo, L. Dendrimer biocompatibility and toxicity. *Adv Drug Del Rev*, 2005, 57(15), 2215-37.

Dunphy, JE; Udupa, KN. Chemical and histochemical sequences in the normal healing of wounds. *N Engl J Med*, 1955, 253(20), 847–51.

Durgaprasad, S; Pai, CG; Vasanthkumar, Alvres JF; Namitha, S. A pilot study of the antioxidant effect of curcumin in tropical pancreatitis. *Indian J Med Res*, 2005, 122(4), 315-18.

Eamlamnam, K; Patumraj, S; Visedopas, N; Thong-Ngam, D. Effects of aloe vera and sucralfate on gastric microcirculatory changes, cytokine levels and gastric ulcer healing in rats. *World J Gastroenterol*, 2006, 12(13), 2034–9.

Esquenazi, MD; Wigg, MM; Miranda, Rodrigues HM; Tostes, JBF; Rozental, S; da Silva, AJ; Alviano, CS. Antimicrobial and antiviral activities of polyphenolics from *Cocos nucifera Linn.* (Palmae) husk fiber extract. *Res Microbiol*, 2002, 153(10), 647–52.

Esteves, I; Souza, IR; Rodrigues, M; Cardoso, LG; Santos, LS; Sertic, JA; et al. Gastric antiulcer and anti-inflammatory activities of the essential oil from *Casearia sylvestris Sw. J Ethnopharmacol*, 2005, 101(1-3), 191-6.

Ferreira, FB; Torres, SA; Rosa, OP; Ferreira, CM; Garcia, RB; Marcucci, CM; Gomes, BP. Antimicrobial effect of propolis and other substances against selected endodontic pathogens. *Oral Surg Oral Med Oral Pathol Oral Radiol Endod*, 2007, 104(5), 709-16.

Ferreira, SH; Lorenzetti, BB; Poole, S. Bradykinin initiates cytokine mediated inflammatory hyperalgesia. *Br J Pharmacol*, 1993, 110(3), 1127-31.

Franzotti, EM; Santos, CVF; Rodrigues, HMSL; Mourão, RHV; Andrade, MR; Antoniolli, AR. Antiinflammatory, analgesic activity and acute toxicity of *Sida cordifolia* L. (malva-branca). *J Ethnopharmacol*, 2000, 72(1-2), 273-278.

Frasson, APZ; Bittencourt, CF; Heinzmann, BM. Caracterização físico-química e biológica do caule de *Caesalpinia ferrea* Mart. *Rev Bras Farmacogn*, 2003, 13, 35–39.

Freshney, RI. Culture of animal cells: a manual of basic technique. 3rd ed. New York, 1994, 732p.

Gaddi, A; Cícero, AFG; Pedro, EJ. Clinical perspectives of anti-inflammatory therapy in the elderly: the lipoxigenase

(LOX)/cycloxigenase (COX) inhibition concept. *Arch Gerontol Geriatr*, 2004, 38(3), 201-12.

Garcia, AR; Amaral, ACF; Azevedo, MMB; Corte-Real, S; Lopes, RC; Alviano, CS; Pinheiro, AS; Vermelho, AB; Rodrigues, IA. Cytotoxicity and anti-Leishmania amazonensis activity of Citrus sinensis leaf extracts. *Pharm Biol*, 2017, 55(1), 1780-6.

Gehlen, ML; Moreira, H; Moreira, L; Sabag, FP; Repka, JCD. Spectrophotometric evaluation of Evans blue in inflammatory cornea reaction: experimental study in rabbits. *Arq Bras Oftalmol*, 2004, 67(0), 219-25.

Goel, A; Kunnumakkara, AB; Aggarwal, BB. Curcumin as 'curecumin", from kitchen to clinic. *Biochem Pharmacol*, 2008, 75, 787-809.

Gomes, LAP. Avaliação da biocompatibilidade e atividade antimicrobiana *in vitro* da matriz de Hidrogel associada ao extrato glicólico do *Punica granatum L.* (romã) [dissertação] [Evaluation of biocompatibility and antimicrobial action *in vitro* of a hydrogel scaffolds Hydromatrix associated to glycolic extract of Punica granatum (pomegranate)] [dissertation]. São José dos Campos (SP): São Paulo State University (Unesp), Institute of Science and Technology, 2017.

Graham, J; Barberio, M; Wang, GS. Capsaicin Cream for Treatment of Cannabinoid Hyperemesis Syndrome in Adolescents: A Case Series. *Pediatrics*, 2017, 140(6), e20163795.

Graham, JG; Fabricant, MLQDS; Farnsworth, NR. Plants used against cancer - an extension of the work of Jonathan Hartwell. *J Ethnopharmacol*, 2000, 73, 347–77.

Gupta, M; Mazumder, UK; Gomathi, P; Selvan, VT. Anti-inflammatory evaluation of leaves of *Plumeria acuminata*. *BMC Complement Altern Med*, 2006, 2, 6–36.

Hagiu, A; Attin, T; Schmidlin, PR; Ramenzoni, LL. Dose-dependent green tea effect on decrease of inflammation in human oral gingival epithelial keratinocytes: *in vitro* study. *Clin Oral Investig*, 2019, Epub ahead of print.

Haroutounian, S; Finnerup, NB. Recommendations for pharmacologic therapy of neuropathic pain. *Essent Pain Medic*, 2018, 445-56.

Harrison, RG. Observations on the living developing nerve fiber. *Proc Soc Exp Biol Med*, 1970, 4, 140-3.

Hashemi, SA; Madani, SA; Abediankenari, S. The review on properties of aloe vera in healing of cutaneous wounds. *Biomed Res Int*, 2015, 2015, 714216.

Heggars, JP; Pelley, RP; Robson, MC. Beneficial effects of *Aloe* in wound healing. *Phytot Res*, 1993, 7, 48–52.

Holt, CI; Hutchins, MO; Pileggi, R. A real time quantitative PCR analysis and correlation of COX-1 and COX-2 enzymes in inflamed dental pulps following administration of three different NSAID. *J Endod*, 2005, 31(11), 799-804.

Honma, T; Itagaki, T; Nakamura, M; Kamakura, S; Takahashi, I; Echigo, S; Sasano, Y. Bone formation in rat calvaria ceases within a limited period regardless of completion of defect repair. *Oral dis*, 2008, 14(5), 457-64.

Im, I; Park, KR; Kim, SM; Kim, C; Park, JH; Nam, D; Jang, HJ; Shim, BS; Ahn, KS; Mosaddik, A; Sethi, G; Sho, SK; Ahn, KS. The butanol fraction of guava (*Psidium cattleianum* Sabine) leaf extract suppresses MMP-2 and MMP-9 expression and activity through the suppression of the ERK1/2 MAPK signaling pathway. *Nutr Cancer*, 2012, 64(2), 255-66.

International Organization for Standardization. ISO 7405, dentistry – preclinical evaluation of biocompatibility of medical devices used in dentistry – test methods for dental materials. Genève, ISO, 1997.

Jaiarj, P; Khoohaswan, P; Wongkrajang, Y; Peungvicha, P; Suriyawong, P; Saraya, ML; et al. Anticough and antimicrobial activities of *Psidium guajava* Linn. leaf extract. *J Ethnopharmacol*, 1999, 67(2), 203-12.

Jittapiromsak, N; Sahawat, D; Banlunara, W; Sangvanich, P; Thunyakitpisa, P. Acemannan, an extracted product from Aloe vera, stimulates dental pulp cell proliferation, differentiation, mineralization, and dentin formation. *Tissue Eng Part A*, 2010, 16(6), 1997–2006.

Jobin, C; Bradham, CA; Russo, MP; Juma, B; Narula, AS; Brenner, DA; Sartor, RB. Curcumin blocks cytokine-mediated NF-kappa B activation and proinflammatory gene expression by inhibiting inhibitory factor I-kappa B kinase activity. *J Immunol*, 1999, 163(6), 3474-3483.

Jurenka, JS. Anti-inflammatory properties of Curcumin, a major constituent of Curcuma longa: a review of preclinical and clinical research. *Altern Med Ver*, 2009, 14(2), 141-153.

Karyakina, EE; Vokhmyanina, DV; Sizova, NV; Sabitov, NA; Borisova, AV; Sazontova, TG; Arkhipenko, YV; Tkachuk, VA; Zolotov, YA; Karyakin, AA. Kinetic approach for evaluation of total antioxidant activity. *Talanta*, 2009, 80(2), 749–53.

Kaur, M; Singh, RP; Gu, M; Agarwal, R; Agarwal C. Grape seed extract inhibits *in vitro* and *in vivo* growth of human colorectal carcinoma cells. *Clin Cancer Res*, 2006, 12(20), 6194-202.

Kawagishi, E; Nakakura-Ohshima, K; Nomura, S; Ohshima, H. Pulpal responses to cavity preparation in aged rat molars. *Cell. Tissue Res*, 2006, 326(1), 111-22.

Khan, RA; Mallick, N; Feroz, Z. Anti-inflammatory effects of *Citrus sinensis* L., *Citrus paradisi* L. and their combinations. *Pak J Pharm Sci*, 2016, 29(3), 843-52.

Knipping, K; van Esch, EC; Wijering, SC; van der Heide, S; Dubois, AE; Garssen, J. *In vitro* and *in vivo* anti-allergic effects of *Arctium lappa L. Exp Biol Med (Maywood)*, 2008, 233(11), 1469-77.

Knudson, CB; Toole, BP. Changes in the pericellular matrix during differentiation of limb bud mesoderm. *Dev Biol*, 1985, 112(2), 308–18.

Kobayashi, Y; Nakano, Y; Inayama, K; Sakai, A; Kamiya, T. Dietary intake of the flower extracts of German chamomile (*Matricaria recutita* L.) inhibited compound 48/80-induceditch-scratch responses in mice. *Phytomedicine*, 2003, 10(8), 657–664.

Kondo, H; Abe, K; Emori, Y; Arai, S. Gene organization of oryzacystatin-II, a new cystatin superfamily member of plant origin, is closely related to that of oryzacystatin-I but different from those of animal cystatins. *FEBS Lett*, 1991, 278(1), 87-90.

Kren, V; Martinkove, L. Glycosides in medicine: "The role of glycosidic residue in biological activity". *Curr Med Chem*, 2001, 8(11), 1303–28.

Lapa, AJ; Souccar, C; Lima-Landman, MTR; Godinho, RO; Nogueira TCML. Farmacologia e toxicologia de produtos naturais. *In*: Simões CMO, et al. Farmacognosia: da planta ao medicamento. 5ª Ed. Porto Alegre/Florianópolis: *Editora Da UFRGS/Editora Da UFSC* [Pharmacology and toxicology of natural products. In*: Pharmacognosy: from plant to medicine.* 5th Ed.] UFRGS and UFSC publishers, 2003, 247-262.

Leguizamón, NDP; Rodrigues, EM; de Campos, ML; Nogueira, AVB; Viola, KS; Schneider, VK; Neo-Justino, DM; Tanomaru-Filho, M; Zambuzzi, WF; Henrique-Silva, F; Soares-Costa, A; Faria, G; Cirelli, JA. *In vivo* and *in vitro* antiinflammatory and pro-osteogenic effects of citrus cystatin CsinCPI-2. *Cytokine*, 2019, 123, 154760.

Liu, K; Chen, Q; Liu, Y; Zhou, X; Wang, X. Isolation and biological activities of decanal, linalool, valencene, and octanal from sweet orange oil. *J Food Sci*, 2012, *77*(11), 1156-61.

Loki, AL; Rajamohan, T. Hepatoprotective and antioxidant effect of tender coconut water on carbon tetrachloride induced liver injury in rats. *Indian J Biochem Biophys*, 2003, 40(5), 354–357.

Lope, ER; Chapadeiro, E; Raso, P; Tafuri, WL. Bogliolo – Patologia. 4ª Ed. [Pathology 4th Ed.] *Belo Horizonte: Guanabara Koogan*, 1987, 67-112.

Lopes-Rocha, R; Miranda, JL; Ferreira, FO; Marinho, AS; Verli, FD. Effect of topical propolis and dexamethasone on the healing of oral surgical wounds. *Wound Healing Southern Africa*, 2012, 5(1), 25-30.

Lorenzi, H; Matos, FJA. Plantas Medicinais no Brasil: nativas e exóticas [*Medicinal Plants in Brazil: natives and exotics*] São Paulo: Nova Odessa, 2008, 576p.

Lozoya, X; Meckes, M; Aboud-Zaid, M; Tortoriello, J; Nozzolillo, C; Arnason, JT. Quercetin glycosides in *Psidium guajava L.* leaves and determination of spasmolytic principle. *Arch Med Res*, 1994, 25(1), 11-5.

Lyss, G; Knorre, A; Schmidt, TJ; Pahl, HL; Merfort, I. The antiinflammatory sesquiterpene lactone helenalin inhibits the transcription factor NF-kB bdirectly targeting p65. *J Biol Chem*, 1998, 273(50), 33508-16.

Madarova, L. Antibacterial properties of propolis. *Cesk Stomatol*, 1980, 80, 304-7.

Magro-Filho, O; Carvalho, ACP. Application of propolis to dental sockets and skin wounds. *J Nihon Univ Sch Dent*, 1990, 32(1), 4-13.

Magro-Filho, O; Carvalho, ACP. Topical effect of propolis in the repair of sulcoplasties by the modified kazanjian technique. *J Nihon Univ Sch Dent*, 1994, 36(2), 102-111.

Mangaiyarkarasi, SP; Manigandan, T; Elumalai, M; Cholan, PK; Kaur, RP. Benefits of *Aloe vera* in dentistry. *J Pharm Bioallied Sci*, 2015, 7(1), 255-9.

Marcucci, MC. Propolis: chemical composition, biological properties and therapeutic activity. *Apidologie*, 1995, 26, 83–99.

Margis, R; Reis, EM; Villeret, V. Structural and phylogenetic relationships among plant and animal cystatins. *Arch Biochem Biophys*, 1998, 359(1), 24–30.

Martin, MP; Pileggi, R. A quantitative analysis of propolis: a promising new storage media following avulsion. *Dent Traumatol*, 2004, 20(2), 85-9.

Martins, MD; Marques, MM; Bussadori, SK; Mesquita-Ferrari, RA; Pavesi, VCS; Wadt, NS; Fernandes, KP. *In vitro* cytotoxicity of arnica brasileira (*Solidago microglossa*) and arnica paulista (*Porophyllum ruderale*). *ConScientiae Saúde*, 2009, 8(1), 99-104.

Matias, R. Contribuição para o estudo químico e atividade antibacteriana e cicatrizante das plantas *Equisetum giganteum*, *Piper amalago* e *Piper aduncum*. Maringá: Universidade Estadual de Maringá. Tese de Doutorado em Química. [Contribution to the chemical study and antibacterial and healing activity of the plants *Equisetum giganteum*, *Piper amalago* and *Piper aduncum*. Maringa: State University of Maringa Chemistry Thesis], 2010.

McKay, DL; Blumberg, JB. A review of the bioactivity and potential health benefits of chamomile tea (*Matricariarecutita L.*). *Phytother Res*, 2006, 20(7), 519–30.

Medina-Remón, A; Casas, R; Tressserra-Rimbau, A; Ros, E; Martínez-González, MA; Fitó, M; Corella, D; Salas-Salvadó, J; Lamuela-Raventos, RM; Estruch, R. Polyphenol intake from a Mediterranean diet decreases inflammatory biomarkers related to atherosclerosis: a substudy of the PREDIMED trial. *Br J Clin Pharmacol*, 2017, 83(1), 114-28.

Miller, MB; Koltai, PJ. Treatment of experimental frostbite with pentoxifylline and *Aloe* T*era* cream. *Arch of Otolaryngol Head Neck Surg*, 1995, 121(6), 678-80.

Moon, EJ; Lee, YM; Lee, OH; Lee, MJ; Lee, SK; Chung, MH; Park, YI; Sung, CK; Choi, JS; Kim, KW. A novel angiogenic factor derived from *Aloe vera* gel: beta-sitosterol, a plant sterol. *Angiogenesis*, 1999, 3(2), 117-123.

Moreira, AS; Spitzer, V; Schapoval, EES; Schnekel, EP. Antiinflammatory activity of extracts and fractions from the leaves of *Gochnatia polymorpha*. *Phytother Res*, 2000, 14(8), 638-40.

Moreira-Neto, JJS; Gondim, JO; Raddi, MSG; Pansani, CA. Viability of human fibroblasts in coconut water as a storage. *Int Endod J*, 2009, 42(9), 827-30.

Mourão, RH; Santos, FO; Franzotti, EM; Moreno, MP; Antoniolli, AR. Anti inflammatory activity and acute toxicity (LD50) of the juice of *Kalanchoe brasiliensis* (Comb.) leaves picked before and during blooming. *Phytother Res*, 1999, 13(4), 352–354.

Mukherjee, PK; Rai, S; Bhattacharyya, S; Debath, PK; Biswas, TK; Jana, U; Pandit, S; Saha, BP; Paul, PK. Clinical study of 'Triphala'- A Well Known Phytomedicine from India. *IJPT*, 2006, 5, 51-4.

Naczk, M; Shahidi, F. Extraction and analysis of phenolics in food. *J Chromatogr A*, 2004, 1054(1-2), 95–111.

Naito, Y; Yasumuro, M; Kondou, K; Ohara, N. Antiinflammatory effect of topically applied propolis extract in carrageenan-in-duced rat hind paw edema. *Phytother Res*, 2007, 21(5), 452-6.

Najjar, T; Kahn, D. Comparative study of healing and remodeling in various bones. *J Oral Surgery*, 1977, 35(5), 375-9.

Ndhlala, AR; Amoo, SO; Stafford, GI; Finnie, JF; Van Staden, J. Antimicrobial, anti-inflammatory and mutagenic investigation of the South African tree aloe (*Aloe barberae*). *J Ethnopharmacol*, 2009, 124 (3), 404-8.

Nichols, JA; Katiyar, SK. Skin photo protection by natural polyphenols: anti-inflammatory, antioxidant and DNA repair mechanisms. *Arch Dermatol Res*, 2010, 302(2), 71-83.

Niedner, R. Influence of epithelialization by a complex of active ingredients from Symphytum. *Acta Ther*, 1989, 15, 289-97.

Nossa, PM; Guenka, LC; Couto, LB; da-Cruz-Perez, DE. Effects of the *Serjania erecta* and *Zeyheria montana* ethanol extracts in experimental pulpitis in rats: a histological study. *Med Oral Patol Oral Cir Bucal*, 2013, 18(2), 337-42.

Novais, RZ. Evaluation of the tissue answer from the watery vegetable and hydro alcoholic extract of araça (*Psidium cattleianum*) according to edemogenic and morphological analysis in mice [dissertation]. Araçatuba: Dentistry College – São Paulo State University "Júlio de Mesquita Filho" – Unesp, 2008.

Okamoto, T; Russo, MC. Wound healing following tooth extraction. Histochemical study in rats. *Rev Facul Odontol Araça*, 1973, 2(0), 153-63.

Okasala, O; Salo, T; Tammi, R; Hakkinen, L; Jalkanen, M; Inki, P; Larjava, H. Expression of proteoglycans and hyaluronan during wound healing. *J Histochem Cytoch*, 1995, 43(2), 125–135.

Oliskovicz, K; Facco, G; Fávero, S; Jardim, MIA; Dourado, DM; Sarragiotto, MH; Matias, R. Morfologia da reparação tecidual de feridas cutâneas de ratos Wistar tratados durante sete e catorze dias com extrato de *Equisetum pyramidale* cultivado. [Tissue repair morphology of skin wounds of Wistar rats treated for seven and fourteen days with cultured Equisetum pyramidale extract] *Ensaios e Ciência: Ciências Biológicas, Agrárias e da Saúde*, 2006, 10(1), 153-166.

Ortiz, MI; Fernández-Martínez, E; Soria-Jasso, LE; Lucas-Gómez, I; Villagómez-Ibarra, R; González-García, MP; Castañeda- Hernández,

G; Salinas-Caballero M. Isolation, identification and molecular docking as cyclooxygenase (COX) inhibitors of the main constituents of *Matricaria chamomilla* L. extract and its synergistic interaction with diclofenac on nociception and gastric damage in rats. *Biomed Pharmacother*, 2016, 78, 248–256.

Öztürk, A; Ilman, AA; Saglam, H; Yalçinkaya, U; Aykut, S; Akgöz, S; Ozkan, Y; Yanik, K; Kivçak, B; Yalçin, N; Ozdemir, RM. The effects of phytoestrogens on fracture healing: experimental research in New Zealand white rabbits. *Turk J Trauma & Emerg Surg*, 2008, 14(1), 21-7.

Padumadasa, C; Dharmadana, D; Abeysekera, A; Thammitiyagodage, M. *In vitro* antioxidant, anti-inflammatory and anticancer activities of ethyl acetate soluble proanthocyanidins of the inflorescence of Cocos nucifera L. *BMC Complementary Alterm Med*, 2016, 16(1), 345-351.

Padumadasa, C; Dharmadana, D; Abeysekera, AM; Thammitiyagoda, MG. Investigation of ethyl acetate soluble proanthocyanidins in the inflorescence of *Cocos nucifera L. J Pharmacogn Phytochem*, 2015, 4(2), 107–11.

Pan, SY; Litscher, G; Gao, SH; Zhou, SF; Yu, ZL; Chen, HQ; et al. Historical perspective of traditional indigenous medical practices: the current renaissance and conservation of herbal resources. *Evid Based Complement Alternat Med*, 2014, 2014, 525340.

Park, YK; Koo, H; Rosalen, PL; Cury, JA; Gomes, BPFA; Ambrosano, GMB. *In-vitro* antimicrobial activity of propolis and *Arnica Montana* against oral pathogens. *Arch Oral Biol*, 2000, 45(2), 141–8.

Parolia, A; Thomas, MS; Kundabala, M. Propolis and its potential uses in oral health. *Int J Med Sci*, 2010, 2, 210-15.

Paulino, N; Teixeira, C; Martins, R; Scremin, A; Dirsch, VM; Vollmar, AM; Abreu, SR; de Castro, SL; Marcucci, MC. Evaluation of the analgesic and antiinflammatory effects of a Brazilian green propolis. *Planta Med.*, 2006, 72(10), 899-906.

Pepe, G; Pagano, F; Adesso, S; Sommella, E; Ostacolo, C; Manfra, M; Chieppa, M; Sala, M; Russo, M; Marzocco, S; Campiglia, P.

Bioavailable *Citrus sinensis* Extract: Polyphenolic Composition and Biological Activity. *Molecules*, 2017, 22(4), 623-38.

Perde-Schrepler, M; Chereches, G; Brie, I; Tatomir, C; Postescu, ID; Soran, L; Filip, A. Grape seed extract as photochemopreventive agent against UVB-induced skin cancer. *J Photochem Photobiol B*, 2013, 118(5), 16–21.

Poi, WR; de Carvalho Júnior, JAR; de Carvalho, PSP; Okamoto, T. Influência da pasta Sultan sobre o processo de reparo em alvéolo dental infectado. Análise histológica em ratos. *Rev Odontol Bras Cent*, 2000, 9(28), 9-13.

Pott, A; Pott, VJ. Plantas do Pantanal [Pantanal Plants]. Brasília, DF: *Embrapa*, 1994, 320 p.

Pott, VJ; Pott, A. Plantas aquáticas do Pantanal [Pantanal Aquatic Plants]. Brasília: *Embrapa Comunicação para Transferência de Tecnologia*, 2000, 404 p.

Raina, K; Tyagi, A; Kumar, D; Agarwal, R; Agarwal, C. Role of oxidative stress in cytotoxicity of grape seed extract in human bladder cancer cells. *Food Chem Toxicol*, 2013, 61, 187–95.

Rajeshwi, HR; Dhamecha, D; Jagwani, S; Patil, D; Hegde, S; Potdar, R; Metgud, R; Jalalpure, S; Roy, S; Jadhav, K; Tiwari, NK; Koduru, S; Hugar, S; Dodamani, S. Formulation of thermoreversible gel of cranberry juice concentrate: Evaluation, biocompatibility studies and its antimicrobial activity against periodontal pathogens. *Mater Sci Eng C Mater Biol Appl*, 2017, 75(1), 1506–14.

Rinaldi, S; Silva, DO; Bello, F; Alviano, CS; Alviano, DS; Matheus, ME; Fernandes, PD. Characterization of the antinociceptive and anti-inflammatory activities from *Cocos nucifera* L. (Palmae). *J Ethnopharmacol*, 2009, 122(3), 541–546.

Robson, MC; Hill, DP; Woodske, ME; Steed, DL. Wound healing trajectories as predictors of effectiveness of therapeutic agents. *Arch Surg*, 2000, 135(7), 773-7.

Romero, V; Lara, JR; Otero-Espinar, F; Salgado, MH; Modolo, NSP; Barros, GAM. Capsaicin topical cream (8%) for the treatment of myofascial pain syndrome. *Rev Bras Anestesiol*, 2019, 69(5), 432-8.

Roy, AM; Baliga, MS; Elmets, CA; Katiyar, SK. Grape seed proanthocyanidins induce apoptosis throughp53, Bax, and Caspase 3 pathways. *Neoplasia*, 2005, 7(1), 24–36.

Rutberg, M; Spangberg, E; Spangberg, L. Evaluation of enhanced vascular permeability of endodontic medicaments *in vivo*. *J Endod*, 1977, 3(9), 347-51.

Ruviére, DB; Machado, AC; Novais, RZ; Gaetti Jardim-Junior, E; Dezan-Junior, E. Evaluation of the tissue response to inactivated microorganisms associated with aqueous and hydroalcoholic araça (*Psidium cattleianum*) solutions. *J Appl Oral Sci*, 2008, 20(2), 93-101.

Sabino, KCC; Castro, FA; Oliveira, JCR; Dalmau, SRA; Coelho, MGP. Successful treatment of collagen- induced arthritis in mice with a hydroalcohol extract of seeds of *Pterodon pubescen*. *Phytother Res*, 1999, 13, 613-15.

Salil, G; Rajamohan, T. Hypolipidemic and antiperoxidative effect of coconut protein in hypercholesterolemic rats. *Indian J Exp Biol*, 2001, 39(10), 1028-34.

Salvemini, D; Wang, ZQ; Bourdon, DM; Stern, MK; Currie, MG; Manning, PT. Evidence of peroxynitrite involvement in the carrageenan induced rat paw edema. *Eur J Pharmacol*, 1996, 303(3), 217-20.

Scheller, S; Ilewics, L; Luciak, M; Skrobidurska, D; Matuga, W. Biological properties and clinical application of Propolis IX. Investigation of the influence of EEP on dental pulp regeneration. *Arzneim Forsch*, 1978, 28, 289–91.

Schmidt, CA; Murillo, R; Heinzmann, B; Laufer, S; Wray, V; Merfort, I. Structural and conformational analysis of proanthocyanidins from *Parapipta- denia rigida* and their wound-healing properties. *J Nat Prod*, 2011, 74(6), 1427-36.

Scott, JE. Proteoglycan fibrillar collagen interactions. *Biochem J*, 1988, 252, 313–323.

Seneviratne, KN; Dissanayake, DMS. Variation of phenolic content in coconut oil extracted by two conventional methods. *Inter J Food Sci Technol*, 2008, 43(4), 597–602.

Shafer, WG; Hine, MK; Levy, BM. Tratado de Patologia Bucal 4ª Ed. [Oral Pathology 4th Ed.] Rio de Janeiro: *Guanabara Koogan*, 1987, 555-9.

Shelton, RM. Aloe vera: its chemical and therapeutic properties. *Int J Dermatol*, 1991, 30, 679–83.

Shipochliev, T; Dimitrov, A; Aleksandrova, E. Anti-inflammatory action of a group of plant extracts. *Vet Med Nauki*, 1981, 18(6), 87– 94.

Shukla, AAM; Rasik, GK; Jain, R; Shankar, DK. Kulshrestha and Dhawan. *In vitro* and *in vivo* wound healing activity of asiaticoside isolated from Centella asiatica. *J Ethnopharmacol*, 1999, 65(1), 1-11.

Siddique, S; Javed, S; Nawaz, S; Khan, RA; Shahzad, K. Volatile components and antimicrobial activity of *Citrus sinensis* var. mosammi leaves oil. *Electron J Environ Agric Food Chem*, 2012, 11, 172–9.

Silva, FB; Almeida, JM; Sousa, SM. Natural medicaments in endodontics – a comparative study of the anti-inflammatory action. *Braz Oral Res*, 2004, 18(2), 174-9.

Silva, LCR; Nunes-Pinheiro, DCS; Morais, SM; Lopes-Neto, BE; Santos, GJL; Campello; et al. Toxicological evaluation and effect of ethyl acetate extract of the fiber of *Cocos nucifera* L. (Palmae) on inflammatory response *in vivo*. *Rev Bras Plantas Med*, 2009, 11(4), 429-34.

Silva, RR; Oliveira, e Silva; Fontes, HR; Alviano, CS; Fernandes, PD; Alviano, DS. Antiinflammatory, antioxidant, and antimicrobial activities of *Cocos nucifera* var. typica. *BMC Complement Altern Med*, 2013, 13, 107.

Singla, RK; Jaiswal, N; Bhat, GV; Jagani, H. Antioxidant and antimicrobial activities of *Cocos nucifera* Linn. (Arecaceae) endocarp extracts. *Indo Global J Pharm Sci*, 2011, 1(4), 354–361.

Sosa, S; Balick, MJ; Arvigo, R; Esposito, RG; Pizza, C; Altinier, G; Tubaro, A. Screening of the topical anti-inflammatory activity of some Central American plants. *J Ethnopharmacol*, 2002, 81(2), 211-5.

Souza, BD; Lückemeyer, DD; Reyes-Carmona, JF; Felippe, WT; Simões, CM; Felippe, MC. Viability of human periodontal ligament fibroblasts in milk, Hank's balanced salt solution and coconut water as storage media. *Int Endod J*, 2011, 44(2), 111-15.

Souza, GC; Haas, APS; Van Poser, GL; Elisabetsky, E. Farmácias caseiras comunitárias do município de Maquiné (RS): uma avaliação etnofarmacológica [Community home-made pharmacies in the municipality of Maquiné (RS): an ethnopharmacological evaluation]. *Rev Bras Plantas Med*, 2004, 6(2), 83-91

Staiger, C. Comfrey: ancient and modern uses. *Pharm J*, 2007, 279, 22-9.

Stankovic, M; Tesevic, V; Vajs, V; Todorovic, N; Milosavljevic, S; Godevac, D. Antioxidant properties of grape seed extract on human lymphocyte oxidative defence. *Planta Med*, 2008, 74(7), 730–5.

Stanley, HR. Biological evaluation of dental material. *Int Dent J*, 1992, 42(1), 37-46.

Starzonek, J; Roscher, K; Blüher, M; Blaue, D; Schedlbauer, C; Hirz, M; Raila, J; Vervuert, I. Effects of a blend of green tea and curcuma extract supplementation on lipopolysaccharide-induced inflammation in horses and ponies. *PeerJ*, 2019, 12, 7, e8053.

Steinke, S; Gutknecht, M; Zeidler, C; et al. Cost-effectiveness of an 8% cap-saicin patch in the treatment of brachioradial pruritus and notalgiaparaesthetica, two forms of neuropathic pruritus. *Acta Derm Venereol*, 2017, 97, 71-6.

Stickel, F; Seitz, HK. The efficacy and safety of comfrey. *Public Health Nutr*, 2000, 3(4A), 501-8.

Surh, YJ; Chun, KS; Cha, HH; Han, SS; Keum, YS; Park, KK; Lee, SS. Molecular mechanisms underlying chemopreventive activities of anti-inflammatory phytochemicals, down-regulation of COX-2 and iNOS through suppression of NF-kappa B activation. *Mutat Res*, 2001, (1), 243- 268.

Suyenaga, ES; Reche, E; Farias, FM; Schapoval, EE; Chaves, CG; Henriques, AT. Anti-inflammatory investigation of some species of Mikania. *Phytother Res*, 2002, 16(6), 519–23.

Tan-No, K; Nakajima, T; Shoji, T; Nakagawasai, O; Niijima, F; Ishikawa, M; Endo, Y; Sato, T; Satoh, S; Tadano, T. Antiinflammatory effect of propolis through inhibition of nitric oxide production on carrageenin-induced mouse paw edema. *Biol Pharm Bull*, 2006, 29(1), 96-9.

Teske, M; Trentini, AMM. Compêndio de fitoterapia [Herbal Medicine Compendium]. 4th Ed. Herbarium Publisher, 2001, 317 p.

Tona, L; Kambu, K; Ngimbi, N; Mesia, K; Penge, O; Lusakibanza, M; Cimanga, K; De Bruyne, T; Apers, S; Totte, J; Pieters, L; Vlietinck, AJ. Antiamoebic and spasmolytic activities of extracts from some antidiarrhoeal traditional preparations used in Kinshasa, Congo. *Phytomedicine*, 2000, 7(1), 31-38.

Torneck, CD. Reaction of rat connective tissue to polyethylene tube implants part I. *Oral Surg Oral Med Oral Pathol*, 1966, 21(3), 379-87.

Tresvenzol, LMF; Parente, LML; Lino Júnior, RS; Fiuza, TS; Bara, MTF; Cunha, LC; Laxor, LP; Miguel, MP; Paula, JR. Evaluation of acute and healing activity of ethanol extracts of *Memora nodosa* (Silva Manso) Miers (Bignoniaceae) leaves and roots. *Rev Bras Plantas Med*, 2013, 15(3), 423-30.

Tripoli, E; La Guardia, M; Giammanco, S; Di Majo, D; Giammanco, M. Citrus flavonoids: Molecular structure, biological activity and nutritional properties: A review. *Food Chem*, 2007, 104, 466–79.

Tubaro, A; Zilli, C; Redaelli, C; Della Loggia, R. Evaluation of antiinflammatory activity of a chamomile extract after topical application. *Planta Med*, 1984, 50(4), 359.

Tudose, A; Celia, C; Cardamone, F; Vono, M; Molinaro, R; Paolino, D. Regenerative properties of *Aloe vera* juice on human keratinocyte cell culture. *Farmacia*, 2009, 57, 590–7.

Turley, EA. The role of cell-associated hyaluronan- binding protein in fibroblast behaviour. *Ciba Found Symp*, 1989, 143, 121–33.

Underhill, CB; Toole, BP. Binding of hyaluronate to the surface of cultured cells. *J Cell Biol*, 1979, 82(2), 475–84.

Uribe-Fentanes, LK; Soriano-Padilla, F; Pérez-Frutos, JR; Veras-Hernández, MA. Action of Calendula officinalis essence on bone preservation after the extraction. *Rev Med Inst Mex Seguro Soc*, 2018, 56(1), 98-105.

Valentim, D; Bueno, CRE; Marques, VAS; Vasques, AMV; Cury, MTS; Cintra, LTA; Dezan-Junior, E. Calcium hydroxide associated with a new vehicle: *Psidium cattleianum* leaf extracts. Tissue response evaluation. *Braz Oral Res*, 2017, 31, 43-51.

Vasconcelos, CF; Maranhao, HM; Batista, TM; Carneiro, EM; Ferreira, F; Costa, J; Soares, LA; Sa, MD; Souza, TP; Wanderley, AG. Hypoglycaemic activity and molecular mechanisms of *Caesalpinia ferrea* Martius bark extract on streptozotocin-induced diabetes in Wistar rats. *J Ethnopharmacol.*, 2011, 137(3), 1533–1541.

Veit, M; Beckert, C; Höhne, C; Bauer, K; Geiger, H. Interspecific and intraspecific variation of phenolics in the genus *Equisetum* subgenus *Equisetum. Phytochemistry*, 1995, 38(4), 881-91.

Wahedi, HM; Jeong, M; Chae, JK; Do, SG; Yoon, H; Kim, SY. Aloesin from Aloe vera accelerates skin wound healing by modulating MAPK/Rho and Smad signaling pathways *in vitro* and *in vivo. Phytomedicine*, 2017, 28, 19-26.

Wheeler, DS; Catravas, JD; Odoms, K; Denenberg, A; Malhotra, V; Wong,HR. Epigallocatechin-3-gallate, a green tea-derived polyphenol, inhibits IL-1 beta-dependent proinflammatory signal transduction in cultured respiratory epithelial cells. *J Nutr*, 2004, 134(5), 1039-1044.

Winter, CA; Risley, EA; Nuss, GW. Carrageenin-induced edema in hind paw of the rat as an assay for anti-inflammatory drugs. *Proc Soc Exp Biol Med*, 1962, 111, 544-7.

Yahara, N; Tofani, I; Maki, K; Kojima, K; Kojima, Y; Kimura, M. Mechanical assessment of effects of grape seed proanthocyanidins extract on tibial bone diaphysis in rats. *J Musculoskelet Neuronal Interact*, 2005, 5(2), 162–9.

Ye, X; Krohn, RL; Liu, W; Joshi, SS; Kuszynski, CA; McGinn, TR; Bagchi, M; Preuss, HG; Stohs, SJ; Bagchi, D. The cytotoxic effects of a novel IH636 grape seed proanthocy-anidin extract on cultured human cancer cells. *Mol Cell Biochem*, 1999, 196(1-2), 99–108.

Yong, JW; Ge, L; Ng, YF; Tan, SN. The chemical composition and biological properties of coconut (*Cocos nucifera* L.) water. *Molecules*, 2009, 14(12), 5144–64.

Zakaria, ZA; Reezal, E; Mat Jais, AM; Somchit, MN; Sulaiman, MR; Marmin, AHI; Sidek, H; Husin, SH; Rahim, MHA; Abdul Rahman, L. The anti-inflammatory, anti-pyretic and wound healing activities of *Coco nucifera* (MATAG Types) fresh juice and kernel extract in experimental animals. *J Pharmacol Toxicol*, 2006, 1(6), 516-526.

Zhao, F; Wang, L; Liu, K. *In vitro* antiinflammatory effects of arctigenin, a lignan from *Arctium lappa L.*, through inhibition on iNOS pathway. *J Ethnopharmacol*, 2009, 122(3), 457-62.

Zhong, Y; Chiou, YS; Pan, MH; Shahidi, F. Antiinflammatory activity of lipophilic epigallocatechin gallate (EGCG) derivatives in LPS-stimulated murine macrophages. *Food Chem*, 2012, 134(2), 742–8.

In: Contemporary Use of Plant Extracts … ISBN: 978-1-53617-650-6
Editor: C. R. Emerenciano Bueno

Chapter 4

PHYTOTHERAPY IN CARIOLOGY AND RESTORATIVE DENTISTRY

Victor Eduardo de Souza Batista[1,5,*], Anderson Catelan[1], Aljomar José Vechiato-Filho[2], Christine Men Martins[3], Ana Maria Veiga Vasques[4], Marina Tolomei Sandoval Cury[4] and Carlos Roberto Emerenciano Bueno[4]

[1]Department of Dentistry, Presidente Prudente Dental School, University of Western São Paulo - UNOESTE, Presidente Prudente, São Paulo, Brazil
[2]Dental Oncology Service, Institute of Cancer of São Paulo São Paulo (ICESP), São Paulo, Brazil
[3]Department of Endodontics, University of Western Sao Paulo (UNOESTE), Presidente Prudente, Sao Paulo, Brazil
[4]Department of Endodontics, São Paulo State University (UNESP), Araçatuba School of Dentistry, Araçatuba, SP, Brazil
[5]Department of Dental Materials and Prosthodontics, São Paulo State University (UNESP), Araçatuba School of Dentistry, Araçatuba, SP, Brazil

[*] Corresponding Author's Email: victor_edsb@hotmail.com.

ABSTRACT

The use of plant extract for health treatment has been reported over the years. The treatment of diseases that affect the oral cavity is not different, specifically for dental caries treatment. The American Academy of Cariology (AAC) defines the cariology as "the science and art of understanding the etiology, mechanisms of the disease known as dental caries including initiation, reversal, progression, diagnosis, prognosis, risk management, prevention, non-surgical and surgical therapies, and oral health-focused outcomes." The use of herbal therapy is proposed in different stages of the mechanism of the dental caries disease, mainly in the diagnosis, prevention and treatment outcomes.

This chapter will show the application of herbal therapy in the diagnosis and prevention as well as its application of herbal therapy regarding the treatment of the dental caries disease by restorative dentistry.

Keywords: dental caries, dentistry, operative, ethnopharmacology, phytotherapy

INTRODUCTION

As is well described in previous chapters, the use of plant extract for health treatment has been reported over the years. The treatment of diseases that affect the oral cavity is not different, specifically for dental caries treatment.

Dental caries is an infectious disease, considered one of the most prevalent chronic diseases – among several diseases that may affect the oral cavity – in the world (Raphael et al. 2018, Tomczyk et al. 2011). It is a localized destruction of the dental hard tissues by acidic by-products from bacterial fermentation of dietary carbohydrates and it is estimated that three billion people worldwide have this infectious disease. Moreover, it is estimated 60–100% of children and adults suffer from dental caries in their lifetime (Selwitz et al. 2007, Delimont & Carlson 2019). For this reason, a specific area of dentistry destined to study this pathology was defined: the Cariology. The American Academy of Cariology (AAC) defines the cariology as "*the science and art of understanding the etiology, mechanisms of the disease known as dental caries including initiation, reversal, progression, diagnosis, prognosis, risk management, prevention, non-surgical and surgical therapies, and oral health-focused outcomes*."

In this context, several studies have reported the use of herbal therapy in the different stages of the mechanism of the dental caries disease, mainly in the diagnosis, prevention and treatment outcomes (Peters et al. 2010, Prabhakar et al. 2015, Aldana et al. 2013, Dos Santos et al. 2011a). The aim of this chapter is to show the application of herbal therapy in the diagnosis and prevention (as described in the following cariology section 1) as well as its application of herbal therapy regarding the treatment of the dental caries disease by restorative dentistry (as reported in the following restorative dentistry section 2).

1. Application of Phytotherapy in Cariology

1.1. Disclosing Solution Using Natural Agents

The control of biofilm (dental plaque) through periodic professional dental prophylaxis is necessary to avoid the dental caries as well as other problems in the oral cavity (Fasoulas et al. 2019). The dentist uses disclosing solution as an auxiliary method to visualize and to assess the amount of biofilm on the surfaces of the teeth. This way, it is possible for both patient and the dentist to see the dental biofilm and, finally, they elaborate a strategy of improvement in the oral hygiene of the patient (de Alencar et al. 2019; Fasoulas et al. 2019).

Several substances are purposed in the literature as disclosing solution. This solution may contain the combination of brilliant green and crystal violet, iodine, erythrosine, bismarck brown, gentian violet, basic fuchsin and other substances (Datta et al. 2017). Few studies using natural solution are reported in the literature. Interestingly, Brazilian researchers proposed the use of *Euterpe oleracea* (extracted from açai fruit) and *Bixa orellama* (extract from urucum) as disclosing solution (Ribeiro Nazaré et al. 2007), described along the book (chapter 7 - Other applications of plants extracts in dentistry).

1.2. Toothpastes and Mouthwash Using Natural Agents

Currently, the population have become more conscious about the side-effects of fluoride toothpastes and herbal products have drawn attention as options in the struggle against caries since the use of oral care products containing natural agents has become a common practice worldwide for being considered healthy and safe (Karadağlıoğlu et al. 2019; Braga et al. 2019). Furthermore, herbal products have been suggested as an economic, safe and probably effective alternative for prevention and control of various oral diseases (Bhat et al. 2015). For this reason, in recent years, an uncounted number of toothpaste preparations containing herbal products have been found useful for oral and dental health (Korkmaz et al. 2019) and in the next paragraphs it will show the evidence about its applications.

Researchers have studied for herbal alternative to enhance antibacterial activity against the *Streptococcus mutans (S. mutans),* one of the most effective cariogenic bacteria in the initial formation of caries. Recently, the antibacterial activity of *Origanum dubium* and *Cinnamomum cassia* oils combined with herbal toothpastes against *S. mutans* was assessed and this combination exhibited the largest inhibition zones after the addition of the essential oils (Karadağlıoğlu et al. 2019).

Also, the effect of herbal agents on the prevention of enamel demineralization has been studied in toothpastes and mouthwash and the results showed that two commercial products containing natural agents were effective as antimicrobial agents and protection against enamel demineralization: a toothpaste containing *Commiphora myrrha* (mirra) and propolis; and a mouth rinse containing *Malva sylvestris* (malow) (Braga et al. 2019).

The antimicrobial activity against *S. mutans* and *Staphylococcus aureus (S. aureus)* of toothpastes containing *Aloe vera L.* and *Fragaria vesca L.* extracts was assessed by Korkmaz and collaborators. The authors reported that herbal toothpastes that have *A. vera* and wild strawberry extracts may be suggested similar to the conventional contents (Korkmaz et al. 2019).

Toothpastes of various compositions were formulated using the ethanolic extracts of *Dennettia tripetala* (pepper fruit) seeds, buds of *Syzygium aromaticum* with *Jatropha curcas* latex as the active ingredients in order to assess the antimicrobial activity – against *E. coli, Bacillus sp., S. aureus, S. epidermis, M. luteus, S. mutans, C. albicans, S. pyogenes, L. acidophilus,* and *P. aeruginosa* – and the formulated toothpastes exhibited potent antimicrobial property against the tested pathogens (Oluwasina 2019).

The effect of toothpaste made of the leaf extracts of *Artemisia dracunculus*, *Satureja khuzestanica* (Jamzad), and *Myrtus communis* (Linn) was tested against five microorganisms, including *Streptococcus mutans*, *Lactobaccilus caseie*, *S. sanguis*, *S. salivarius*, and *Candida albicans*, using agar well diffusion method. The results showed that the formulated toothpaste showed potent inhibitory activities against Gram-positive bacteria and *C. albicans* (Sadeghi-Nejad et al. 2018).

Also, herbal extract of stems of *Salvadora persica* tree were incorporated in the toothpastes and the results showed that to brushing teeth with Meswak-based toothpaste may cause a significant drop in plaque score (Varma et al. 2018, Azaripour et al. 2017).

There are trademarks of herbal dental products that use a combination of several kinds of herbal products in its composition, such as the brands Patanjali Dant Kanti Dental – that contain *Azadirachta indica* (Neem) *Acacia nilotica* (Babool) and *Barleria prionitis* (Vajradanti); Himalaya Complete Care Toothpaste – that contain *Punica granatum* (Pomegranate) and Triphala as anti-diabetic substances – and Vicco Vajradanti Toothpaste – that contains *Syzygium cumini* (Jamun), *Cinnamon*, *Glycyrrhiza glabra* (Liquorice), *Hemidesmus indicus* (Anantmul), *Phyllanthus emblica* (Amla) and *Barleria prionitis* (Vajradanti). Researches assessing the Salivary Alkaline Phosphatase (ALP) and salivary Acid Phosphatase (ACP), salivary pH and salivary glucose showed that these brands of herbal toothpastes were effective in reducing the levels of ALP, ACP, salivary levels of glucose and improving pH of the saliva which they are important parameter in the maintaining of oral health (Khairnar et al. 2016, Khairnar et al. 2017).

The Antimicrobial effect of the dentifrice containing extract of *Rosmarinus officinalis* Linn was assessed and the results showed that the toothpaste containing the extract of *Rosmarinus officinalis* had the ability to inhibit the growth of *S. mutans, S. oralis* and *L. rhamnosus*, revealing an antimicrobial activity similar to commercially available toothpastes for inhibition of *S. mutans* and *S. oralis* (Valones et al. 2016).

The effect in the plaque formation of herbal dentifrice containing Propolis compared to *Salvadora persica* and Colgate total also was assessed by a crossover clinical study and the results showed that the use of the propolis as dentifrice is safe and effective in reducing plaque accumulation when compared to Miswak and Colgate total toothpaste (Bhat et al. 2015).

The herbal mouthrinses as an adjuvant to oral hygiene on dental plaque formation also is searched and the studies have shown that most of herbal products used as an adjunct of the oral hygiene achieved better results in comparison to non-use of mouthrinse (Santi et al. 2019). Furthermore, the use of *Camelia sinensis*, *Azadirachta indica*, *Anacardium occidentale* Linn, *Schinustere binthifolius* and *Curcuma Longa* have presented better results in plaque reduction in relation to chlorhexidine – this product is widely used in dentistry and considered gold standard mouthrinse (Santi et al. 2019, Abu-Obaid et al. 2019).

The effectiveness of *Ocimum sanctum* and *Aloa vera* mouthrinses in comparison with chlorhexidine mouthwash was assessed by a randomized controlled comparative clinical study. The *Aloe vera* mouthwash used in the study was commercially obtained from the market (Patanjali™) and the *Ocimum sanctum* mouthwash was prepared in the following way: dried leaves of *O. sanctum* were grounded into a fine powder, thus, three hundred gram of finely powdered *O. sanctum* was macerated with 100% ethanol for a week in a round-bottom flask. After, the extract was filtered through a muslin cloth for coarse residue and finally through Whatman no. 1 filter paper. The filtrate obtained was reduced at a low temperature

<50°C to obtain a solid residue of *O. sanctum* extract. From 300 g of *O. sanctum* powder dissolved in 1 L of ethanol, 18 g of residue was obtained yield 6% w/w. The extract was suspended in polyethylene glycol 400 (20% v/v) and sterile distilled water to give a final concentration of 4% (w/v). Finally, the flavoring agent 0.005% spearmint oil was added. The results of this clinical study indicated that *O. sanctum* and *A. vera* may prove to be as effective as chlorhexidine mouthwash in its ability in reducing the indices as plaque accumulation, gingival inflammation and bleeding when used in the long-term follow-up (Penmetsa et al. 2019).

The antimicrobial effects of herbal mix and cranberry mouthrinses against to *S. mutans* also was researched. The herbal mix mouthrinse (1%) was made mainly from 0.36% pomegranate peel extract, 0.36% myrrh resin extract, 0.18% chamomile flower extract, 0.1% cinnamon bark extract, 0.1 g sodium benzoate, and 0.2 g ascorbic acid; and, the cranberry mouthrinse was made mainly from cranberry extract that was dissolved in sterilized water with other ingredients (0.1 g ZnC12, 0.1 g sodium saccharine, 0.05 g menthol, 0.1 g sodium benzoate and 3 ml of glycerine). These herbal mouthrinses were compared to chlorhexidine digluconate mouthrinse (0.12%) and the results showed that herbal mix and cranberry mouthrinses could be effective natural alternative to chlorhexidine mouthrinse in improving oral health (Abu-Obaid et al. 2019).

1.3. Antibiofilm Formation Effect of the Herbal Extract

Biofilms are highly organized and structured microbial communities enmeshed in an extracellular matrix. In the mouth, the biofilm may be formed in several type of surface as teeth and different kind of prostheses (when present) causing many oral diseases (Feng et al. 2013, Almeida Lde et al. 2016).

14-Deoxy-11,12-didehydroandrographolide is a biologically active molecule present in the extract of *Andrographis paniculata* (Kalmegh) and it has been studied as an inhibitor against biofilm formation (Majumdar et al. 2019, Yen et al. 2019). The studies have reported that this herb may be used as molecule drug against biofilm development by inhibiting the bacterial quorum sensing pathway against microorganisms (Majumdar et al. 2019). Further studies about this molecule is necessary for the application in the clinical routine.

Numerous plant essential oils which act as antibiofilm agents against mouth-inhabiting bacteria – especially *S. mutans* – have been studies (Ashrafi et al. 2019, Kim et al. 2019). *Mentha piperita* essential oils have been studied due to several biological actions, such as antifungal, antibacterial, antiviral and larvicidal activities. Ashrafi and collaborators developed the *Mentha piperita* loaded in a chitosan polymeric nanogel and showed that biofilm formation by *S. mutans* on the dental surface efficiently decreased. The authors explained that the inhibitory effect on the biofilm synthesis was revealed to be at the level of gene expression and it showed a downregulation effect on eight genes involved in biofilm and virulence factors causing bacterial adherence such as exopolysaccharides. Furthermore, the authors reported that this association is an efficient nanoformulation with the greatest inhibitory action against some glycosyltransferase genes, important enzymes involved in extracellular polymers, subsequently inhibition of colonization of the bacterial cells at sub-MIC dose (Ashrafi et al. 2019).

The antimicrobial effect of the mixed herbal powder extract composed by herbal extracts of *Acacia arabica, Terminalia bellerica and Emblica officinalis* on the biofilm of *Streptococcus mutans*, *Lactobacillus casei*, *Actinomyces viscosus* and *Candida albicans* also was studied by Ramalingam and Amaechi (Ramalingam & Amaechi 2018). This association showed anti-adherence and antibiofilm effect as well as the faster killing activity (Ramalingam & Amaechi 2018). Plants extracts effectively inhibited sucrose mediated adherence of *S. mutans* and cariogenic biofilm formation and showed remarkable inhibitory effects on the growth of cariogenic microorganism at very low concentration when compare to chlorhexidine (Ramalingam & Amaechi 2018).

The application of essential oils from *Cinnamon cassia* (cinnamon) and *Cymbopogon winterianus* (citronella) also was tested against the viability of *C. albicans* biofilms (Almeida Lde et al. 2016). Thus, the authors concluded that essential oils from citronella and cinnamon have potential for use as daily denture cleansers due to their anti-Candida and immediate antibiofilm activity and they justified that the antimicrobial effect of cinnamon and citronella likely originates from the natural biological activity of their chemical constituents, such as cinnamaldehyde and citronellal (Almeida Lde et al. 2016).

Houttuynia cordata is a widely used traditional medicine and the literature report that *H. cordata* may exert moderate antimicrobial effects against methicillin-resistant *Staphylococcus aureus* (MRSA) and other oral microorganisms. Additionally, A decoction of dried *Houttuynia cordata* leaves may exhibit antibiofilm effects against MRSA, *Fusobacterium nucleatum* (involved in dental plaque formation), and *Candida albicans* as well as inhibitory effects on interleukin-8, CCL20, IP-10, and GROα productions by human oral keratinocytes stimulated by *Porphyromonas gingivalis* lipopolysaccharide (a cause of periodontal disease), without cytotoxic effects (Sekita et al. 2017).

The antifungal, antimicrobial, and antibiofilm properties of *Zingiber officinale* (ginger) extract against Candida species, some bacterial pathogens and the extract's effects on biofilm formation was assessed by an *in vitro* study. The authors reported that ginger extract has good antifungal and antibiofilm formation by fungi against *C. albicans* and *C. Krusei*, in which concentrations between 0.625 mg/mL and 5 mg/mL had the highest antibiofilm and antifungal effects (Aghazadeh et al. 2016).

1.4. Effect of Plant Extracts on Demineralization

Demineralization is common in dental caries and currently is associated with continuous exposure to acids. In this cases, dental structures may not heal itself by a cellular repair mechanism and must rely on repair by a physicochemical process involving inorganic constituents from saliva or solutions (Chu et al. 2007). Recently, attention was turned to prevention and it includes compounds of plants, as alternatives to promote remineralization in both enamel and dentin (Silva et al. 2015).

Phytotherapy has been developed to overcome this issue specially because plant extracts present polyphenols, triterpernes and flavonoids (Giacaman et al. 2014). Furthermore, proanthocyanidins – polyphenols found in cocoa, grape, and peanuts – which are substances that have been the target of recent studies aiming to control or treat carious lesions, preventing damage caused by reactive oxygen species, inhibiting the glycosyltransferases and possible acid production by *Streptococcus mutans* (Silva et al. 2015).

Studies evaluating the efficacy of a treatment with different phytotherapic, under cariogenic challenge, to minimize or even prevent the onset of caries in the enamel and dentin throughout surface microhardness of blocks obtained from bovine central incisors are widely used. Thus, results are promising to regard the use of phytotherapic.

Chu and collaborators (Chu et al. 2007) analyzed *Galla chinensis*, a natural non-toxic traditional Chinese medicine. According to the results, *Galla chinensis* demonstrated potential to rehardening of artificial carious lesions under dynamic pH-cyclic conditions; and this result is corroborated with Zou and collaborators (Zou et al. 2008) study. Also, Zhang and collaborators (Zhang et al. 2009) observed that its potential seems to be weaker compared to sodium fluoride and the organic matrix of enamel was shown to play a substantial role in the observed mechanism. Cheng et al. (2010) observed that extract could slow down the remineralization of enamel in the surface layer and thereby facilitate ion transport into the lesion body and the action mechanism in enhancing the remineralization of dental caries is different from fluoride. However, Huang and collaborators (Huang et al. 2012) observed that *Galla chinensis* extract's solutions were unstable under neutral and alkaline conditions; they were not effective on polymicrobial biofilms at alkaline pH.

Silva and collaborators (Silva et al. 2015) evaluated the efficacy of grape seed extract in enamel and dentin. For both enamel and dentin, fluoride traditionally used showed the best results; however, grape seed extract also inhibited demineralization of carious lesions even in a smaller scale when compared to fluoride. This result corroborates with previously study performed Xie and collaborators (Xie et al. 2008).

The application of *Myracrodruon urundeuva All.* and *Qualea grandiflora Mart.* leaves isolated or combined were evaluated by Pires and collaborators due to extract showed great properties (Pires et al. 2018). It was observed that both extracts reduce bacteria viability; however, none of the extracts were able to reduce enamel demineralization.

Other natural products were studied. One study observed that apple-derived polyphenols concentrate in low concentrations appears to have a potential anticaries activity on enamel (Giacaman et al. 2014). *Psidium cattleianum* was studied by Brighenti and collaborators and a potential anticariogenic effect was seen, presenting lower surface microhardness than deionized water (Brighenti et al. 2012).

Interestingly that this process of demineralization/remineralization using plants agents is also studied in deciduous teeth (Antonio et al. 2011). In one study was used fragments of primary first molar to stimulated biofilm formation and later on the biofilm was treated with *Coffea canephora* extract compared with chlorhexidine. Microhardness were evaluated and it was observed that dental fragments subjected to the coffee extract and to chlorhexidine were not significant.

1.5. Treatment of Toothache by Using of Herbal Extract

Toothache may be defined as an orofacial pain originated from a dental element and/or adjacent structures in consequence of several diseases or conditions, such as dental caries, periodontal disease, trauma, occlusal dysfunction, and abscess (Megersa et al. 2019). Toothache is a common problem that occurring in the human population throughout the world, thus, the use of plant species as a chewing stick is proposed in order to reduce the pain, mainly in lower socioeconomic status groups and in populations where dental caries is untreated since to visit the dentists is not possible and the toothache need to be treat at home (Megersa et al. 2019). A several medicinal plants such as *Acmella caulirhiza*, *Allium sativum*, *Capparis tomentosa*, *Clausena anisata*, *Datura stramonium*, *Ehretia cymosa*, *Euclea racemosa*, *Premna schimperi*, *Asiasari radix*,

Zanthoxylum armatum, Zanthoxylum bungeanum Maxim, Kirkia acuminate, and *Solanum incanum* were suggested for toothache treatment, however, the studies about the field present low level of scientific evidence (Kunwar et al. 2013, Jeong et al. 2014, Zhang et al. 2017, Maroyi et al. 2017, Megersa et al. 2019).

1.6. Other Application

1.6.1. Toothbrushes

The tooth cleaning with chewing sticks prepared from twigs stems or roots has been practiced in several places around the world, such as Asia, Africa, the Middle East and United States for thousands of years. This type of toothbrush is performed from the plants *Acacia arabica* and *Salvadora persica* and it is used for cleaning purpose. Researchers have shown antimicrobial effect important for the risk reduction of the dental caries (Almas 2001, Almas & Al-Zeid 2004, Baeshen et al. 2008).

1.6.2. Herbal Lollipop

The control of the dietary habits in very important to decrease the occurrence of dental caries. An herbal lollipop contains 15mg extract of *Glycyrrhiza uralensis* (liquorice root) was developed in order to avoid cariogenic dietary and its application showed to be effective to reduce the number of *S. mutans* in high-risk children (Peters et al. 2010, Almaz et al. 2017, Krishnakumar et al. 2018, Chen et al. 2019).

1.6.3. Incorporation of Herbal Extract in Dental Materials

Herbal extracts have recently gained even more attention as active agents to be incorporated into dental materials (Shahriari et al. 2019). The glass-ionomer cement (GIC) is applied in dentistry as base, liner, or direct restorative material, mainly in atraumatic restorative technique (Shahriari et al. 2019).

The *Salvia officinalis* extract powder was incorporated into the powder component of GIC and this new modified GIC showed a direct antibacterial property against *S. mutans* and *L. casei* (Shahriari et al. 2019).

Proanthocyanidin-rich extract – polyphenols found in cocoa, grape, and peanuts – was added to glass ionomer cement, with an improved remineralization rate after pH cycling compared to group restored only with GIC, without significantly compromising the hardness (Prabhakar et al. 2012). Dentin biomodification with proanthocyanidin application effectively stabilizes collagen and increases its caries resistance (Walter et al. 2008), decreasing demineralization rate and when combined with fluorides can be used to prevent dental caries (Pavan et al. 2011), being considered as a minimally invasive method for treating caries disease by inhibiting demineralization and/or promoting remineralization (Xie et al. 2008).

2. Application of Phytotherapy in Restorative Dentistry

2.1. Effect of Herbal in the Dental Adhesion

2.1.1. Dental Adhesive Restorations

Adhesive Dentistry has provided minimally invasive restorative procedures, restoring the shape, function, and esthetic of teeth; replacing the loss of dental structure, either by carious process or trauma, through direct and indirect restorations. During adhesive protocol, primers and/or fluid resins are applied, penetrating into enamel microporosities and interfibrillary spaces, involving collagen fibrils of three-dimensional collagen structure with resinous monomers after dentin demineralization, and then polymerized, resulting in micromechanical retention of restorative materials (Maciel et al. 1996).

Although adhesion to dental enamel is established and stable over time when considering the dentin substrate, it is still critical due to the structural characteristics and composition of this substrate (Van Meerbeek et al.

2003), being highly dependent of an adequate impregnation of resin monomers in demineralized dentin and its longevity depends on formation of a compact and homogeneous hybrid layer (Marshall et al. 1997). Adequate conversion of monomers to polymers of adhesive systems is a fundamental prerequisite for the stability of tooth-restoration bonding interface over time (Navarra et al. 2009). However, new therapies should focus not only on the stability of resin-based materials, but also on the content of dentin organic matrix involved in restorative and restorative treatments (Castellan et al. 2011).

Collagen is the major constituent of the vast majority of connective tissues, such as tendons, skin, blood vessels, bones, and dentin (Kjaer et al. 2005). Collagen disorganization within hybrid layer is one of the major degradation patterns found in failed adhesive restorations (Hashimoto et al. 2000, Castellan et al. 2011), in addition to the loss of resinous materials from interfibrillary spaces (Hashimoto et al. 2000). Type I collagen represents approximately 90% organic content of dentin (Veis & Schlueter 1964, Kjaer et al. 2005), being the predominant component of the extracellular matrix and constituting about 20-25% of total human body protein (Castellan et al. 2010b).

Proanthocyanidin has been reported to stabilize and to increase crosslinks of collagen-based tissues (Masquelier et al. 1981). This compound occurs naturally in plant metabolites and is widely available in fruits, vegetables, nuts, seeds, flowers, and bark (Fine 2000). Although proanthocyanidin is primarily known for its antioxidant activity, this compound has also been reported to demonstrate antibacterial, antiviral, anticarcinogenic, antiinflammatory, antiallergic, and vasodilatory actions (Fine 2000). More recently, it has been recognized as a dentin collagen crosslinking agent in restorative and preventive dentistry treatments [Bedran-Russo 2009 (US Patent # 2009/0123581)].

Since the dentin collagen matrix is a vital component in restoring lost dental structure, modeling of a demineralized dentin stronger and with improved mechanical properties will provide a more stable and healthier substrate, which is desirable for today's adhesive restorative procedures (Castellan et al. 2010b). Natural proanthocyanidin-based extracts have reduced cytotoxicity compared to effects of synthetic agents (Han et al. 2003), and are able to improve and stabilize human dentin collagen matrices by inducing exogenous crosslinking (Castellan et al. 2011), mainly by hydrogen bonds between phenolic hydroxyl and the carbonyl groups and amide compound of protein (Han et al. 2003).

Proanthocyanidin-rich grape seed extract increased the mechanical properties of demineralized dentin, such as elastic modulus (Bedran-Russo et al. 2008, Castellan et al. 2010a, dos Santos et al. 2011a, dos Santos et al. 2011b, de Siqueira et al. 2019), nanohardness (dos Santos et al. 2011a, dos Santos et al. 2011b, de Siqueira et al. 2019), stiffness (Zhou et al. 2016) and ultimate bond strength (Bedran-Russo et al. 2007, Liu et al. 2011). Dentin pretreatment using 5-30% proanthocyanidin solution from 30 s to 60 min increased tooth-restoration bond strength (Al-Ammar et al. 2009, Macedo et al. 2009, Castellan et al. 2010a, Fang et al. 2012, Srinivasulu et al. 2012, Castellan et al. 2013, Srinivasulu et al. 2013; Bacelar-Sá et al. 2017, Gajjela et al. 2017, Autieri et al. 2018, Bharti et al. 2018), and adhesive interface remained stable, improving bonding durability over time (Castellan et al. 2013, Verma et al. 2013, Liu et al. 2014, Hass et al. 2016a, Leme-Kraus et al. 2019), including eroded dentin after 2 years of water storage (de Siqueira et al. 2019). Moreover, it did not interfere on degree of conversion during adhesive polymerization (Fang et al. 2012, Hass et al. 2016b, de Siqueira et al. 2019, Siqueira et al. 2019) and decreased the nanoleakage (de Siqueira et al. 2019, Siqueira et al. 2019). Dentin treated with proanthocyanidin sealed the dentin with minimum permeability at bonded interface and it remained stable after 6-months of water storage (Bacelar-Sá et al. 2017).

A previous study (Epasinghe et al. 2012) evaluated the bond strength after the incorporation proanthocyanidin-rich extract in a simplified adhesive system with prior acid conditioning at concentrations of 0 (control), 1, 2 and 3%. The authors showed that up to 2% concentration there was no difference in immediate bond strength values (24 h), showing more mixed failures, besides presenting lower nanoleakage; at 3% concentration, there was a decrease on bond strength, more adhesive failures, and higher nanoleakage. Two percent proanthocyanidin extract incorporation in 5-10% phosphoric acid seems to be a viable alternative for produce stable resin-dentin and enamel-resin interfaces, without requiring additional steps during bonding procedure and jeopardizing adhesive polymerization (Hass et al. 2016a, Paludo et al. 2019, Siqueira et al. 2019).

In addition, the interaction of three different proanthocyanidin-rich extracts (two extracted from grape seed and one from cocoa seed) with polar solvents and type I collagen fibrils from demineralized dentin tissue was studied. It was verified that all extracts increased dentin stiffness, but they presented different behaviors, concluding that extraction process and pharmacognostic parameters may influence on solubility of extracts and their constitution and, consequently, the proanthocyanidin interaction with dentin. Grape seed extract containing proanthocyanidin extracted from *Vitis vinifera* (Mega-Natural, Madera, CA, USA), which has been shown to have the best interaction with human dentin (Castellan et al. 2010b).

Proanthocyanidin-rich extract from grape seed also increases the enzymatic biodegradation resistance of tooth-restoration interface collagen when extract was added in a simplified dental adhesive with previous acid conditioning and submitted to enzymatic degradation with 0.1% collagenase during 0 (control), 1 or 6 days (Green et al. 2010). Similar results were obtained by previous investigations (Macedo et al. 2009, Castellan et al. 2010a, Liu et al. 2014, Hass et al. 2016b, Zhou et al. 2016, Balalaie et al. 2019, Leme-Kraus et al. 2019), in which a higher resistance to enzymatic degradation of dentin was observed for groups that had this substrate pretreated with proanthocyanidin. However, in addition to bacterial enzymes, endogenous enzymes such as matrix metalloproteinases (MMPs) can be released and activated through adhesive procedures, exposing dentin to gelatinolytic activity (Pashley et al. 2004, Nishitani et al. 2006, Mazzoni et al. 2012).

Human dentin has at least MMP-2, -9 (gelatinases), -8 (collagenase), -3 (stromelysin) and -20 (enamelisin) (Mazzoni et al. 2012, Epasinghe et al. 2013). Application of acidic conditioners followed by etch-and-rinse adhesives application (De Munck et al. 2009, Mazzoni et al. 2012) and acid self-conditioning procedures (Nishitani et al. 2006, Tay et al. 2006) may lead to activation and increased expression of MMPs (Green et al.

2010). These enzymes can hydrolyze the collagen of hybrid layer and compromise the durability of tooth-restoration bonding interface (De Munck et al. 2009, Botta et al. 2012), together with cysteine cathepsins (Epasinghe et al. 2013), being involved in the degradation of extracellular matrix components during normal and pathological conditions (Ramamurthy et al. 2002, Epasinghe et al. 2013). Cysteine cathepsin B is the main cathepsin found in carious and sound dentin, and it cleaves non-helical telopeptide extensions of collagen like cathepsin L, while cathepsin K cleaves triple helical region of collagen (Epasinghe et al. 2013).

Degradation of bonding interface demonstrates increased collagen zone exposed (Sanabe et al. 2011). In addition, *in situ* zymography demonstrated that the hybrid layer formed with adhesives with previous acid conditioning exhibits intense gelatinolytic activity and that the adhesive procedures increase MMPs activity (Mazzoni et al. 2012).

To minimize these problems, proanthocyanidin application has shown the ability to inhibit proteolytic activity on demineralized dentin matrix and to stabilize the resin-dentin interface against enzymatic degradation (Liu et al. 2014, Scheffel et al. 2014, Seseogullari-Dirihan et al. 2015, Hass et al. 2016b), without promoting deleterious structural changes to triple helix of collagen (Botta et al. 2012) and no reducing on cell viability in cytotoxicity test (Hass et al. 2016b). Proanthocyanidin biomodification inactivates 75-90% of B and K cysteine cathepsins and more than 90% of MMP-2, -8, and -9, resulting in lower collagen solubilization from dentin matrix by collagen-bound proteases established by lower loss of dry mass and reduced hydroxyproline release (Epasinghe et al. 2013).

Epigallocatechin-3-gallate is other well-known collagen crosslinker extracted from green tea, *Camellia sinensis* plant. Green tea contains several polyphenols named catechin compounds such as epicatechin, epigallocatechin, epicatechin gallate, and epigallocatechin gallate, which are chemical antioxidants with capacity to destroy free radicals. Epigallocatechin is most active and abundant catechin of green tea, it is water soluble and no cytotoxic (Khamverdi et al. 2013). Some studies have assessed the effect of green tea extract (Carvalho et al. 2016, Khamverdi et al. 2013, Monteiro et al, 2013) and epigallocatechin-3-gallate

(Albuquerque et al. 2019, Du et al. 2012, Kalaiselvam et al. 2018, Khamverdi et al. 2015, Santiago et al. 2013, Singh et al. 2017, Yang et al. 2016, Yu et al. 2017a) on bond strength over time.

Biomodification of demineralized dentin with pretreatment using solution of 0.05-2% green tea extract for 60 s, revealed no significant difference on immediate bond strength (Khamverdi et al. 2013, Carvalho et al. 2016), while in another study the application of a green tea solution reduced adhesion to dentin (Monteiro et al. 2013). However, the bond strength remained stable over the long term (Carvalho et al. 2016; Khamverdi et al. 2013, Monteiro et al. 2013). Green tea has been reported as a natural inhibitor of MMPs, being the epicatechin gallate and epigallocatechin gallate strongly related to MMP inhibition (Carvalho et al. 2016).

Some investigations have showed that dentin pretreatment with 0.02% epigallocatechin-3-gallate/ethanol (Yang et al. 2016), 0.02 M epigallocatechin-3-gallate, and 0.02 M catechin (Kalaiselvam et al. 2018) solutions can effectively improve the immediate bond strength and bonding stability of adhesive systems. However, in others investigations the experimental aqueous solutions containing 0.1% (Albuquerque et al. 2019, Santiago et al. 2013, Singh et al. 2017) and 0.02% (Santiago et al. 2013) epigallocatechin-3-gallate have no significant effect on immediate bond strength, but all experimental solutions were effective in preserving the bonding after water storage (Santiago et al. 2013). The 0.05 epigallocatechin solution decreased the immediate adhesion (Santiago et al. 2013).

Similarly, the incorporation of epigallocatechin to adhesive systems was also evaluated and it was found that 200 and 300 μg/mL epigallocatechin-3-gallate provided increase in immediate bond strength values and enhanced bonding stability (Du et al. 2012). Meanwhile, the incorporation of 50 and 100 μM epigallocatechin-3-gallate (Khamverdi et al. 2015), 200-600 μg/mL epigallocatechin-3-gallate and epigallocatechin-3-O-(3-O-methyl)-gallate (Yu et al. 2017a), and 1.0% microparticles aqueous solution of epigallocatechin-3-gallate-loaded/poly (D-L lactide-co-glycolide) acid (Albuquerque et al. 2019) did not affect the immediate bond strength, but preserved the durability of resin-dentin bond over time, without affecting the degree of conversion of monomer into polymer (Du et al. 2012, Khamverdi et al. 2015, Yu et al. 2017a).

Aloe barbadensis miller named *Aloe vera* is a succulent herb with green fleshy and filled with a clear viscous gel (Sinha et al. 2016), which contains aloins and barbadoins as main chemical constituents (Sinha et al. 2018). *Aloe vera* has potent antibacterial, antifungal, antiviral properties (Sinha et al. 2016), and it exhibits anti-proteolytic activity with inhibitory effect against MMP-2 and -9 (Kudalkar et al. 2014, Sinha et al. 2016, Sinha et al. 2018). Application of *Aloe vera* solution on phosphoric acid-etched dentin for 30 s improved the bond strength of a two-step etch-and-rinse adhesive immediately and for 6-month water storage (Sinha et al. 2018).

Therefore, the use of natural phytochemical bioactive agents, which simultaneously can reduce the activity of proteolytic enzymes and crosslink the demineralized collagen matrix; it is essential to stabilize the resin-dentin adhesive interface and increase durability of dental resin-based restorations (Balalaie et al. 2018).

2.1.2. Bond Strength after Bleaching Procedure

Bleaching agents are hydrogen peroxide-based and when applied on dental enamel the hydrogen peroxide dissociates in free radicals such as nascent oxygen, hydroxyl radical, per-hydroxyl, and superoxide anions (Minoux et al. 2008) These products of bleaching reaction have been reported decrease the bond strength of adhesive resin-based restoration to enamel due to presence of residual oxygen that inhibit resin polymerization (Vidhya et al. 2011, Nair et al. 2019). General approach recommends the waiting period from 24 h to 4 weeks for bonding procedures after bleaching (Vidhya et al. 2011). However, in some clinical situations it is not possible to wait for this period, so the use of antioxidants prior to restorative procedure has been recommended (Vidhya et al. 2011, Abraham et al. 2013, Berger et al. 2013, Arumugam et al. 2014, Kadiyala et al. 2015, Manoharan et al. 2016, Mukka et al. 2016, Subramonian et al.

2015, Xu et al. 2018, Bansal et al. 2019, Nair et al. 2019, Nari-Ratih et al. 2019, Rana et al. 2019).

Teeth pretreatment by application of solution containing 5-10% proanthocyanidin-rich extracts from grape seed (Vidhya et al. 2011, Abraham et al. 2013, Arumugam et al. 2014, Subramonian et al. 2015, Manoharan et al. 2016, Mukka et al. 2016, Xu et al. 2018, Bansal et al. 2019, Nair et al. 2019) and pine bark (Subramonian et al. 2015, Mukka et al. 2016) has shown promising results, the antioxidant effect of proanthocyanidin was able to minimize the deleterious effects of hydrogen peroxide by neutralizing free radicals such as nascent oxygen that negatively interferes with polymerization of resinous materials; increasing the bond strength of dental enamel immediately after bleaching procedure (Vidhya et al. 2011). Furthermore, 600-1,000 μmol of epigallocatechin gallate (Khamverdi et al. 2013), 5-10% green tea (Berger et al. 2013, Bansal et al. 2019, Nari-Ratih et al. 2019, Rana et al. 2019), 5% white tea (Rana et al. 2019), 5% lycopene (Arumugam et al. 2014), 10-50% *Aloe vera* (Kadiyala et al. 2015; Nair et al. 2019, Nari-Ratih et al. 2019), and 5% pomegranate (Mukka et al. 2016) extracts can be also used as alternative natural antioxidants in improving the bond strength of dental enamel (Rana et al. 2019).

2.1.3. Bond Strength after Endodontic Treatment

After endodontic tooth treatment completed has been recommended the immediate sealing using restorative materials to prevent recontamination of root canal, decreasing the microleakage and maintaining the health of dental apical tissues (Cecchin et al. 2018, Chandrashekhar et al. 2018). Thus, it has been suggested the restoration of nonvital teeth using composite resin-based materials (Schwartz 2006).

However, during cleaning and shaping of root canal chemical substances are used and dentin surface may change, affecting the interaction of dental adhesive and dentin (Cecchin et al. 2018, Chandrashekhar et al. 2018, Wang et al. 2019). Sodium hypochlorite is the most commonly chemical irrigant for endodontic therapy due to antimicrobial activity and ability to dissolve organic substance

(Chandrashekhar et al. 2018, Wang et al. 2019), but its remnants and oxidation products of sodium hypochlorite can interfere negatively on adhesive polymerization (Chandrashekhar et al. 2018).

In this sense, studies have been conducted for neutralization of sodium hypochlorite using antioxidant agents (Cecchin et al. 2018, Chandrashekhar et al. 2018, Dikmen et al. 2015, Manimaran et al. 2011, Nagpal et al. 2013, Wang et al. 2019). Natural antioxidants application as noni fruit juice for 10 min (Dikmen et al. 2015), 10% tannic acid and 10% green tea for 5 min (Cecchin et al. 2018), and 5-30% solution of proanthocyanidin-rich extract from grape seed for 1-10 min has significant reversal effects for improving the bond strength of self-etch (Cecchin et al. 2018, Dikmen et al. 2015, Manimaran et al. 2011, Nagpal et al. 2013, Wang et al. 2019) and etch-and-rinse (Cecchin et al. 2018, Chandrashekhar et al. 2018) adhesive systems to hypochlorite-treated pulp chamber dentin, allowing adhesive restorations to be immediately performed after endodontic treatment.

2.1.4. Luting of Fiber Glass Posts

Glass fiber posts have been indicated for the restoration of endodontically treated teeth mainly because of their similar elastic modulus to human radicular dentin (Cecchin et al. 2015). However, luting of fiber posts is considered critical due to unfavorable conditions of root canal for bonding, such as chemical agents used during endodontic treatment, high cavity configuration factor, difficulties in adequately solvent evaporation, low irradiance in deeper portions of canal to adequate polymerization of resin cement, and contamination of dentin walls by root canal filling material (Alonso et al. 2018).

As with adhesive restorations, the loss of integrity of resin-dentin bonding over time occurs by combined effect of hydrolytic deterioration of resin-based components and enzymatic degradation of collagen fibrils by endogenous proteases (Cecchin et al. 2015). So, the use of proanthocyanidin solution prior adhesive luting has been recommended to increase the bond strength of fiber glass post to root dentin (Alandia-Román et al. 2017), to reduce/inhibit the activity of proteolytic enzymes

(Cecchin et al. 2015, Alonso et al. 2018), and to improve the bonding stability of adhesive interface in root canal (Cecchin et al. 2015, Alonso et al. 2018). As well as the epigallocatechin-3-gallate that improves the dentin compromised sodium hypochlorite-treated and bonding properties of fiber glass post to root canal (Yu et al. 2017b).

2.1.5. Bond Strength of Glass Ionomer Cements

As with adhesive restorations, the loss of integrity of resin-dentin bonding over time occurs by combined effect of hydrolytic deterioration of resin-based components and enzymatic degradation of collagen fibrils by endogenous proteases (Cecchin et al. 2015). So, the use of proanthocyanidin solution prior adhesive luting has been recommended to increase the bond strength of fiber glass post to root dentin (Alandia-Román et al. 2017), to reduce/inhibit the activity of proteolytic enzymes and to improve the bonding stability of adhesive interface in root canal (Cecchin et al. 2015, Alonso et al. 2018). As well as the epigallocatechin-3-gallate that improves the dentin compromised sodium hypochlorite-treated and bonding properties of fiber glass post to root canal (Yu et al. 2017b).Glass ionomer cements bond to tooth hard tissues by an ionic interaction between carboxylic components of polyacrylic acid and the calcium of enamel and dentin, after polyacrylic acid conditioning step to remove the smear layer and to expose the collagen fibrils at 0.5-1 μm depth (Shafiei et al. 2017). Thus, some collagen fibrils at base of hybrid layer may remain unprotected after polyacrylic acid conditioning step (Tay et al. 2001) and compromise the adhesion glass ionomer restorations over time.

Resin-modified glass ionomer cements and dentin has been reported to prone to degradation by endogenous MMPs (Shafiei et al. 2017). Application of proanthocyanidin extract solution to dentin surface increased its bonding to conventional glass ionomer cement (Atabek & Özden et al. 2019) and it no affected the immediate bond strength and maturation of resin-modified glass ionomer, so it can be recommended as proteolytic inhibitor before bonding of resin-modified glass ionomer to dentin (Shafiei et al. 2017).

2.2. Treatment of Dentinal Hypersensitivity by Using of Herbal Extract

Dentinal hypersensitivity (DH) is a common painful condition that affects the teeth. herbal dentrifices have been formulated for the treatment of this condition. Clinical studies have showed that herbal dentifrice containing *Spinacia oleracea* is able to reduce the DH symptoms (Kumari et al. 2013, Kumari et al. 2016).

A propolis varnish was developed to treatment of DH and, although it presents only *in vitro* studies, it was possible to obtain a significant reduction in the number of open dental tubules after application this new varnish (Kripal et al. 2019). In fact, further research will be necessary to introduce it as a clinical protocol for DH treatment.

2.3. Prevention of Enamel and Dentin Erosion

Dental erosion is defined as the loss of dental hard tissue (with histological changes) through chemical etching and dissolution by acids of nonbacterial origin (Mirkarimi et al. 2012, Sales-Peres Ade et al. 2013). For this type of alteration, the use of herbal extract has been proposed in order to reduce the enamel and dentin erosion, improved the texture of eroded dentine as well as increase the microhardness of erode dentin (Wiegand et al. 2007, Mirkarimi et al. 2012, Sales-Peres Ade et al. 2013).

An in vitro study showed that the use olive oil offered protection against enamel and dentin erosion when applied as 2% emulsion or 2% olive-oil-containing mouthrinse (composition: 2% extra virgin olive oil, 2% betaine, xylitol, 0.5% pro-vitamin B5, 0.5% pro-vitamin E, 0.24% lemon aroma, 0.2% allantoin, 0.07% potassium fluoride, aqua, PEG-40 hydrogenated castor oil, parsley seed oil, benzoic acid, sodium saccharin, sodium benzoate) (Wiegand et al. 2007).

The impact of green tea (*Camellia sinensis*) on dentin erosion was assessed by an *in vitro* study using extracted human premolars (Mirkarimi et al. 2012). The authors showed that green tea increases the surface microhardness of eroded dentin, improving the microhardness values before and after immersion of 46.5±2.79 to 54.5±4.4, respectively (Mirkarimi et al. 2012). Furthermore, other researchers showed that the green tea extract solution was able to reduce the wear and roughness caused in the dentin erosion as well as to have protective effects on dentin loss (De Moraes et al. 2016, Passos et al. 2018).

Also, the use of *Azadirachta indica* (Neem) was tested as dentin erosion prevention. The association of 10% Neem extract and 1.23% NaF (defined as Neem-containing fluoride gel) was be able to reduce dentin erosion (Sales-Peres Ade et al. 2013).

2.4. Cleaning of Dental Cavities

Atraumatic restorative treatment (ART) is defined as a minimally invasive treatment the uses only hand instruments to excavate soft, demineralized dental tissue followed by placement of adhesive restorative material that creates an environment for arresting caries progression with minimum invasive intervention. The problematic step of this technique is the permanence of bacteria in the cavity after the excavation that may result in the ART restorations fail due to secondary caries development subsequently (Prabhakar et al. 2015, Patri & Sahu 2017). Thus, the use of some herbal extract is proposed to reduce the ART restorations fail.

The effect of *Aloe vera* and propolis as cavity disinfecting agents after minimally invasive hand excavation of dental caries was assessed by a randomized clinical trial and the results showed that ethanolic extracts of *Aloe vera* or propolis may be used as effective cavity disinfectants, which in turn may help to reduce secondary caries thus contributing to long-term restorative success (Prabhakar et al. 2015).

Patri & Sahu (2017) evaluated the *Melaleuca alternifolia* (Tea Tree Oil) and *Aloe vera* as cavity disinfectant in comparison with 2% chlorhexidine and proposed that natural antibacterial agents like tea tree oil and *Aloe vera* could be effectively used as cavity disinfectants which will help in minimizing secondary caries and rendering a long-term restorative success (Patri & Sahu 2017).

REFERENCES

Abraham S, Ghonmode WN, Saujanya KP, Jaju N, Tambe VH, Yawalikar PP. Effect of grape seed extracts on bond strength of bleached enamel using fifth and seventh generation bonding agents. *J Int Oral Health* 2013;5(6):101-7.

Abu-Obaid E, Salama F, Abu-Obaid A, Alanazi F, Salem M, Auda S. Comparative Evaluation of the Antimicrobial Effects of Different Mouthrinses against Streptococcus Mutans: An in Vitro Study. *J Clin Pediatr Dent* 2019;43(6):398-407.

Aghazadeh M, Zahedi Bialvaei A, Aghazadeh M, Kabiri F, Saliani N, Yousefi M, Eslami H, Samadi Kafil H. Survey of the Antibiofilm and Antimicrobial Effects of Zingiber officinale (in Vitro Study). *Jundishapur J Microbiol* 2016;9(2):e30167.

Al-Ammar A, Drummond JL, Bedran-Russo AK. The use of collagen cross-linking agents to enhance dentin bond strength. *J Biomed Mater Res B Appl Biomater* 2009;91(1):419-424.

Alandia-Román CC, Vincenti SA, Silami FD, Silveira RE, Pinto GC, Pires-de-Souza FC. The effect of proanthocyanidins and chlorhexidine on the bond strength of glass fiber posts to root dentin. *Gen Dent* 2017;65(2):23-27.

Albuquerque N, Neri JR, Lemos M, Yamauti M, de Sousa F, Santiago SL. Effect of polymeric microparticles loaded with catechin on the physicochemical properties of an adhesive system. *Oper Dent* 2019;44(4):E202-E211.

Aldana J, Téllez N, Gamboa F. Antimicrobial activity of fractions and subfractions of Elaeagia utilis against microorganisms of importance in dental caries. *Acta Odontol Latinoam* 2013;26(2):104-11.

Almas K, Al-Zeid Z. The immediate antimicrobial effect of a toothbrush and miswak on cariogenic bacteria: a clinical study. *J Contemp Dent Pract* 2004;5(1):105-14.

Almas K. The antimicrobial effects of seven different types of Asian chewing sticks. *Odontostomatol Trop* 2001;24(96):17-20.

Almaz ME, Sönmez IŞ, Ökte Z, Oba AA. Efficacy of a sugar-free herbal lollipop for reducing salivary Streptococcus mutans levels: a randomized controlled trial. *Clin Oral Investig* 2017;21(3):839-845.

Almeida Lde F, Paula JF, Almeida RV, Williams DW, Hebling J, Cavalcanti YW. Efficacy of citronella and cinnamon essential oils on Candida albicans biofilms. *Acta Odontol Scand* 2016;74(5):393-8.

Alonso JRL, Basso FG, Scheffel DLS, de-Souza-Costa CA, Hebling J. Effect of crosslinkers on bond strength stability of fiber posts to root canal dentin and in situ proteolytic activity. *J Prosthet Dent* 2018;119(3):494.e1-494.e9.

Antonio AG, Iorio NL, Pierro VS, Candreva MS, Farah A, dos Santos KR, Maia LC. Inhibitory properties of Coffea canephora extract against oral bacteria and its effect on demineralisation of deciduous teeth. *Arch Oral Biol* 2011;56(6):556-64.

Arumugam MT, Nesamani R, Kittappa K, Sanjeev K, Sekar M. Effect of various antioxidants on the shear bond strength of composite resin to bleached enamel: An in vitro study. *J Conserv Dent* 2014;17(1):22-6.

Ashrafi B, Rashidipour M, Marzban A, Soroush S, Azadpour M, Delfani S, Ramak P. Mentha piperita essential oils loaded in a chitosan nanogel with inhibitory effect on biofilm formation against S. mutans on the dental surface. *Carbohydr Polym* 2019;(15)212:142-149.

Atabek Ş, Özden AN. Comparison of the effect of proanthocyanidin surface treatments on shear bond strength of different cements. *Materials (Basel)* 2019;12(17):E2676.

Autieri G, Mussano F, Petruzzi M, Carossa M, Genova T, Corsalini M, Carossa S. Proanthocyanidin may improve the shear bond strength at the composites/dentine interface. *J Biol Regul Homeost Agents* 2018;32(4):1021-1025.

Azaripour A, Mahmoodi B, Habibi E, Willershausen I, Schmidtmann I, Willershausen B. Effectiveness of a miswak extract-containing toothpaste on gingival inflammation: a randomized clinical trial. *Int J Dent Hyg* 2017;15(3):195-202.

Bacelar-Sá R, Giannini M, Ambrosano GMB, Bedran-Russo AK. Dentin sealing and bond strength evaluation of Hema-free and multi-mode adhesives to biomodified dentin. *Braz Dent J* 2017;28(6):731-737.

Baeshen HA1, Kjellberg H, Lingström P, Birkhed D. Uptake and release of fluoride from fluoride-impregnated chewing sticks (miswaks) in vitro and in vivo. *Caries Res* 2008;42(5):363-8.

Balalaie A, Rezvani MB, Basir MM, Rezadoost H, Balalaie S. A New Approach for Determining the minimum concentration of proanthocyanidin for preservation of collagen in H dentin. *Eur J Prosthodont Restor Dent* 2019;27(4):154-163.

Balalaie A, Rezvani MB, Mohammadi Basir M. Dual function of proanthocyanidins as both MMP inhibitor and crosslinker in dentin biomodification: A literature review. *Dent Mater J* 2018;37(2):173-182.

Bansal M, Kaur P, Cyriac AR, Kadian N, Jaiswal P, Rathee K. Impact of Different Antioxidants on the bond strength of resin based composite on bleached enamel-an in vitro study. *J Contemp Dent Pract* 2019;20(1):64-70.

Bedran-Russo AK, Pashley DH, Agee K, Drummond JL, Miescke KJ. Changes in stiffness of demineralized dentin following application of collagen crosslinkers. *J Biomed Mater Res B Appl Biomater* 2008;86(2):330-334.

Bedran-Russo AK, Pereira PN, Duarte WR, Drummond JL, Yamauchi M. Application of crosslinkers to dentin collagen enhances the ultimate tensile strength. *J Biomed Mater Res B Appl Biomater* 2007;80(1):268-272.

Bedran-Russo AK. Collagen cross-linking agents on dental restorative treatment and preventive dentistry 2009 (*US Patent Application Publication #2009/01233581*).

Berger SB, De Souza Carreira RP, Guiraldo RD, Lopes MB, Pavan S, Giannini M, Bedran-Russo AK. Can green tea be used to reverse compromised bond strength after bleaching? *Eur J Oral Sci* 2013;121(4):377-81.

Bharti N, Chandra A, Tikku AP, Verma P, Bharti R, Shakya VK, Bains R. An ex vivo evaluation of effect of dentin pretreatment with various agents for varying time intervals on the shear bond strength of resin. *J Conserv Dent* 2018;21(1):37-41.

Bhat N, Bapat S, Asawa K, Tak M, Chaturvedi P, Gupta VV, George PP. The antiplaque efficacy of propolis-based herbal toothpaste: A crossover clinical study. *J Nat Sci Biol Med* 2015;6(2):364-8.

Botta SB, Ana PA, Santos MO, Zezell DM, Matos AB. Effect of dental tissue conditioners and matrix metalloproteinase inhibitors on type I collagen microstructure analyzed by fourier transform infrared spectroscopy. *J Biomed Mater Res Part B Appl Biomater* 2012;100(4):1009-1016.

Braga AS, Girotti LD, de Melo Simas LL, Pires JG, Pelá VT, Buzalaf MAR, Magalhães AC. Effect of commercial herbal toothpastes and mouth rinses on the prevention of enamel demineralization using a microcosm biofilm model. *Biofouling* 2019;35(7):796-804.

Brighenti FL, Gaetti-Jardim E Jr, Danelon M, Evangelista GV, Delbem AC. Effect of Psidium cattleianum leaf extract on enamel demineralisation and dental biofilm composition in situ. *Arch Oral Biol* 2012;57(8):1034-40.

Carvalho C, Fernandes FP, Freitas Vda P, França FM, Basting RT, Turssi CP, Amaral FL. Effect of green tea extract on bonding durability of an etch-and-rinse adhesive system to caries-affected dentin. *J Appl Oral Sci* 2016;24(3):211-7.

Castellan CS, Bedran-Russo AK, Antunes A, Pereira PN. Effect of dentin biomodification using naturally derived collagen cross-linkers: one-year bond strength study. *Int J Dent* 2013;2013:918010.

Castellan CS, Bedran-Russo AK, Karol S, Pereira PN. Long-term stability of dentin matrix following treatment with various natural collagen cross-linkers. *J Mech Behav Biomed Mater* 2011;4(7):1343-1350.

Castellan CS, Pereira PN, Grande RH, Bedran-Russo AK. Mechanical characterization of proanthocyanidin-dentin matrix interaction. *Dent Mater* 2010a;26(10)968-973.

Castellan CS, Pereira PN, Viana G, Chen SN, Pauli GF, Bedran-Russo AK. Solubility study of phytochemical cross-linking agents on dentin stiffness. *J Dent* 2010b;38(5):431-436.

Cecchin D, Farina AP, Bedran-Russo AK. Efficacy of Natural Collagen Crosslinkers on the Compromised Adhesive Bond Strength to NaOCl-treated Pulp Chamber Dentin. *J Adhes Dent* 2018;20(4):365-369.

Cecchin D, Pin LC, Farina AP, Souza M, Vidal Cde M, Bello YD, Ferraz CC, Bedran-Russo A. Bond strength between fiber posts and root dentin treated with natural cross-linkers. *J Endod* 2015;41(10):1667-71.

Chandrashekhar S, Patil S, Abraham S, Mehta D, Chaudhari S, Shashidhar J. A comparative evaluation of shear bond strength of composite resin to pulp chamber dentin treated with sodium thiosulfate and proanthocyanidin: An in vitro study. *J Conserv Dent* 2018;21(6):671-675.

Chen Y, Agnello M, Dinis M, Chien KC, Wang J, Hu W, Shi W, He X, Zou J. Lollipop containing Glycyrrhiza uralensis extract reduces Streptococcus mutans colonization and maintains oral microbial diversity in Chinese preschool children. *PLoS One* 2019;14(8):e0221756.

Cheng L, ten Cate JM. Effect of Galla chinensis on the in vitro remineralization of advanced enamel lesions. *Int J Oral Sci* 2010;2(1):15-20.

Chu JP, Li JY, Hao YQ, Zhou XD. Effect of compounds of Galla chinensis on remineralisation of initial enamel carious lesions in vitro. *J Dent* 2007;35(5):383-7.

Datta D, Ramesh Kumar SG, Aswath Narayanan MB, Leena Selvamary A, Sujatha A. Disclosing solutions used in dentistry. *World Journal of Pharmaceutical Research* 2017;6(6):1648-1656.

de Alencar CR, de Oliveira GC, Tripodi CD, Gonçalves PS, Ionta FQ, Honorio HM, Oliveira TM, Rios D. Dental Plaque Disclosing as an

Auxiliary Method for Professional Dental Prophylaxis in Early Childhood. *Int J Clin Pediatr Dent* 2019;12(3):189-193.

De Moraes MD, Carneiro JR, Passos VF, Santiago SL. Effect of green tea as a protective measure against dental erosion in coronary dentine. *Braz Oral Res* 2016;30. pii: S1806-83242016000100213.

De Munck J, Van den Steen PE, Mine A, Van Landuyt KL, Poitevin A, Opdenakker G, Van Meerbeek B. Inhibition of enzymatic degradation of adhesive-dentin interfaces. *J Dent Res* 2009;88(12):1101-1106.

de Siqueira FSF, Hilgemberg B, Araujo LCR, Hass V, Bandeca MC, Gomes JC, Reis A, Loguercio AD, Cardenas AFM. Improving bonding to eroded dentin by using collagen cross-linking agents: 2 years of water storage. *Clin Oral Investig* (in press). doi: 10.1007/s00784-019-02918-9.

Delimont NM, Carlson BN. Prevention of dental caries by grape seed extract supplementation: A systematic review. *Nutr Health* 2019 doi: 10.1177/0260106019887890. [Epub ahead of print].

Dikmen B, Gurbuz O, Ozsoy A, Eren MM, Cilingir A, Yucel T. Effect of Different Antioxidants on the Microtensile Bond Strength of an Adhesive System to Sodium Hypochlorite-treated Dentin. *J Adhes Dent* 2015;17(6):499-504.

dos Santos PH, Karol S, Bedran-Russo AK. Long-term nano-mechanical properties of biomodified dentin-resin interface components. *J Biomech* 2011a;44(9):1691-1694.

dos Santos PH, Karol S, Bedran-Russo AK. Nanomechanical properties of biochemically modified dentin bonded interfaces. *J Oral Rehabil* 2011b;38(7):541-546.

Du X, Huang X, Huang C, Wang Y, Zhang Y. Epigallocatechin-3-gallate (EGCG) enhances the therapeutic activity of a dental adhesive. *J Dent* 2012;40(6):485-92.

Epasinghe DJ, Yiu CK, Burrow MF, Hiraishi N, Tay FR. The inhibitory effect of proanthocyanidin on soluble and collagen-bound proteases. *J Dent* 2013;41(9):832-9.

Epasinghe DJ, Yiu CK, Burrow MF, Tay FR, King NM. Effect of proanthocyanidin incorporation into dental adhesive resin on resin-dentin bond strength. *J Dent* 2012;40(3):173-180.

Fang M, Liu R, Xiao Y, Li F, Wang D, Hou R, Chen J. Biomodification to dentin by a natural crosslinker improved the resin-dentin bonds. *J Dent* 2012;40(6):458-466.

Fasoulas A, Pavlidou E, Petridis D, Mantzorou M, Seroglou K, Giaginis C. Detection of dental plaque with disclosing agents in the context of preventive oral hygiene training programs. *Heliyon* 2019;5(7):e02064.

Feng G, Klein MI, Gregoire S, Singh AP, Vorsa N, Koo H. The specific degree-of-polymerization of A-type proanthocyanidin oligomers impacts Streptococcus mutans glucan-mediated adhesion and transcriptome responses within biofilms. *Biofouling* 2013;29(6):629-40.

Fine AM. Oligomeric proanthocyanidin complexes: history, structure, and phytopharmaceutical applications. *Alter Med Rev* 2000;5(2):144-151.

Gajjela RS, Satish RK, Sajjan GS, Varma KM, Rambabu T, Vijaya Lakshmi BH. Comparative evaluation of chlorhexidine, grape seed extract, riboflavin/chitosan modification on microtensile bond strength of composite resin to dentin after polymerase chain reaction thermocycling: An in vitro study. *J Conserv Dent* 2017;20(2):120-124.

Giacaman RA, Contzen MP, Yuri JA, Muñoz-Sandoval C. Anticaries effect of an antioxidant-rich apple concentrate on enamel in an experimental biofilm-demineralization model. *J Appl Microbiol* 2014;117(3):846-53.

Green B, Yao X, Ganguly A, Xu C, Dusevich V, Walker MP, Wang Y. Grape seed proanthocyanidins increase collagen biodegradation resistance in the dentin/adhesive interface when included in an adhesive. *J Dent* 2010;38(11):908-915.

Han B, Jaurequi J, Tang BW, Nimni ME. Proanthocyanidin: a natural crosslinking reagent for stabilizing collagen matrices. *J Biomed Mater Res A* 2003;65(1):118-124.

Hashimoto M, Ohno H, Kaga M, Endo K, Sano H, Oguchi H. In vivo degradation of resin-dentin bonds in human over 1 to 3 years. *J Dent Res* 2000;79(6):1385-1391.

Hass V, Luque-Martinez I, Muñoz MA, Reyes MF, Abuna G, Sinhoreti MA, Liu AY, Loguercio AD, Wang Y, Reis A. The effect of proanthocyanidin-containing 10% phosphoric acid on bonding properties and MMP inhibition. *Dent Mater* 2016a;32(3):468-75.

Hass V, Luque-Martinez IV, Gutierrez MF, Moreira CG, Gotti VB, Feitosa VP, Koller G, Otuki MF, Loguercio AD, Reis A. Collagen cross-linkers on dentin bonding: Stability of the adhesive interfaces, degree of conversion of the adhesive, cytotoxicity and in situ MMP inhibition. *Dent Mater* 2016b;32(6):732-41.

Huang X, Cheng L, Exterkate RA, Liu M, Zhou X, Li J, ten Cate JM. Effect of pH on Galla chinensis extract's stability and anti-caries properties in vitro. *Arch Oral Biol* 2012;57(8):1093-9.

Jeong SH, Lee JE, Jin SH, Ko Y, Park JB. Effects of Asiasari radix on the morphology and viability of mesenchymal stem cells derived from the gingiva. *Mol Med Rep* 2014;10(6):3315-9.

Kadiyala A, Saladi HK, Bollu IP, Burla D, Ballullaya SV, Devalla S, Maroli S, Jayaprakash T. Effect of Different Anti-Oxidants on Shear Bond Strength of Composite Resins to Bleached Human Enamel. *J Clin Diagn Res* 2015;9(11):ZC40-3.

Kalaiselvam R, Ganesh A, Rajan M, Kandaswamy D. Evaluation of bioflavonoids on the immediate and delayed microtensile bond strength of self-etch and total-etch adhesive systems to sound dentin. Indian *J Dent Res* 2018;29(2):133-136.

Karadağlıoğlu Öİ, Ulusoy N, Başer KHC, Hanoğlu A, Şık İ. Antibacterial Activities of Herbal Toothpastes Combined with Essential Oils against Streptococcus mutans. *Pathogens* 2019;8(1). pii: E20.

Khairnar M, Dodamani A, Karibasappa GN, Deshmukh M, Naik R. Comparative Evaluation of Efficacy of Three Different Herbal Toothpastes on Salivary Alkaline Phosphatase and Salivary Acid Phosphatase - A Randomized Controlled Trial. *J Clin Diagn Res* 2016;10(9):ZC69-ZC73.

Khairnar MR, Dodamani AS, Karibasappa GN, Naik RG, Deshmukh MA. Efficacy of herbal toothpastes on salivary pH and salivary glucose - A preliminary study. *J Ayurveda Integr Med* 2017;8(1):3-6.

Khamverdi Z, Rezaei-Soufi L, Kasraei S, Ronasi N, Rostami S. Effect of Epigallocatechin Gallate on shear bond strength of composite resin to bleached enamel: an in vitro study. *Restor Dent Endod* 2013;38(4):241-7.

Khamverdi Z, Rezaei-Soufi L, Rostamzadeh T. The Effect of Epigallocatechin Gallate on the Dentin Bond Durability of Two Self-etch Adhesives. *J Dent (Shiraz)* 2015;16(2):68-74.

Kim BS, Park SJ, Kim MK, Kim YH, Lee SB, Lee KH, Choi NY, Lee YR, Lee YE, You YO. Inhibitory Effects of Chrysanthemum boreale Essential Oil on Biofilm Formation and Virulence Factor Expression of Streptococcus mutans. E*vid Based Complement Alternat Med* 2015;2015:616309. doi: 10.1155/2015/616309.

Kjaer M, Langberg H, Miller BF, Boushel R, Crameri R, Koskinen S, Heinemeier K, Olesen JL, Døssing S, Hansen M, Pedersen SG, Rennie MJ, Magnusson P. Metabolic activity and collagen turnover in human tendon in response to physical activity. *J Musculoskelet Neuronal Interact* 2005;5(1):41-52.

Korkmaz FM, Ozel MB, Tuzuner T, Korkmaz B, Yayli N. Antimicrobial activity and volatile constituent analysis of three commercial herbal toothpastes containing Aloe vera L. and Fragaria vesca L. extracts. *Niger J Clin Pract* 2019;22(5):718-726.

Kripal K, Chandrasekaran K, Chandrasekaran S, Kumar VR, Chavan SKD, Dileep A. Treatment of dentinal hypersensitivity using propolis varnish: A scanning electron microscope study. *Indian J Dent Res* 2019;30(2):249-253.

Krishnakumar G, Gaviappa D, Guruswamy S. Anticaries Efficacy of Liquorice Lollipop: An ex vivo Study. *J Contemp Dent Pract* 2018;19(8):937-942.

Kudalkar MD, Nayak A, Bhat KS, Nayak RN. Effect of Azadirachta indica (Neem) and Aloe vera as compared to subantimicrobial dose doxycycline on matrix metalloproteinases (MMP)-2 and MMP-9: An in-vitro study. *Ayu* 2014;35(1):85-9.

Kumari M, Naik SB, Martande SS, Pradeep AR, Singh P. Comparative efficacy of a herbal and a non-herbal dentifrice on dentinal hypersensitivity: a randomized, controlled clinical trial. *J Investig Clin Dent* 2016;7(1):46-52.

Kumari M, Naik SB, Rao NS, Martande SS, Pradeep AR. Clinical efficacy of a herbal dentifrice on dentinal hypersensitivity: a randomized controlled clinical trial. *Aust Dent J* 2013;58(4):483-90.

Kunwar RM, Mahat L, Acharya RP, Bussmann RW. Medicinal plants, traditional medicine, markets and management in far-west Nepal. *J Ethnobiol Ethnomed* 2013;9:24.

Leme-Kraus AA, Phansalkar RS, Dos Reis MC, Aydin B, Sousa ABS, Alania Y, McAlpine J, Chen SN, Pauli GF, Bedran-Russo AK. Dimeric proanthocyanidins on the stability of dentin and adhesive biointerfaces. *J Dent Res* 2019 (in press). doi: 10.1177/0022034519892959. [Epub ahead of print].

Liu R, Fang M, Xiao Y, Li F, Yu L, Zhao S, Shen L, Chen J. The effect of transient proanthocyanidins preconditioning on the cross-linking and mechanical properties of demineralized dentin. *J Mater Sci Mater Med* 2011;22(11):2403-2411.

Liu RR, Fang M, Zhang L, Tang CF, Dou Q, Chen JH. Anti-proteolytic capacity and bonding durability of proanthocyanidin-biomodified demineralized dentin matrix. *Int J Oral Sci* 2014;6(3):168-74.

Macedo GV, Yamauchi M, Bedran-Russo AK. Effects of chemical cross-linkers on caries-affected dentin bonding. *J Dent Res* 2009;88(12)1096-1100.

Maciel KT, Carvalho RM, Ringle RD, Preston CD, Russel CM, Pashley DH. The effects of acetone, ethanol, HEMA, and air on the stiffness of human decalcified dentin matrix. *J Dent Res* 1996;75(11):1851-1858.

Majumdar M, Misra TK, Roy DN. In vitro anti-biofilm activity of 14-deoxy-11,12-didehydroandrographolide from Andrographis paniculata against Pseudomonas aeruginosa. *Braz J Microbiol* 2019. doi: 10.1007/s42770-019-00169-0. [Epub ahead of print].

Manimaran VS, Srinivasulu S, Rajesh Ebenezar A, Mahalaxmi S, Srinivasan N. Application of a proanthocyanidin agent to improve the bond strength of root dentin treated with sodium hypochlorite. *J Conserv Dent* 2011;14(3):306-308.

Manoharan M, Shashibhushan KK, Poornima P, Naik SN, Patil D, Shruthi AS. Effect of newer antioxidants on the bond strength of composite on bleached enamel. J *Indian Soc Pedod Prev Dent* 2016;34(4):391-6.

Maroyi A. Kirkia acuminata oliv.: a review of its ethnobotany and pharmacology. *Afr J Tradit Complement Altern Med* 2017;14(2):217-226.

Marshall GW, Jr. Marshall SJ, Kinney JH, Balloch M. The dentin substrate: structure and properties related to bonding. *J Dent* 1997;25(6):441-58.

Masquelier J, Dumon MC, Dumas J. Stabilization of collagen by procyanidolic oligomers. *Acta Therap* 1981;7:101-5.

Mazzoni A, Nascimento FD, Carrilho M, Tersariol I, Papa V, Tjäderhane L, Di Lenarda R, Tay FR, Pashley DH, Breschi L. MMP activity in the hybrid layer detected with in situ zymography. *J Dent Res* 2012;91(5):467-72.

Megersa M, Jima TT, Goro KKn.The Use of Medicinal Plants for the Treatment of Toothache in Ethiopia. *Evid Based Complement Alternat Med* 2019;2019:2645174.

Minoux M, Serfaty R. Vital tooth bleaching: biologic adverse effects-a review. *Quintessence Int* 2008;39(8):645-59.

Mirkarimi M, Toomarian L. Effect of green tea extract on the treatment of dentin erosion: an in vitro study. *J Dent (Tehran)*. 2012;9(4):224-8.

Monteiro TM, Basting RT, Turssi CP, França FM, Amaral FL. Influence of natural and synthetic metalloproteinase inhibitors on bonding durability of an etch-and-rinse adhesive to dentin. *Int J Adhes Adhes* 2013;47:83-8.

Mukka PK, Komineni NK, Pola S, Soujanya E, Karne AR, Nenavath B, Shiva S, Vuppunuthula P. An in-vitro comparative study of shear bond strength of composite resin to bleached enamel using three herbal antioxidants. *J Clin Diagn Res* 2016;10(10):ZC89-92.

Nagpal R, Manuja N, Pandit IK. Effect of proanthocyanidin treatment on the bonding effectiveness of adhesive restorations in pulp chamber. *J Clin Pediatr Dent* 2013;38(1):49-53.

Nair R, Bandhe S, Ganorkar OK, Saha S, Sial S, Nair A. A comparative evaluation of the three different antioxidant treatments on the bond strength of composite resin to bleached enamel: An in vitro study. *J Conserv Dent* 2019;22(1):82-86.

Nari-Ratih D, Widyastuti A. Effect of antioxidants on the shear bond strength of composite resin to enamel following extra-coronal bleaching. *J Clin Exp Dent* 2019;11(2):e126-e132.

Navarra CO, Cadenaro M, Armstrong SR, Jessop J, Antoniolli F, Sergo V, Di Lenarda R, Breschi L. Degree of conversion of filtek silorane adhesive and clearfil SE bond within the hybrid layer and adhesive layer: an in situ Raman analysis. *Dent Mater* 2009;25(9):1178-1185.

Nishitani Y, Yoshiyama M, Wadgaonkar B, Breschi L, Mannello F, Mazzoni A, Carvalho RM, Tjäderhane L, Tay FR, Pashley DH. Activation of gelatinolytic/collagenolytic activity in dentin by self-etching adhesives. *Eur J Oral Sci* 2006;114(2):160-166.

Oluwasina OO, Ezenwosu IV, Ogidi CO, Oyetayo VO. Antimicrobial potential of toothpaste formulated from extracts of Syzygium aromaticum, Dennettia tripetala and Jatropha curcas latex against some oral pathogenic microorganisms. *AMB Express* 2019;9(1):20.

Paludo T, Marcondes ML, Souto AA, Lopes GC, Loguércio AD, Spohr AM. Effect of grape seed extract-containing phosphoric acid formulations on bonding to enamel and dentin. *Braz Oral Res* 2019;33:e098.

Pashley DH, Tay FR, Yiu C, Hashimoto M, Breschi L, Carvalho RM, Ito S. Collagen degradation by host-derived enzymes during aging. *J Dent Res* 2004;83(3):216-221.

Passos VF, Melo MAS, Lima JPM, Marçal FF, Costa CAGA, Rodrigues LKA, Santiago SL. Active compounds and derivatives of camellia sinensis responding to erosive attacks on dentin. *Braz Oral Res* 2018;32:e40.

Patri G, Sahu A. Role of Herbal Agents - Tea Tree Oil and Aloe vera as Cavity Disinfectant Adjuncts in Minimally Invasive Dentistry-An In vivo Comparative Study. *J Clin Diagn Res* 2017;11(7):DC05-DC09.

Pavan S, Xie Q, Hara AT, Bedran-Russo AK. Biomimetic approach for root caries prevention using a proanthocyanidin-rich agent. *Caries Res* 2011;45(5):443-447.

Penmetsa GS, Pitta SR. Efficacy of Ocimum sanctum, Aloe vera and chlorhexidine mouthwash on gingivitis: A randomized controlled comparative clinical study. *Ayu* 2019;40(1):23-26.

Peters MC, Tallman JA, Braun TM, Jacobson JJ. Clinical reduction of S. mutans in pre-school children using a novel liquorice root extract lollipop: a pilot study. *Eur Arch Paediatr Dent* 2010;11(6):274-8.

Pires JG, Zabini SS, Braga AS, de Cássia Fabris R, de Andrade FB, de Oliveira RC, Magalhães AC. Hydroalcoholic extracts of Myracrodruon urundeuva All. and Qualea grandiflora Mart. leaves on Streptococcus mutans biofilm and tooth demineralization. *Arch Oral Biol* 2018;91:17-22.

Prabhakar AR, Karuna YM, Yavagal C, Deepak BM. Cavity disinfection in minimally invasive dentistry - comparative evaluation of Aloe vera and propolis: A randomized clinical trial. *Contemp Clin Dent* 2015;6(Suppl 1):S24-31.

Prabhakar AR, Sharma D, Sugandhan S. Comparative evaluation of the remineralising effects and surface microhardness of glass ionomer cement containing grape seed extract and casein phosphopeptide – amorphous calcium phosphate: An in vitro study. *Eur Arch Paediatr Dent* 2012;13(3):138-143.

Ramalingam K, Amaechi BT. Antimicrobial effect of herbal extract of Acacia arabica with triphala on the biofilm forming cariogenic microorganisms. *J Ayurveda Integr Med* 2018. doi: 10.1016/j.jaim.2018.01.005. [Epub ahead of print].

Ramamurthy NS, Xu JW, Bird J, Baxter A, Bhogal R, Wills R, Watson B, Owen D, Wolff M, Greenwald RA. Inhibition of a alveolar bone loss by matrix metalloproteinase inhibitors in experimental periodontal disease. *J Periodontal Res* 2002;37(1)1-7.

Rana R, Kaushik M, Sharma R, Reddy P, Mehra N. Comparative evaluation of effects of natural antioxidants on the shear bond strength of composite resin to bleached enamel. *Indian J Dent Res* 2019;30(1):112-116.

Raphael SL, Foster Page LA, Hopcraft MS, Dennison PJ, Widmer RP, Evans RW. A survey of cariology teaching in Australia and New Zealand. *BMC Med Educ* 2018;18(1):75.

Ribeiro Nazaré RF, Emmi DT, Barroso RFF, da Rocha PO. Bacterial plaque evidencing composition based on natural corants. *U.S. Patent 7,182,935 B2* 2007; filed February 27.

Sadeghi-Nejad B, Moghimipour E, Yusef Naanaie S, Nezarat S. Antifungal and antibacterial activities of polyherbal toothpaste against oral pathogens, in vitro. *Curr Med Mycol* 2018;4(2):21-26.

Sales-Peres Ade C, Marsicano JA, Garcia RP, Forim MR, Silva MF, Sales-Peres SH. Effect of natural gel product on bovine dentin erosion in vitro. *J Appl Oral Sci* 2013;21(6):597-600.

Sanabe ME, Costa CA, Hebling J. Exposed collagen in aged resin-dentin bonds produced on sound and caries-affected dentin in the presence of chlorhexidine. *J Adhes Dent* 2011;13(2):117-124.

Santi SS, Casarin M, Grellmann AP, Chambrone L, Zanatta FB. Effect of herbal mouthrinses on dental plaque formation and gingival inflammation: A systematic review. *Oral Dis* 2019. doi: 10.1111/odi.13254. [Epub ahead of print].

Santiago SL, Osorio R, Neri JR, Carvalho RM, Toledano M. Effect of the flavonoid epigallocatechin-3-gallate on resin-dentin bond strength. *J Adhes Dent* 2013;15(6):535-40.

Scheffel DL, Hebling J, Scheffel RH, Agee K, Turco G, de Souza Costa CA, Pashley D. Inactivation of matrix-bound matrix metalloproteinases by cross-linking agents in acid-etched dentin. *Oper Dent* 2014;39(2):152-8.

Schwartz RS. Adhesive dentistry and endodontics. Part 2: bonding in the root canal system-the promise and the problems: a review. *J Endod* 2006;32(12):1125-34.

Sekita Y, Murakami K, Yumoto H, Hirao K, Amoh T, Fujiwara N, Hirota K, Fujii H, Matsuo T, Miyake Y, Kashiwada Y. Antibiofilm and Anti-Inflammatory Activities of Houttuynia cordata Decoction for Oral Care. *Evid Based Complement Alternat Med* 2017;2017:2850947.

Selwitz RH, Ismail AI, Pitts NB. Dental caries. *Lancet* 2007;369(9555):51-9.

Seseogullari-Dirihan R, Mutluay MM, Vallittu P, Pashley DH, Tezvergil-Mutluay A. Effect of pretreatment with collagen crosslinkers on dentin protease activity. *Dent Mater* 2015;31(8):941-7.

Shafiei F, Firouzmandi M, Zamanpour M. The effect of two cross-linking agents on dentin bond strength of resin-modified glass ionomer. *Eur J Dent* 2017;11(4):486-490.

Shahriari S, Barekatain M, Shahtalebi MA, Farhad SZ. Evaluation of Preventive Antibacterial Properties of a Glass-Ionomer Cement Containing Purified Powder of Salvia officinalis: An In vitro Study. *Int J Prev Med* 2019;10:110.

Silva APP, Gonçalves RS, Borges AFS, Bedran-Russo AK, Shinohara MS. Effectiveness of plant-derived proanthocyanidins on demineralization on enamel and dentin under artificial cariogenic challenge. *J Appl Oral Sci* 2015;23(3):302-9.

Singh P, Nagpal R, Singh UP. Effect of dentin biomodifiers on the immediate and long-term bond strengths of a simplified etch and rinse adhesive to dentin. *Restor Dent Endod* 2017;42(3):188-199.

Sinha DJ, Jaiswal N, Vasudeva A, Garg P, Tyagi SP, Chandra P. Comparative evaluation of the effect of chlorhexidine and Aloe barbadensis Miller (Aloe vera) on dentin stabilization using shear bond testing. *J Conserv Dent* 2016;19(5):406-9.

Sinha DJ, Jandial UA, Jaiswal N, Singh UP, Goel S, Singh O. Comparative evaluation of the effect of different disinfecting agents on bond strength of composite resin to dentin using two-step self-etch and etch and rinse bonding systems: An in-vitro study. *J Conserv Dent* 2018;21(4):424-427.

Siqueira FSF, Hilgemberg B, Araujo LCR, Hass V, Bandeca MC, Reis A, Gomes JC, Cardenas AFM, Loguercio AD. Effect of phosphoric acid containing mmp-inactivator on the properties of resin bonding to eroded dentin. *J Adhes Dent* 2019;21(2):149-158.

Srinivasulu S, Vidhya S, Sujatha M, Mahalaxmi S. Effect of collagen cross-linkers on the shear bond strength of a self-etch adhesive system to deep dentin. *J Conserv Dent* 2013;16(2):135-8.

Srinivasulu S, Vidhya S, Sujatha M, Mahalaxmi S. Shear bond strength of composite to deep dentin after treatment with two different collagen cross-linking agents at varying time intervals. *Oper Dent* 2012;37(5):485-91.

Subramonian R, Mathai V, Christaine Angelo JB, Ravi J. Effect of three different antioxidants on the shear bond strength of composite resin to bleached enamel: An in vitro study. *J Conserv Dent* 2015;18(2):144-8.

Tay FR, Pashley DH, Loushine RJ, Weller RN, Monticelli F, Osorio R. Self-etching adhesives increase collagenolytic activity in radicular dentin. *J Endod* 2006;32(9):862-868.

Tay FR, Smales RJ, Ngo H, Wei SH, Pashley DH. Effect of different conditioning protocols on adhesion of a GIC to dentin. *J Adhes Dent* 2001;3(2):153-67.

The American Academy of Cariology (AAC) https://aacariology.org/about/.

Tomczyk M, Wiater A, Pleszczyńska M. In vitro anticariogenic effects of aerial parts of Potentilla recta and its phytochemical profile. *Phytother Res* 2011;25(3):343-50.

Valones MA, Higino JS, Souza PR, Crovella S, Caldas AF Júnior, Carvalho AA. Dentifrice Containing Extract of Rosmarinus officinalis Linn.: An Antimicrobial Evaluation. *Braz Dent J* 2016;27(5):497-501.

Van Meerbeek B, De Muncj J, Yoshida Y, Inoue S, Vargas M, Vijay P, Van Landuyt K, Lambrechts P, Vanherle G. Buonocore memorial lecture. Adhesion to enamel and dentin: current status and future challenges. *Oper Dent* 2003;28(3):215-235.

Varma SR, Sherif H, Serafi A, Fanas SA, Desai V, Abuhijleh E, Al Radaidah A. The Antiplaque Efficacy of Two Herbal-Based Toothpastes: A Clinical Intervention. J *Int Soc Prev Community Dent* 2018;8(1):21-27.

Veis A, Schlueter RJ. The macromolecular organization of dentine matrix collagen. I. Characterization of dentin collagen. *Biochemistry* 1964;3:1650-1657.

Verma R, Singh UP, Tyagi SP, Nagpal R, Manuja N. Long-term bonding effectiveness of simplified etch-and-rinse adhesives to dentin after different surface pre-treatments. *J Conserv Dent* 2013;16(4):367-70.

Vidhya S, Srinivasulu S, Sujatha M, Mahalaxmi S. Effect of grape seed extract on the bond strength of bleached enamel. *Oper Dent* 2011;36(4):433-438.

Walter R, Miguez PA, Arnold RR, Pereira PN, Duarte WR, Yamauchi M. Effects of natural cross-linkers on the stability of dentin collagen and the inhibition of root caries in vitro. *Caries Res* 2008;42(4):263-268.

Wang Y, Chen C, Zang HL, Liang YH. The recovery effect of proanthocyanidin on microtensile bond strength to sodium hypochlorite-treated dentine. *Int Endod J* 2019;52(3):371-376.

Wang Y, Spencer P. Quantifying adhesive penetration in adhesive/dentin interface using confocal Raman microspectroscopy. *J Biomed Mater Res* 2002; 59(1):46-55.

Wiegand A, Gutsche M, Attin T. Effect of olive oil and an olive-oil-containing fluoridated mouthrinse on enamel and dentin erosion in vitro. *Acta Odontol Scand* 2007;65(6):357-61.

Xie Q, Bedran-Russo AK, Wu CD. In vitro remineralization effects of grape seed extract on artificial root caries. *J Dent* 2008;36(11):900-6.

Xu Y, Zhou J, Tan J. Use of grape seed extract for improving the shear bond strength of total-etching adhesive to bleached enamel. *Dent Mater J* 2018;37(2):325-331.

Yang H, Guo J, Deng D, Chen Z, Huang C. Effect of adjunctive application of epigallocatechin-3-gallate and ethanol-wet bonding on adhesive-dentin bonds. *J Dent* 2016;44:44-9.

Yen CC, Liu YT, Lin YJ, Yang YC, Chen CC, Yao HT, Chen HW, Lii CK. Bioavailability of the diterpenoid 14-deoxy-11,12-didehydroandrographolide in rats and up-regulation of hepatic drug-metabolizing enzyme and drug transporter expression. *Phytomedicine* 2019;61:152841.

Yu HH, Zhang L, Xu S, Li F, Yu F, Liu ZY, Huang L, Chen JH. Effects of Epigallocatechin-3-gallate (EGCG) on the bond strength of fiber posts to Sodium hypochlorite (NaOCl) treated intraradicular dentin. *Sci Rep* 2017b;7(1):4235.

Yu HH, Zhang L, Yu F, Li F, Liu ZY, Chen JH. Epigallocatechin-3-gallate and Epigallocatechin-3-O-(3-O-methyl)-gallate Enhance the Bonding Stability of an Etch-and-Rinse Adhesive to Dentin. *Materials (Basel)* 2017a;10(2).

Zhang L, Xue J, Li J, Zou L, Hao Y, Zhou X, Li W. Effects of Galla chinensis on inhibition of demineralization of regular bovine enamel or enamel disposed of organic matrix. *Arch Oral Biol* 2009;54(9):817-22.

Zhang M, Wang J, Zhu L, Li T, Jiang W, Zhou J, Peng W, Wu C. Zanthoxylum bungeanum Maxim. (Rutaceae): A Systematic Review of Its Traditional Uses, Botany, Phytochemistry, Pharmacology, Pharmacokinetics, and Toxicology. *Int J Mol Sci* 2017;18(10).

Zhou J, Chiba A, Scheffel DL, Hebling J, Agee K, Tagami J, Tan J, Abuelenain D, Nawareg MA, Hassan AH, Breschi L, Tay FR, Pashley DH. Cross-linked dry bonding: A new etch-and-rinse technique. *Dent Mater* 2016;32(9):1124-32.

Zou L, Zhang L, Li J, Hao Y, Cheng L, Li W, Zhou X. Effect of Galla chinensis extract and chemical fractions on demineralization of bovine enamel in vitro. *J Dent* 2008;36(12):999-1004.

In: Contemporary Use of Plant Extracts … ISBN: 978-1-53617-650-6
Editor: C. R. Emerenciano Bueno

Chapter 5

PHYTOTHERAPY IN ENDODONTICS

Francine Benetti[1,2,*], Alexandre Henrique dos Reis-Prado[1], Gabriel Pereira Nunes[2], Leopoldo Cosme-Silva[3], Luciano Tavares Angelo Cintra[2], Eloi Dezan Junior[2] and Carlos Roberto Emerenciano Bueno[2]

[1]Department of Restorative Dentistry, Federal University of Minas Gerais (UFMG), School of Dentistry, Belo Horizonte, Minas Gerais, Brazil

[2]Department of Endodontics, São Paulo State University (UNESP), Araçatuba School of Dentistry, Araçatuba, São Paulo, Brazil

[3]Department of Restorative Dentistry, Faculty of Dentistry, Federal University of Alagoas (UFAL), Maceió, Alagoas, Brazil

ABSTRACT

Studies of the herbal therapies applicability in dentistry field increase prevention and treatment of several diseases. The natural products show anti-inflammatory, antioxidant, and antimicrobial properties. According

[*] Corresponding Author's Email: francine-benetti@ufmg.br.

to the World Health Organization, phytotherapy is the use of herbal substances with therapeutic values, involving minimal or no industrial processing. Some endodontic materials may cause defects on the dentin and/or being an irritant to the tissues, besides of limited antimicrobial effectiveness. The herbal alternatives can prevent adverse effects of synthetic drugs as toxicity and microbial resistance. In addition, herbal products include cost-effectiveness, increase quality of life, nutritional values, easy availability and increased service life.

This chapter will present studies of the several herbal alternatives with different potential in endodontic applications: irrigating solutions, intracanal medication, addition in endodontic sealer and for repair materials, and other applications.

Keywords: bioactive materials, dentin, enamel, remineralization, teeth hard tissues

1. The Use of Phytotherapy in Dentistry

Currently, investigations in dentistry have been increasing in search of herbal therapies, as well as their applicability for prevention, control and treatment of diseases. The use of natural products through extracts is closely related to their properties such as anti-inflammatory, antioxidant, antimicrobial and especially low cytotoxic potential (Gunjan Kumar et al. 2013, Seal et al. 2016).

Several studies report that herbal medicines present biological and pharmacological activities and also highlight the efficacy, safety and quality of these new agents (Calixto 2000, Groppo et al. 2008, Albano et al. 2013). Overall, the herbal dentistry has been applied as anti-inflammatories, analgesics, antibiotics, sedatives and, particularly, as irrigants and intracanal medication in endodontics. Natural products have been considered alternative or adjuvant in dentistry, and their choice is linked to the characteristics of botanically derived molecules, as they have more benefits and advantages over their synthetic derivatives, as a result of their natural evolution and decreased probability of resistance (Jeon et al. 2011).

Different studies have shown the effectiveness of natural products in controlling the oral cavity biofilm, as well as preventing disease or stagnating its evolution (Khan et al. 2009, Sun et al. 2016, Huang et al. 2017). Results have shown that the flavonoids present in pomegranate (*punic granatun*) juice have antibacterial action against etiologic pathogens of gingivitis, as well as pomegranate mouthwash was effective against periodontal microorganisms such as *A. actinomycetemcomitans*, *P. gingivalis* and *P. intermedica* (Prasad et al. 2014). In addition, the use of 10% pomegranate topical gel relieved the pain of recurrent aphthous stomatitis and reduced the time for complete healing of these (Ghalayani et al. 2013). To prove the effectiveness of herbal medicine use in periodontal treatment, a systematic review and updated meta-analysis concluded that local use of herbal medicine as an adjunct to conventional periodontal treatment may promote additional benefits in reducing periodontal disease (Moro et al. 2018).

Cariology is the area of dentistry that relentlessly seeks the prevention of the dental caries. The use of herbal medicines in the mouthwash as a preventive auxiliary of caries has also shown promising results. *Triphala*, a basic element of Ayurvedic medicine, when added to the mouthwash has been shown to have significant anti-caries activity, enabling a similar comparison to chlorhexidine, especially highlighting its advantages of not promote teeth discoloration and having a lower cost (Tandon et al. 2010), as well as *Aloe vera* and propolis phytotherapics showed potentials as disinfectants in cavity after minimally invasive excavation of the dental caries. Prabhakar et al. (2015) in a randomized clinical study reported that there was a significant reduction in bacterial counts after cavity disinfection with these natural products. Similarly, Fani & Kohanteb (2012) suggested that optimal concentration of *A. vera* in a gel vehicle could be used as an antiseptic to prevent dental caries and periodontal disease.

In relation to their sedative and anxiolytic applicability, herbal medicines are used in surgical procedures, especially in third molar extractions (Gonçalves & França, 2007). In the literature it is reported the use of compounds extracted from the plants *Melissa officinalis*

(*Lamiaceae*), *Valeriana officinalis* (*Valerianaceae*), *Passiflora incarnata* (*Passifloraceae*) and *Piper methysticum* (*Piperaceae*) (Groppo et al. 2008). Pinheiro et al. (2014) evaluated the efficacy of *Valeriana officinalis L.* in controlling anxiety during surgery found that patients remained more relaxed during the operation and that the use of a single oral dose of 100 mg of valerian had a greater effect on maintaining controlled systolic blood pressure and heart rate after surgery. Likewise, Farah et al. (2019) observed that valerian provided the necessary comfort and relaxation without sedation and less drowsiness than benzodiazepine midazolam during molar extraction.

Futhermore, the inflammatory process is always an inconvenience of the treatment in dental procedures and the control of the exacerbated inflammatory response is made by the use of drugs that tend to cause allergic reactions or make the healing process postoperative difficult. Thus, phytotherapy has also been used to contain inflammation (Dioguardi et al. 2019). Mayouf et al. (2019) confirmed that *Asphoelus microcarpus* extract has anti-inflammatory and antioxidant properties. The anti-inflammatory power and antioxidant capacity of this plant make it a potential weapon for reducing risk factors for acute and chronic inflammatory diseases (local inflammation in the course of stomatitis or acute and chronic periapical endodontic lesions). This study was conducted in animal model (rats and mice) and showed significant results in the second phase of the inflammatory process (3 to 6 h), with similar effect to a non-steroidal anti-inflammatory drug. Likewise, when the methanolic extract of the medicinal plant *Plumeria acuminata* was tested in models of acute and chronic inflammation developed in rats, its anti-inflammatory activity similar to indomethacin was noted in the two phases analyzed (Gupta et al. 2006). Regarding the inflammatory process in the pulp tissue, Sabir et al. (2005) when analyzed propolis in inflamed dental pulp of rats, observed that the use of this flavonoid has the potential to stimulate tertiary dentin and delay the inflammatory reaction of the pulp tissue.

2. PHYTOTHERAPY IN ENDODONTICS

In ancient history, people searched for drugs in nature to heal from diseases. As a result of lack of information and scientific evidence, everything was based on experience. The Sumerian clay tablet from Nagpur has been one of the oldest evidence of medicinal plants' as drugs (Petrovska et al. 2012). According to the World Health Organization, phyththerapy is defined as the use of herbal substances with therapeutic values, involving minimal or no industrial processing (Tilburt & Kaptchuk 2008). Around 85% of global population relies on medical treatments based on phytotherapy, and approximately 25% of the medicines are derived from plants (Machado et al. 2012).

For thousands of years, natural products have been applied into dental practice and have become even more popular today due to their high biocompatibility, antimicrobial and anti-inflammatory properties (Oncag et al. 2006). Microorganisms have been associated in the literature as the major cause of endodontic infections and failure of primary treatment. Anatomically complex the root canal system facilitates the proliferations of these microbes. For this reason, the rationale for endodontic therapy is to eradicate the infection and to prevent reinfection of root and/or periapical area by biomechanical preparation (Akpata 1976, Haapasalo et al. 2010, Kandaswamy et al. 2010, Narayanan & Vaishnavi 2010).

Some conventional endodontic materials may be connected with some defects on the dentin and/or being an irritant to the periradicular tissues. Moreover, limited antimicrobial effectiveness of these substances may be related to difficulty in penetration to the most peripheral areas of the root-canal system.

Then, researchers have been looking for herbal alternatives to prevent side effects of synthetic drugs as toxicity and microbial resistance. Other advantages include cost-effectiveness, increase quality of life, nutritional values, easy availability and increased service life (Parle & Bansal 2006, Prabhakar et al. 2010, Pujar & Makandar 2011). This chapter will offer a review of several herbal alternatives with different potential of endodontic applications.

2.1. Irrigating Solutions Derived from Phytotherapic Medicine

The existence of remaining bacteria in the root canal system may affect the outcome of the endodontic therapy (Lopes & Siqueira 2015). For many years, several chemical substances have been used in endodontics as an adjunct to increase the antimicrobial effect during cleaning and shaping phase (Prabhakar et al. 2010). The most commonly irrigant used in the root canal preparation is sodium hypochlorite (NaOCl) in concentrations ranging from 0.5 to 6%. Other examples of conventional intracanal solutions are chlorhexidine digluconate (CHX), MTAD (Dentsply Tulsa Dental, Tulsa, OK, USA) and Ethylenediaminetetraacetic acid (EDTA).

Irrigation has also a role in dissolving organic tissues, helping to remove debris and reducing instrument friction during mechanical preparation (Siqueira & Rôças 2008, Hargreaves & Cohen 2011). Despite of these benefits, some traditional irrigating solutions also have some cytotoxicity potential and they may be related to pain episodes and injuries to the periapical tissues. As a result of these clinical and biological problems, herbal compounds have been preferred as an alternative of irrigating substances (Agrawal et al. 2016, Aydin et al. 2018).

2.1.1. Morinda Citrifolia

Morinda citrifolia is a traditional medicinal plant discovered in Polynesia. Commercially namely as Noni, it has been used for over 2000 years (Murray et al. 2008, Neelakantan et al. 2011). Noni is a tree distributed throughout the warm areas of the Pacific (Levand & Larson 1979). It is also identified as Nono or Nonu, Indian Mulberry, Ba Ji Tian, Cheese Fruit and Nhan in different cultures around the world (Agrawal et al. 2016).

Its juice (MCJ) has been reported to have a broad spectrum of nutritional and therapeutic values. Researches on the use of different solvent extracts of Noni identified antibacterial, anti-inflammatory and antifungal properties (Sunder et al. 2011). According to Podar et al. (2015), MCJ appears to be the first herbal solution identified as a possible natural alternative to NaOCl.

Some components having antibacterial properties of *M. citrifolia* are scopoletin, octoanoic acid, potassium, vitamin C, terpenoids, alkaloids, anthraquinones, G-sitosterol, carotene, linoleic acid, caproic acid, vitamin A, flavone glycosides, Alizarin, amino acids, acubin, L-asperuloside, caprylic acid, ursolic acid, rutin, and a putative proxeronine (Neelakantan et al. 2011).

In a study conducted by Sunder et al. (2011), two components extracted from the Noni's fruit and leaves vary in their efficacy in controlling Ralstonia solancearum growth; the results from the chloroform extracted from the leaf were found better than the acetone extracts. When compared to CHX, *M. citrifolia* showed lesser antibacterial activity against *E. faecalis*, but none of these solutions had any effect on micro-hardness of root dentin (Prabhakar et al. 2013). Another *in vitro* survey compared the effectiveness of MCJ, NaOCl and CHX in conjunction with EDTA in removing the smear layer from instrumented root canals. The efficiency of *M. citrifolia* was similar to NaOCl with EDTA (Murray et al. 2008).

2.1.2. Propolis

Propolis or bee glue is a natural substance collected by bees (*Apis mellifera L.*) from various plants and mixed with wax and other materials. Its chemical composition varies with the plant species, seasonality, food availability, luminosity, collector type and altitude (Koru et al. 2007, Agrawal et al. 2016). Due to immunomodulation, anti-inflammatory and antibacterial activity (Hu et al. 2005), different studies involving propolis have been developed in dentistry. The literature describes effective antibacterial and antifungal compounds of Propolis against *Actinomyces naeslundii*, *Fusobacterium nucleatum*, *Lactobacillus acidophilus*, *Peptostreptococcus anaerobius*, *Prevotella oralis*, *Prevotella melaninogenica*, *Porphyromonas gingivalis*, *Veillonella parvula*, *S. aureus*, *E. coli* and *C. Albicans* (Kujumgiev et al. 1999, Koru et al. 2007).

Flavonoids and cinnamic acid derivatives have been considered as the main pharmacological active components (Neelakantan et al. 2011). The inhibition of topoisomerase enzyme by propolis avoids DNA damage in the human cells (Montoro et al. 2012). However, when used in high concentrations can be linked to cytotoxic and genotoxic activity on the human lymphocytes due to hydrogen peroxide produced (Tsai et al. 2012).

Cytotoxicity and oxidative DNA damage of propolis, chitosan and NaOCl were evaluated on the fibroblast cell line (Aydin et al. 2018). The authors stated that chitosan and propolis are more reliable in terms of biocompatibility than NaOCl. A comparative evaluation on microbial efficacy of propolis, NaOCl and saline solution when used as intracanal irrigants indicated that the propolis has antimicrobial activity similar to that of NaOCl (Agrawal et al. 2016).

Kandaswamy et al. (2010) investigated the antimicrobial activity of 2% CHX gel, propolis, MCJ, 2% povidone iodine, and calcium hydroxide on *E. faecalis*. The results demonstrated a superior inhibition of *E. faecalis* by propolis and MCJ over calcium hydroxide. Nevertheless, another laboratory study found no effective antibacterial activity of propolis against *E. faecalis* compared to 3% NaOCl and 0.2% CHX (Gupta et al. 2007). Thus, it is important to develop more *in vitro* and *in vivo* studies to provide more information about its real effectiveness.

2.1.3. Triphala, Green Tea Polyphenols and Tumeric

Triphala is an Indian ayurvedic herbal formulation. It is derived from the fruits of three medicinal plants namely *Terminalia Bellerica*, *Terminalia Chebula*, and *Emblica Officinalis*. While, green tea polyphenols (GTP) is a popular drink in Japan and China, which comes from tea plant *Camellia sinensis*. Polyphenolic compounds from the leaves of tea plant have antioxidant effect in the human plasma and act against various microorganisms (Dou 2009, Agrawal et al. 2016), preventing the formation of biofilm (Vishnuvardhini et al. 2018).

An experimental survey evaluated the antibacterial efficacy of *Triphala*, green tea polyphenols, MTDA, GTP and 5% NaOCl against *E. faecalis* biofilm. According to the results, *Triphala*, GTP and MTDA reduced substantively the biofilm after 6-week (Prabhakar et al. 2010).

Another phytotherapic component is tumeric or curcumin. It is a typical herb from India, China and South East Asia. Tumeric, also known as *Curcuma longa*, it is a rhizomatous herbaceous perennial plant from the ginger family (Priyadarsini 2014). Diferuloylmethane, the main natural polyphenol of the curcumin's rhizome, has antioxidant, anti-inflammatory, antimutagenic and antimicrobial functions (Neelakantan et al. 2013). Its active components also include curcuminoids, tumerone, atlantone and zingiberone (Vishnuvardhini et al. 2018).

When associated with photodynamic therapy, aqueous preparation of tumeric reveals a toxic effect against gram-positive and gram-negative bacteria (Haukvik et al. 2010). Neelakantan et al. (2013) observed an eradication of *E. faecalis* biofilm when using 3% NaOCl and *Curcuma longa*. Thus, tumeric can be applied as an interesting alternative of irrigant and intracanal medicament.

2.1.4. Neen and King of Bitter

Neen or *Azadirachta indica* is a medicinal tree. It is commonly called as Nin, "Indian neem/Margosa tree" or "Indian lilac". Several portions of the plant are used to obtain more than 140 compounds, as the isoprenoid group of neem leaf. It appears to have immune modulatory, antimicrobial antioxidant, and anti-carcinogenic characteristics (Podar et al. 2015). A study evaluated the disinfection of dentinal tubules using *Azadirachta indica*, propolis, 2% CHX gel and calcium hydroxide against *Candida albicans*, and reveled similar antifungal efficacy of *A. indica*, propolis and 2% CHX. Moreover, a study conducted by Rosaline et al. (2013) proved that Neen is effective in preventing adhesion of *E. faecalis* to dentin. Also, when compared to 5.25% NaOCl, Neen leaf extract has outstanding activity against *E. faecalis* and *C. albicans* (Vinothkumar et al. 2013). These findings confirm the notable potential of its bioactive compounds as an endodontic irrigant.

Another herbal medicine with a similar property is *Andrographis paniculata*. It is an annual herbaceous plant typical in southern Asia. *A. paniculata* is also known as "king of bitter" or Bhui-neem ("neem of the ground"). This specie is a strong stimulator of the immune system and it is effective against a large range of infections, involving bacteria and viruses (Dedhia et al. 2018). Its most significant antimicrobial compounds are diterpenoids and flavonoids (Rajalakshmi & Cathrine 2016). Dedhia et al.

(2018) observed higher inhibition of *C. albicans* and similar antibacterial effect against *S. aureus* when compared to NaOCl.

2.1.5. Tea Tree Oil and Aloe Vera

Melaleuca alternifolia or Tea tree is a native Australian plant. It presents mild solvent action, being useful for dissolving necrotic pulp tissue (Neelakantan et al. 2011). Its main antimicrobial component is terpinen-4-ol (typically 30–40%) (Parle & Bansal 2006). An *in vitro* comparison among Tea tree oil, 3% NaOCl and 2% CHX against *E. faecalis* found maximum antibacterial action of CHX, followed by tea tree oil and NaOCl (Kamath et al. 2013). This observation represents the divergence in the literature between those standard irrigants.

One of the oldest medicinal plants is *Aloe vera* (*Aloe barbadenis*). It has been applied for management of many infections (Jain et al. 2016), as a result of its active ingredients Aloin and aloe-emodin (Vishnuvardhini et al. 2018). As an example, various studies have been shown a significant antimicrobial activity against various species such as *Streptococcus pyogen*, *E. faecalis*, *Candida albicans* and *Staphylococcus aureus* (Sahebi et al. 2014). Different researches have been developed to determine the efficacy of *Aloe vera* in killing microorganisms. For instance, evaluation of effectiveness in decontaminating gutta-percha cones (Athiban et al. 2012) and as a natural solution activated with passive ultrasonic irrigation (Bhardwaj et al. 2013). However, the latter established that 1% NaOCl was more effective in removing *E. faecalis* biofilm compared to natural irrigants (Aloe Vera, MCJ and Propolis).

2.1.6. Aroeira-Da-Praia, Quixabeira and German Chamomile

Aroeira-da-praia and *Quixabeira* are native species from South America. An *in vitro* study developed in Brazil by Costa et al. (2012), accessed both antimicrobial and root canal cleaning potential of *Aroeira-da-praia*, *Quixabeira*, 2.5% NaOCl and 0.12% CHX. Although *Quixabeira* demonstrated the highest efficiency in removing the smear layer in the apical third, none was able to totally remove it from the dentinal surface.

Futhermore, all solutions demonstrated antimicrobial activity against *E. faecalis*.

Besides *Aroeira-da-praia* and *Quixabeira*, *German chamomile* (*Marticaria recutita L.*) is native plant from Europe and Western Asia. It has been used as a medicinal herb because of its anti-inflammatory, antimicrobial and sedative activities from chemical compounds of the chamomile's flower (Sadr Lahijani et al. 2006). When compared the cleaning efficacy of chamomile hydroalcoholic extract, tea tree oil and 2.5% NaOCl, Sadr Lahijani et al. (2006) concluded that the capability of chamomile to remove smear layer was superior to NaOCl without EDTA.

2.1.7. Salvadora Persica, Syzigium Aromaticum, Garlic

Salvadora persica, popularly known as Miswak or Meswak, has a wide geographic distribution. Its roots and trunk have been used for oral hygiene, including the root canal cleaning. Studies have proved its antimicrobial effect agains *Candida albicans*, *Streptococcus sp.*, *Staphylococcus aureus* and *E. faecalis* (Halawany 2012). Al-Sabawi et al. (2007) compared the antibacterial effect of alcoholic extract of *Salvadora persica* with 5.25% NaOCl, 0.2% CHX and saline solution. The results exhibited similar action among the irrigants.

Oils like eugenol, isoeugenol and vanillin are derived from *Syzigium aromaticum* (clove). These compounds have antioxidant and antibacterial effects (Vishnuvardhini et al. 2018). When applied to the endodontic therapy, some authors stated that *Syzigium aromaticum* along EDTA was the most successful in removing smear layer compared to other natural irrigants like *Ocimum sanctum* and *Cinnamum zeylanicum*.

It is documented the historical use of garlic (*Allium sativum*) to treat infections by Louis Pasteur (Reuter et al. 1996), especially in reason of large spectrum of inhibitory effect against gram-positive and gram-negative bacteria (Birring et al. 2015). Allicin, active metabolite for garlic extract (Vishnuvardhini et al. 2018), is able to destroy the cell wall and plasma membrane of the bacteria, turning this bulbous plant into a promising alternative to NaOCl (Agrawal et al. 2016). Two studies have been evaluated the antimicrobial potential of garlic extract against *E.*

faecalis. The first revealed that 70% concentration of garlic extract exhibited equal effectiveness of 5.25% NaOCl (Birring et al. 2015). The other investigation found complete inhibition of *E. faecalis* between groups 5.25% NaOCl and 2% CHX, whereas garlic and cinnanom resulted in lower inhibition compared to those groups (Gopalakrishnan et al. 2014). When related to the ability to allow debris evacuation along root canals, *A. sativum* had lower removal capacity compared to NaOCl and EDTA. In addition, dentin integrity was maintained but not statistically significant between groups (Prabhakaran & Mariswamy 2018).

2.1.8. Other Herbal Extracts

Nutmeg, *Liquorice*, *Myrtus Communis*, *Spilanthes Calva DC*, and *Jieeryin* solution have been also briefly described in the literature as natural alternatives for root canals irrigation and disinfection. Antibacterial effect of *Nutmeg* or *Myristica fragrans* has been correlated to its element myristic acid (Agrawal et al. 2016). Moreover, some researchers indicate that *Glycyrrhiza glabra* or *liquorice* (flavouring and sweetening agent) has important antimicrobial, anti-adherence and anti-inflammatory properties. When compared the cytotoxic effect of *liquorice* and *Triphala* on human fibroblasts and its antibacterial efficacy against *E. faecalis*, Satti et al. (2019) do not noticed any toxicity. On the other side, *Triphala* provided the highest antimicrobial activity among all irrigants, including NaOCl.

Myrtus communis is a small tree, which is distributed around tropical regions, cultivated mainly in Iran. The oil extracted from the plant has demonstrated antimicrobial activity against persistent endodontic microorganisms, such as *E. faecalis*, *S. aureus* and *C. albicans* (Nabavizadeh et al. 2014). Furthermore, *Spilanthes* (medicinal herb from tropical areas) and *Jieeryin* (Chinese plant) have been known by its antifungal, anti-inflammatory and antibacterial property against *E. faecalis* (Dube et al. 2013, Vishnuvardhini et al. 2018). Ultrasonic root canal irrigation with 30% *Jieeryin* solution has an equal cleaning effect to NaOCl (Wang et al. 2006).

2.2. Phytotherapic Medicine as Intracanal Medication in Endodontics

When endodontic treatment cannot be completed in one session, intracanal dressing is used between therapy sessions, after root canal preparation, to eliminate and inhibit the proliferation of microorganisms (Hargreaves & Cohen 2011). Natural biocomponents with antimicrobial activity on endodontic microbiota have been also investigated as intracanal medication. Some examples are described below.

2.2.1. Articum Lappa and Propolis

Arctium lappa is an herbaceous plant with many therapeutic applications due to its antimicrobial, antioxidative, antiplatelet, diuretic and anxiolytic effects (Vishnuvardhini et al. 2018). It has been brought from Japan to be grown in Brazil. When it was applied as an intracanal medicament, its main agent extracted was able to inhibit microbial proliferation better than calcium hydroxide (Gentil et al. 2006).

Propolis is known mainly by its antibacterial, antifungal and anti-inflammatory action. Caffeic acid phenethyl ester (CAPE) is an active ingredient of propolis (Ang et al. 2009). CAPE is capable of inhibiting the activation of nuclear factor kappa B, reducing cyclooxygenase-2 expression and may inhibit osteoclast differentiation through increased release of osteoprotegerin (Yuanita et al. 2019). Then, bone resorption is supressing in favor of ethanolic preparation of propolis.

2.2.2. Lemon Solution, Garlic and Agaricus Bisporus

Lemon solution has a lower pH, acting as a chelating agent to the dentin and it is wide efficient against *E. faecalis* when used as intracanal medication (Vishnuvardhini et al. 2018). Recent studies have investigated the efficacy of garlic as an endodontic irrigant in reducing *E. faecalis* proliferation in the root canal. In contrast, a study using real-time polymerase chain reaction (RT-PCR) analyzed the efficacy of garlic extract as an intracanal dressing with 2% CHX and calcium hydroxide and reported maximum efficacy of garlic compared to calcium hydroxide in disinfecting dentinal tubules (Eswar et al. 2013).

Another herbal medicament is *Agaricus bisporus*, popularly known as mushroom. *A. bisporus* is known by its antiviral, antioxidant, anti-inflammatory and antimicrobial potential against gram-positive bacteria (Kurian et al. 2016). Its active compounds are plectasin, confuentin, grifolin and neogrifolin (Alves et al. 2012). These low molecular weight components have the ability to penetrate deeply in the dentinal tubules, being applied as an intracanal dressing in the gel form. The preparation of the gel involves sun drying, grinding and boiling with distilled water, followed by adding hydroxyl ethyl cellulose as thickening agent in 2:1 ratio and injected with a syringe (Vishnuvardhini et al. 2018). A laboratory study comparing the antibacterial activity of mushroom, *Aloe vera* and calcium hydroxide against *E. faecalis* observed better results provided by mushroom extract at all experimental periods.

2.2.3. Psidium Cattleianum and Myracrodruon Urundeuva

Psidium cattleianum is typical in the American continent and it is well-known as "araçá-do-campo" or "araçá comum". The leaf extract has demonstrated biocompatibility and antibacterial property against *S. mutans* (Brighenti et al. 2008, Ruviére et al. 2008). Flavonoids (kaempferol, quercetin, and cyanidin) and ellagic acid (tannin) from phenolic compounds of *P. cattleianum* are considered its bioactive ingredients (Valentim et al. 2017). When the leaf extracts are associated with another medicament as calcium hydroxide, it is capable of producing similar tissue response over time (Valentim et al. 2017).

Ethanolic Leaf extracts of *P. cattleianum* was also investigated, *in vitro*, against *Enterococcus faecalis* and *Candida albicans* biofilm. The extracts were associated with calcium hydroxide pastes as: *Psidium cattleianum* ethanolic, and *Psidium cattleianum* propylene glycolic vehicles, besides group calcium hydroxide with distilled water (positive control) and saline as negative control. While all medications were effective against *C. albicans*, the *P. cattleianum* ethanolic extract presented the fastest and highest antimicrobial activity against *E. faecalis*, significantly reducing the microbial load in 24 h (Sangalli et al. 2018).

Those results evidencing biological biocompatibility and potent antimicrobial activity indicates the *p. cattleianum* as a promising plant extract in the field of dentistry, especially in endodontics.

Myracrodruon urundeuva or "aroeira-do-sertão" is a native tree from South America. The aqueous and ethanolic leaf extracts of aroeira were described to offer analgesic and antimicrobial effects, also presenting an adequate tissue recovery (Machado et al. 2012, Bueno et al. 2018).

2.2.4. Allium Sativum

Oil of natural agents has also been tested directly on pulp tissue during pulpotomy. Mohammad et al. (2015) evaluated the histopathology effects of formocresol and *Allium sativum* oil during a pulpotomy procedure. Allicin and other thiosulfinates are considered to be in charge of therapeutic effects of garlic. The histologic examination showed inflammatory changes solved in the end of the study in the *Allium sativum* group, while formocresol caused severe chronic inflammation of dental pulp and presence of necrosis. The authors concluded that *Allium sativum* oil is a biocompatible material, which offers a good healing potential.

2.2.5. Proanthocyanidins (PACs)

Proanthocyanidins (PACs) also named condensed tannins, are the result of flavanols condensation and have been investigated in the areas of medical and nutritional health for various biological effects. They have a putative role as antioxidants, and they affect the inflammatory process via calcium-dependent release of nitric oxide and protect against $H_{(2)}O_{(2)}$-induced lipid peroxidation. Also, they are able to produce antiadhesive actions against *Streptococcus mutans* in dental infections (de la Iglesia et al. 2010).

Grape seed extract has been preferred as a source of PACs, with a concentration of 95% of PACs. In this view, grape seed extracts were used to evaluate biostimulatory effects on a primary culture of human molars pulp cells. Treatment with grape seed extract, even at the highest concentration and longest period, caused neither direct nor transdentinal cytotoxic effects on human pulp cells. When in direct contact, grape seed extract may play a biostimulatory role, increasing cell metabolism and collagen synthesis and protect dental pulp cells (dos Santos et al. 2019).

In order to assess antimicrobial properties, PACs has been analyzed *in vitro* showing antibacterial capacity against *E. faecalis* using agar diffusion test. Authors tested PACs derived from neem leaf extracts and grape seed extracts. Neem leaf extracts and grape seed extracts showed zones of inhibition indicating anti-microbial properties. Neem leaf extracts showed significantly greater zones of inhibition than 3% sodium hypochlorite. Grape seed extracts showed zones of inhibition but were not as significant as of neem extracts (Ghonmode et al. 2013).

2.3. Phytotherapics in Endodontic Sealer and Repair Material

In Endodontics, there are disagreements regarding the selection of the ideal repair material. It is known that the required properties of these agents are: biocompatibility, antimicrobial activity, easy handling, prevention of micro leaks, and induction of mineralized tissue formation (Song et al. 2017).

Conservative techniques, such as pulpotomy, have been applied in some cases to preserve the remaining vital portion of the pulp tissue exposed by dental caries or trauma in the deciduous or primary teeth. Various materials have been proposed for capping the radicular pulp after pulpotomy. For example, formocresol, glutaraldehyde, calcium hydroxide and mineral trioxide aggregate (MTA). However, cytotoxicity, carcinogenicity, mutagenic and teratogenic changes possibly caused by some materials have been a concern. In this regard, natural medicaments have been studied as alternative pulpotomy agents, such as garlic, also providing economic benefits.

Studies have shown its efficacy after pulpotomy procedure, by avoiding the occurrence of clinical symptoms of pain and mobility, providing a healing ability and leading to tertiary dentin formation (Gala-

García et al. 2008, Gupta et al. 2010). These results are attributed to the several bioactive substances such as glycoprotein, polysaccharides and beta-sitosterol in the stimulation of injury healing, cell proliferation, and growth of blood vessels (Kalra et al. 2017). *Aloe vera* has 75 potentially active compounds such as vitamins, minerals, enzymes, sugars, anthraquinones, hormones, fatty acids and other substances. Moreover, propolis has been described in the literature for exhibit mild or no pulp inflammation compared to traditional repair materials, as MTA (Parolia et al. 2010, Ozório et al. 2012, Balata et al. 2018). Propolis contains flavonoids and caffeic acids which are effective in inhibiting the lipoxygenase pathway of arachidonic acid and promoting phagocytic activities and stimulating cellular immunity (Balata et al. 2018).

Propolis also has been identified in a systematic review as an appropriate material for use in endodontics (Olsson et al. 2006). Analyzing their characteristics and biological responses, Ahangari et al. (2012b) provided evidence in their study that propolis has more beneficial effects than calcium hydroxide in pulp capping therapy for vital teeth.

Besides not causing an inflammatory process, infection or induction of pulp necrosis, the propolis stimulated the deposition of a high quality tubular dentin. In addition, propolis reduces pulp sensitivity, mainly due to the obliteration of dentinal tubules through its good adhesion, as well as its effect in minimizing the pulp inflammation (Ahangari et al. 2018).

As a promising ethnopharmaceutical, propolis has shown potent antimicrobial and anti-inflammatory properties. Propolis has been shown to inhibit prostaglandin synthesis and stimulate the immune system by acting on phagocytic activities, increasing cellular immunity and enhancing therapeutic effects (Ghoddusi et al. 2014). In addition, it can induce formation of transforming growth factor (TGF)-$\beta 1$, which is important for the differentiation of odontoblasts (Ansorge et al. 2003) and can synthesize collagen via pulp cells, mainly because in its composition there are some ions (especially zinc and iron) which are helpers in favoring collagen synthesis (Al-Shaher et al. 2004). A study demonstrated that the pulp response to propolis was comparable to MTA and better than calcium hydroxide (Parolia et al. 2010). The advantages of this material over calcium hydroxide have also been confirmed by Ahangari et al. (2012b). However, to come to a definitive conclusion on these materials, further research is needed, such as randomized controlled clinical trials.

In addition, the use of MTA is also recommended in pulpotomy, due to its excellent biocompatibility, dentin bonding property, satisfactory sealing, and induction of biomineralization (Torabinejad et al. 1997). However, this material has exhibited handling difficulties, extended setting time and possibility of washout (Duarte et al. 2012).

The material used in this endodontic intervention also should be bactericidal, harmless to radicular pulp and surrounding tissues, besides to promote pulp healing and not interfere with the normal physiological process of root resorption (Ohkura et al. 2017, Lopes et al. 2019).

There is an interest regarding the medicinal plants, considering that they may not have any detrimental effect on adjacent living tissues.

However, Kalra et al. (2017) compared the clinical and radiographic results of fresh *Aloe barbadensis* extract and MTA as materials in pulpotomy of primary molars, and found that MTA allowed better success rate compared to fresh extract of *A. barbadensis*, that in this study has unfavorable agent for pulpotomy.

Nevertheless, due to the potent virulence factor of microorganisms and progression of endodontic infections, there is also a need for repair material an optimal antimicrobial property (Kogan et al. 2006). Thus, Cavenago et al. (2017) added extracts from the herbal medications of *Arctium lappa L.* and *Casearia sylvestris Sw* to the MTA and found that all extracts increased the antimicrobial effect of MTA after 24 hours, but only *Casearia sylvestris* extracts significantly reduced bacterial viability after 168 hours.

In addition, the effects of *Aloe Vera* on the physicochemical properties of MTA and Portland cement were evaluated by Borges et al. (2017) concluding that the materials in association with this plant are compliant with American National Standards Institute (ANSI)/American Dental Association (ADA) requirements, except Portland cement that did not showed radiopacity specifications. Moreover, this study also found that the material with *Aloe Vera* was easier to handle, already highlighted as a water-soluble vehicle with viscosity characteristics, which could favor its use in clinical. However, it is not yet known whether the use of *Aloe Vera* as a vehicle would interfere in biological properties of the MTA. Thus, further studies are needed to analyze the biocompatibility, antimicrobial/antibiofilm effect, besides sealing ability of MTA associated with *Aloe Vera*, before any recommendation for clinical use. When mixed with aqueous or propylene glycol extracts of *Arctium lappa L.* and *Casearia sylvestris*, white MTA showed significantly increase of the final setting time and propylene glycol extracts provide higher flowability to MTA, causing changes in the physicochemical properties (Cavenago et al. 2017).

The antimicrobial effect of a calcium hydroxide-based sealer, due to its high pH and release of hydroxyl ions, is well known, but has the disadvantage of low effect on *E. faecalis* biofilms that may result in endodontic treatment failure (Nair et al. 2018). Therefore, Saha et al. (2019) evaluated three herbal extracts (*Glycyrrhiza glabra*, *Tinospora cordifolia* and *Mimusops elengi*) added to three endodontic sealers (eugenol zinc oxide-based sealer, epoxy resin-based sealer and calcium hydroxide-based sealer). The study found that eugenol zinc oxide-based sealer with herbal extracts produced the largest inhibitory zones followed by epoxy resin-based sealer and calcium hydroxide-based sealer with three herbal extracts. The outcomes of this study also anticipated the fact that calcium hydroxide-based endodontic sealer used in combination with the three herbal extracts showed minimal antimicrobial efficacy compared to other tested combinations. This may be explained by not sufficient release of hydroxyl ions to inhibit the growth of microorganisms.

In addition, according to authors, artificial media have a buffer capacity that can provide a reduction in the high pH of calcium hydroxide, making it less effective. In clinical situations, the buffer action of blood and tissue fluid can cause the same effects. However, a limitation of the study is that the efficacy of the extracts was analyzed in a short period of time. In addition, the quantitative analysis of extracts, associated with their qualitative screening, would help elucidate the active principles responsible for the antimicrobial effect. Further studies should be conducted to explore the antimicrobial effectiveness of endodontic materials with herbal extracts for a longer period of time.

3. How Phytotherapics Can Favor Bone Regeneration in Apical Surgery

Apical surgery is used when it is not possible to remove the etiological agent with conventional endodontic treatment, in an attempt to maintain the tooth. The goals of apical surgery are removing inflamed periapical tissue and all pathology, to improve cleaning, shaping and sealing of the apical portion of the root canal (Von Arx et al. 2007). In conventional endodontic treatment, the final phase of treatment consists in filling the root canal system and the space previously occupied by the pulp tissue, promoting the closure of the apical foramen through the deposition of mineralized tissue. In apical surgery, the stimulation of deposition of mineralized tissue also is required.

One of the main clinical concerns in teeth requiring apical surgery is root resorption and periapical bone loss. Normally the calcium hydroxide is used to prevent root resorption, but a study showed that calcium hydroxide is significantly more toxic than propolis (Tronstad et al. 1988).

Regarding bone regeneration, there are no studies that directly evaluate the use of herbal medicines in apical surgery, however, studies evaluated the applicability of natural products in regeneration of bone. Ahangari et al. (2012a) evaluated the effect of propolis in formation and activation of osteoclast cell, and showed that propolis effectively reduces bone loss. In addition, propolis reduced the number of giant cells and positive cells for tartrate resistant acid phosphatase (TRAP), with an inhibitory effect on the early stage of osteoclastogenesis. Propolis also increased osteoprotegerin expression and decreased the number of osteoclasts (Yuanita et al. 2018).

In addition, it has been shown that the caffeic acid phenethyl ester (CAPE), which is an active compound of propolis, has the ability to inhibit osteoclastic activity by suppressing nuclear factor kappa B (Ahangari et al.

2013). This is a product of the cyclooxygenase pathway and is activated in osteoclastogenesis.

A study by Sousa (2010) evaluating *Chenopodium ambrosioides L.*, known as Mastruz, suggested that its extract favored the repair process of reimplanted teeth, reducing polymorphonuclear inflammatory infiltrate, abscess and periodontal ligament necrosis, in addition to stimulate fibroblast proliferation and osteogenesis (Sérvio et al. 2011). The mechanism of action of this herbal drug probably occurs at the cellular level, activating osteoblasts and inhibiting osteoclast activity (Soares et al. 2015).

Although these studies have evaluated the process of bone healing or prevention of bone loss with the use of natural plant extract, there is still a need for standardized studies, especially to directly evaluate the use of herbal medicines in apical surgery.

REFERENCES

Agrawal, V; Kapoor, S; Agrawal, I. Critical Review on Eliminating Endodontic Dental Infections Using Herbal Products. *J Diet Suppl*, 2016, 14(2), 229–40.

Ahangari, Z; Mashhadiabbas, F; Kashefinejad, M; Mansouri, Y. Effect of Propolis on Osteoclasts. 7th *IADR Iranian Division Annual Meeting Tehran*, 2012a.

Ahangari, Z; Mashhadiabbas, F; Kashefinejad, M; Miri, S; tofighi-darian, M. The inhibitory effect of propolis on osteoclast maturation. *Health Med*, 2013, 7(11), 2913–7.

Ahangari, Z; Naseri, M; Vatandoos, F. Propolis: Chemical Composition and Its Applications in Endodontics. *Iran Endod J*, 2018, 13(3), 285–92.

Ahangari, Z; Naseri, M; Jalili, M; Mansouri, Y; Mashhadiabbas, F; Torkaman, A. Effect of Propolis on Dentin Regeneration and the Potential Role of Dental Pulp Stem Cell in Guinea Pigs. *Cell J*, 2012b, 13(4), 223–8.

Akpata, ES. Effect of endodontic procedures on the population of viable microorganisms in the infected root canal. *J Endod*, 1976, 2(12), 369–73.

Al-Sabawi, NA; Al Sheikh, AK; Taha, MY. The antimicrobial activity of salvadora persica solutions (Miswak-Siwak) as root canal irrigant (A comparative study). *J Pure Appl Sci*, 2007, 4, 69-91.

Al-Shaher, A; Wallace, J; Agarwal, S; Bretz, W; Baugh, D. Effect of propolis on human fibroblasts from the pulp and periodontal ligament. *J Endod*, 2004, 30(5), 359–61.

Albano, MN; da Silveira, MR; Danielski, LG; et al. Anti-inflammatory and antioxidant properties of hydroalcoholic crude extract from Casearia sylvestris Sw. (Salicaceae). *J Ethnopharm*, 2013, 147, 612-7.

Alves, MJ; Ferreira, IC; Dias, J; Teixeira, V; Martins, A; Pintado, M. A review on antimicrobial activity of mushroom (Basidiomycetes) extracts and isolated compounds. *Planta Med*, 2012, 78, 1707.

Ang, ES; Pavlos, NJ; Chai, LY; Qi, M; Cheng, TS; Steer, JH; Joyce, DA; Zheng, MH; Xu, J. Caffeic acid phenethyl ester, an active component of honeybee propolis attenuates osteoclastogenesis and bone resorption via the suppression of RANKL-induced NF-kappaB and NFAT activity. *J Cell Physiol*, 2009, 221(3), 642-9.

Ansorge, S; Reinhold, D; Lendeckel, U. Propolis and some of its constituents down-regulate DNA synthesis and inflammatory cytokine production but induce TGF-beta1 production of human immune cells. *Z Naturforsch C*, 2003, 58(7-8), 580–9.

Athiban, PP; Borthakur, BJ; Ganesan, S; Swathika, B. Evaluation of antimicrobial efficacy of Aloe vera and its effectiveness in decontaminating gutta percha cones. *J Conserv Dent*, 2012, 15(3), 246–8.

Aydin, ZU; Akpinar, KE; Hepokur, C; Erdönmez, D. Assessment of toxicity and oxidative DNA damage of sodium hypochlorite, chitosan and propolis on fibroblast cells. *Braz Oral Res*, 2018, 32(8), 1-8.

Balata, GF; Abdelhady, MIS; Mahmoud, GM; Matar, MA; Abd El-Latif, AN. Formulation of Saudi Propolis into Biodegradable Chitosan Chips for Vital Pulpotomy. *Curr Drug Deliv*, 2018, 15(1), 97-109.

Bhardwaj, A; Velmurugan, N; Sumitha, Ballal S. Efficacy of passive ultrasonic irrigation with natural irrigants (*Morinda citrifolia* juice, *Aloe vera* and Propolis) incomparison with 1% sodium hypoclorite for removal of *E. faecalis* biofilm: An *in vitro* study. *Indian J Dent*, 2013, 24, 35-41.

Birring, OJ; Viloria, IL; Nunez, P. Anti-microbial efficacy of Allium sativum extract against Enterococcus faecalis biofilm and its penetration into the root dentin: An *in vitro* study. *Indian J Dent Res*, 2015, 26, 477-82.

Borges, HA; Guedes, OA; Volpato, LER; Filho, GS; Borba, AM; Zina, O; Piva, E; Estrela, C. Physicochemical Properties of MTA and Portland Cement after Addition of Aloe Vera. *Iran Endod J*, 2017, 12(3), 312–7.

Brighenti, FL; Luppens, SB; Delbem, AC; Deng, DM; Hoogenkamp, MA; Gaetti-Jardim Junior, E; et al. Effect of Psidium cattleianum leaf extract on Streptococcus mutans viability, protein expression and acid production. *Caries Res*, 2008, 42(2), 148-54.

Bueno, CRE; Valentim, D; Jardim Junior, EG; Mancuso, DN; Sivieri-Araujo, G; Jacinto, RC; Cintra, LTA; Dezan-Junior, E. Tissue reaction to Aroeira (*Myracrodruon urundeuva*) extracts associated with microorganisms: an *in vivo* study. *Braz Oral Res*, 2018, 32, 1-9.

Calixto, JB. Efficacy, safety, quality control, marketing and regulatory guidelines for herbal medicines (phytotherapeutic agents). *Braz J Med Biol Res*, 2000, 33, 179–89.

Cavenago, BC; Carpio-Perochena, AE; Ordinola-Zapata, R; Estrela, C; Garlet, GP; Tanomaru-Filho, M; Weckwerth, PH; Andrade, FB; Duarte, MAH. Effect of Using Different Vehicles on the Physicochemical, Antimicrobial, and Biological Properties of White Mineral Trioxide Aggregate. *J Endod*, 2017, 43(5), 779-86.

Costa, EM; Evangelista, AP; Medeiros, AC; Dametto, FR; Carvalho, RA. *In vitro* evaluation of the root canal cleaning ability of plant extracts and their antimicrobial action. *Braz Oral Res*, 2012, 26(3), 215-21.

de la Iglesia, R; Milagro, FI; Campión, J; Boqué, N; Martínez, JA. Healthy properties of proanthocyanidins. *Biofactors*, 2010, 36(3), 159-68.

Dedhia, J; Mukharjee, E; Luke, AM; Mathew, S; Pawar, AM. Efficacy of Andrographis paniculata compared to Azadirachta indica, Curcuma longa, and sodium hypochlorite when used as root canal irrigants against Candida albicans and Staphylococcus aureus: An *in vitro* antimicrobial study. *J Conserv Dent*, 2018, 21, 642-5.

Dioguardi, M; Campanella, P; Cocco, A; Arena, C; Malagnino, G; Sovereto, D; Aiuto, Laino RL; Laneve, E; Dioguardi, A; Zhurakivska, K; Muzio, KL. Possible Uses of Plants of the Genus *Asphodelus* in Oral Medicine. *Biomedicines*, 2019, 7(3), 67.

dos Santos, AF; Pacheco, JM; Silva, PAO; Bedran- Russo, AK; Rezende, TMB; Pereira, PNR; Ribeiro, APD. Direct and transdentinal biostimulatory effects of grape seed extract rich in proanthocyanidin on pulp cells. *Int Endod J*, 2019, 52, 424-38.

Dou, QP. Molecular Mechanisms of Green Tea Polyphenols. *Nutr Cancer*, 2009, 61(6), 827–35.

Duarte, MA; Aguiar, KA; Zeferino, MA; Vivan, RR; Ordinola-Zapata, R; Tanomaru-Filho, M; Weckwerth, PH; Kuga, M. Evaluation of the propylene-glycol association on some physical and chemical properties of mineral trioxide aggregate. *Int Endod J*, 2012, 45(6), 565-70.

Duarte, MA; Demarchi, AC; Yamashita, JC; Kuga, MC; Fraga Sde, C. pH and calcium ion release of 2 root-end filling materials. *Oral Surg Oral Med Oral Pathol Oral Radiol Endod*, 2003, 95(3), 345–7.

Dube, M; et al. Comparative evaluation of antibacterial efficacy of spilanthes calva DC root extract, sodium hypochlorite, Chlorhexidine and doxycycline at different concentrations on *Enterococcus faecalis*: an in-vitro study. *Endodontol*, 2013, 25(1), 63–72.

Eswar, K; Venkateshbabu, N; Rajeswari, K; Kandaswamy, D. Dentinal tubule disinfection with 2% chlorhexidine, garlic extract, and calcium hydroxide against Enterococcus faecalis by using real-time polymerase chain reaction: *In vitro* study. *J Conserv Dent*, 2013, 16(3), 194-8.

Fani, M; Kohanteb, J. Inhibitory activity of *Aloe vera* gel on some clinically isolated cariogenic and periodontopathic bacteria. *J Oral Sci*, 2012, 54, 15–21.

Farah, GJ; Ferreira, GZ; Danieletto-Zanna, CF; Luppi, CR; Jacomacci, WP. Assessment of Valeriana officinalis l. (Valerian) for Conscious Sedation of Patients During the Extraction of Impacted Mandibular Third Molars: A Randomized, Split-Mouth, Double-Blind, Crossover Study. *J Oral Maxillofac Surg*, 2019, 77(9), 1796.e1-1796.e8.

Gala-García, A; Teixeira, KIR; Mendes, LL; Sobrinho, APR; Santos, VR; Cortes, ME. Effect of Aloe vera. on Rat Pulp Tissue. *Pharm Biol*, 2008, 46(5), 302–8.

Gentil, M; Pereira, JV; Sousa, YTCS; Pietro, R; Neto, MDS; Vansan, LP; Castro França, S. *In vitro* evaluation of the antibacterial activity ofArctium lappa as a phytotherapeutic agent used in intracanal dressings. *Phytother Res*, 2006, 20(3), 184–6.

Ghalayani, P; Zolfaghary, B; Farhad, AR; Tavangar, A; Soleymani, B. *J Res Pharm Pract*, 2013, 2(2), 88-92.

Ghoddusi, J; Forghani, M; Parisay, I. New Approaches in Vital Pulp Therapy in Permanent Teeth. *Iran Endod J*, 2014, 9(1), 15–22.

Ghonmode, WN; Balsaraf, OD; Tambe, VH; Saujanya, KP; Patil, AK; Kakde DD. Comparison of the antibacterial efficiency of neem leaf extracts, grape seed extracts and 3% sodium hypochlorite against *E. feacalis* - An *in vitro* study. *J Int Oral Health*, 2013, 5(6), 61-6.

Gonçalves, EC; França, FM. Evaluation of the use of homeophatic anxiolytic in dental surgical procedures as alternative drugs to the benzodiazepinics. *Rev Gaúcha Odontol.*, 2007, 55, 175–80.

Gopalakrishnan, S; Rajesh, S; Jotish, R. A comparative evaluation of antimicrobial efficacy of cinnamon and garlic as endodontic irrigants against Enterococcus faecalis-an *in vitro* study. *Endodontol*, 2014, 26(1), 149–57.

Groppo, FC; Bergamaschi, CDEC; Cogo, K; Franz-Montan, M; Motta, RH; de Andrade, ED. Use of phytotherapy in dentistry. *Phytother Res*, 2008, 22(8), 993-8.

Gunjan, Kumar; Md. Jalaluddin; Purnendu, Rout; Rajat, Mohanty; Dileep, CL. Emerging Trends of Herbal Care in Dentistry. *J Clin Diagn Res*, 2013, 7(8), 1827–9.

Gupta, M; Mazumder, UK; Gomathi, P; Selvan, VT. Antiinflammatory evaluation of leaves of Plumeria acuminata. *BMC Complement Altern Med*, 2006, 2, 6–36.

Gupta, N; Bhat, M; Devi, Girish P. Aloe-Vera: A Nature's Gift to Children. *Int J Clin Pediatr Dent*, 2010, 3(2), 87-92.

Gupta, S; Kundabala, M; Acharya, SR; Ballal, V. A Comparative evaluation of antibacterial efficacy of propolis. 3% Sodium Hypochlorite and 2% Chlorhexidine Gluconate against E. Faecalis; An *in vitro* study. *Endodontol*, 2007, 19(2), 31-8.

Haapasalo, M; Shen, Y; Qian, W; Gao, Y. Irrigation in Endodontics. *Dent Clin N Am*, 2010, 54 (2), 291–312.

Halawany, HS. A review on miswak (*Salvadora persica*) and its effect on various aspects of oral health. *Saudi Dent J*, 2012, 24(2), 63–9.

Hargreaves, KM; Cohen, S. Caminhos da Polpa [Pathways of the pulp] 10th ed. Rio de Janeiro: Elsevier 2011, 212-64.

Haukvik, T; Bruzeli, E; Kristensen, S; Tønnesen, H. Photo killing of bacteria by curcumin in selected polyethylene glycol 400 (PEG 400) preparations. Stud Curcumin and Curcuminoids, XLI. *Die Pharm*, 2010, 65, 600-6.

Hu, F; Hepburn, HR; Li, Y; Chen, M; Radloff, SE; Daya, S. Effects of ethanol and water extracts of propolis (bee glue) on acute inflammatory animal models. *J Ethnopharmacol*, 2005, 100, 276-83.

Huang, X; Zhang, K; Deng, M; et al. Effect of arginine on the growth and bioflm formation of oral bacteria. *Arch Oral Biol*, 2017, (82), 256–26.

Jain, S; Rathod, N; Nagi, R; Sur, J; Laheji, A; Gupta, N; Agrawal, P; Prasad, S. Antibacterial Effect of Aloe Vera Gel against Oral Pathogens: An *In-vitro* Study. *J Clin Diagn Res*, 2016, 10(11), ZC41–4.

Jeon, JG; Rosalen, PL; Falsetta, ML; Koo, H. Natural products in caries research: current (limited) knowledge, challenges and future perspective. *Caries Res*, 2011, (45)3, 243–63.

Kalra, M; Garg, N; Rallan, M; Pathivada, L; Yeluri, R. Comparative Evaluation of Fresh *Aloe barbadensis* Plant Extract and Mineral

Trioxide Aggregate as Pulpotomy Agents in Primary Molars: A 12-month Follow-up Study. *Contemp Clin Dent*, 2017, 8(1), 106–11.

Kamath, U; Sheth, H; Ramesh, S; Singla, K. Comparison of the antibacterial efficacy of tea tree oil with 3% sodium hypochlorite and 2% chlorhexidineagainst E. faecalis: An *in vitro* study. *J Contem Dent*, 2013, 3(3), 117–20.

Kandaswamy, D; Venkateshbabu, N; Gogulnath, D; Kindo, AJ. Dentinal tubule disinfection with 2% chlorexidine gel, propolis, Morinda citrifolia juice, 2% povidine iodine and calcium hydroxide. *Int Endod J*, 2010, 43, 419-423.

Khan, R; Islam, B; Akram, M; Shakil, S; Ahmad, A; Ali, SMa. Antimicrobial activity of five herbal extracts against multi drug resistant (MDR) strains of bacteria and fungus of clinical origin. *Molecules*, 2009, 14, 586–97.

Kogan, P; He, J; Glickman, GN; et al. The effects of various additives on setting properties of MTA. *J Endod*, 2006, 32, 569-72.

Koru, O; Toksoy, F; Acikel, CH; Tunca, YM; Baysallar, M; Uskudar Guclu, A; Akca, E; Ozkok Tuylu, A; Sorkun, K; Tanyuksel, M; Salih, B. *In vitro* antimicrobial activity of propolis samples from different geographical origins against certain oral pathogens. *Anaerobe*, 2007, 13(3-4), 140-5.

Kujumgiev, A; Tsvetkova, I; Serkedjieva, Y; Bankova, V; Christov, R; Popov, S. Antibacterial, antifungal and antiviral activity of propolis of different geographic origin. *J Ethnopharmacol*, 1999, 64(3), 235-40.

Kurian, B; Swapna, DV; Nadig, RR; Ranjini, MA; Rashmi, K; Bolar, SR. Efficacy of calcium hydroxide, mushroom, and Aloe vera as an intracanal medicament against Enterococcus faecalis: An *in vitro* study. *Endodontol*, 2016, 28, 137-42.

Levand, O; Larson, HO. Some chemical constituents of *Morinda citrifolia. Planta Med*, 1979, 36(2), 186-7.

Lopes, CS; Junqueira, MA; Cosme-Silva, L; Pegoraro, CAR; Garbelini, CCD; Oliveira, TM; Martins, NS; Neves, JS; Sakai, VT. Initial inflammatory response after the pulpotomy of rat molars with MTA or ferric sulfate. *J Appl Oral Sci*, 2019, 27, e20180550.

Lopes, HP; Siqueira, JF. Endodontia, Biologia e Técnica [Endodontics: Biology and Technique] 4th ed. Rio de Janeiro: Elsevier, 2015, 848 p.

Machado, AC; Dezan Junior, E; Gomes-Filho, JE; Cintra, LT; Ruviére, DB; Zoccal, R; et al. Evaluation of tissue reaction to Aroeira (*Myracrodruon urundeuva*) extracts: a histologic and edemogenic study. *J Appl Oral Sci*, 2012 Jul-Aug, 20(4), 414-8.

Mayouf, N; Charef, N; Saoudi, S; Baghiani, A; Khennouf, S; Arrar, L. Antioxidant and anti-inflammatory effect of asphodelus microcarpus methanolic extracts. *J Ethnopharmacol*, 2019, 239, 111914.

Mohammad, SG; Raheel, SA; Baroudi, K. Histological Evaluation of Allium sativum Oil as a New Medicament for Pulp Treatment of Permanent Teeth. *J Contemp Dent Pract*, 2015, 16(2), 85-90.

Montoro, A; Soriano, JM; Barquinero, JF; Almonacid, M; Montoro, A; Verdú, G; et al. Assessment *in vitro* of cytogenetic and genotoxic effects of propolis on human lymphocytes. *Food Chem Toxicol*, 2012, 50(2), 216-21.

Moro, MG; Silveira Souto, ML; Franco, GCN; Holzhausen, M; Pannuti, CM. Efficacy of local phytotherapy in the nonsurgical treatment of periodontal disease: A systematic review. *J Periodontal Res*, 2018, (3), 288-97.

Murray, PE; Farber, RM; Namerow, KN; Kuttler, S; Garcia Godoy, F. Evaluation of Morinda citrofolia as an endodontic irrigant. *J Endod*, 2008, 34, 66-70.

Nabavizadeh, M; Abbaszadegan, A; Gholami, A; Sheikhiani, R; Shokouhi, M; Shams, MS; Ghasemi, Y. Chemical constituent and antimicrobial effect of essential oil from Myrtus communis leaves on microorganisms involved in persistent endodontic infection compared to two common endodontic irrigants: An *in vitro* study. *J Conserv Dent*, 2014, 17, 449-53.

Nair, N; James, B; Devadathan, A; Minimol, JK; Mathew, J; Jacob, J. Comparative Evaluation of Antibiofilm Efficacy of Chitosan Nanoparticle- and Zinc Oxide Nanoparticle-Incorporated Calcium Hydroxide-Based Sealer: An *In vitro* Study. *Contemp Clin Dent*, 2018, 9(3), 434–9.

Narayanan, L; Vaishnavi, C. Endodontic microbiology. *J Conserv Dent*, 2010, 13(4), 233-9.

Neelakantan, P; Jagannathan, N; Nazar, N. Ethnopharmacological approach in Endodontic Treatment: A Focused Review. *Int J Drug Dev & Res*, 2011, 3(4), 68-77.

Neelakantan, P; Subbarao, C; Sharma, S; Subbarao, CV; Garcia-Godoy, F; Gutmann, JL. Effectiveness of curcumin against Enterococcus faecalis biofilm. *Acta Odontol Scand*, 2013, 71(6), 1453–7.

Ohkura, N; Edanami, N; Takeuchi, R; Tohma, A; Ohkura, M; Yoshiba, Kunihiko Yoshiba N; Ida-Yonemochi, H; Ohshima, H; Okiji, T; Noiri, Y. Effects of pulpotomy using mineral trioxide aggregate on prostaglandin transporter and receptors in rat molars. *Sci Rep*, 2017, 7, 6870.

Olsson, H; Petersson, K; Rohlin, M. Formation of a hard tissue barrier after pulp cappings in humans. A systematic review. *Int Endod J*, 2006, 39(6), 429-42.

Oncag, O; Cogulu, D; Uzel, A; Sorkun, K. Efficacy of propolis as an intracanal medicament against *Enterococcus faecalis*. *Gen Dent*, 2006, 54(5), 319-22.

Ozório, JE; Carvalho, LF; de Oliveira, DA; de Sousa-Neto, MD; Perez, DE. Standardized propolis extract and calcium hydroxide as pulpotomy agents in primary pig teeth. *J Dent Child*, 2012, 79(2), 53-8.

Parle, M; Bansal, N. Herbal Medicine: Are they safe? *Natural Product Radiance*, 2006, 5(1), 6-14.

Parolia, A; Kundabala, M; Rao, NN; Acharia, SR; Agrawal, P. A comparative histological analysis of human pulp following direct pulp capping with propolis, mineral trioxide aggregate and Dycal. *Aust Dent J*, 2010, 55(1), 59-64.

Petrovska, BB. Historical review of medicinal plants' usage. *Pharmacogn Rev*, 2012, 6(11), 1-5.

Pinheiro, ML; Alcântara, CE; de Moraes, M; de Andrade, ED. Valeriana *officinalis* L. for conscious sedation of patients submitted to impacted lower third molar surgery: A randomized, double-blind, placebo-controlled split-mouth study. *J Pharm Bioallied Sci*, 2014, 6(2), 109-14.

Podar, R; Kulkarni, GP; Dadu, SS; Singh, S; Singh, SH. *In vivo* antimicrobial efficacy of 6% Morinda citrifolia, Azadirachta indica, and 3% sodium hypochlorite as root canal irrigants. *Eur J Dent*, 2015, 9, 529-34.

Prabhakar, AR; Basavraj, P; Basappa, N. Comparative evaluation of Morinda citrifolia with Chlorhexidine as antimicrobial endodontic irrigants and their effect on micro-hardness of root canal dentin: an *in vitro* study. *Int J Oral Health Sci*, 2013, 3(1), 5-8.

Prabhakar, AR; Karuna, YM; Yavagal, C; Deepak, BM. Cavity disinfection in minimally invasive dentistry - comparative evaluation of *Aloe vera* and propolis: A randomized clinical trial. *Contemp Clin Dent*, 2015, 6, 24–31.

Prabhakar, J; Senthikumar, M; Priya, MS; et al. Evaluation of antimicrobial efficacy of herbal alternatives (triphala and green tea polyphenols), MTAD, and 5% sodium hypochlorite against Enterococcus faecalis biofilm formed on tooth substrate: An *in vitro* study. *J Endod*, 2010, 36, 83–6.

Prabhakaran, P; Mariswamy, AB. A scanning electron microscope evaluation of efficacy of sodium hypochlorite and Allium sativum in smear layer removal in root canals with the use of modified evacuation system: An ex vivo study. *J Conserv Dent*, 2018, 21, 401-7.

Prasad, D; Kunnaiah, R. Punica granatum: A review on its potential role in treating periodontal disease. *J Indian Soc Periodontol*, 2014, 18, 428–32

Priyadarsini, KI. The chemistry of curcumin: From extraction to therapeutic agent. *Molecules*, 2014, 19, 20091–112.

Pujar, M; Makandar, S. Herbal usage in endodontics-a review. *Int J Contemp Dent*, 2011, 2(1), 34–7.

Rajalakshmi, V; Cathrine, L. Phytochemical screening and antimicrobial activity of ethanolic extract of Andrographis paniculata. *J Pharmacogn Phytochem*, 2016, 5, 175.

Reuter, HD; Koch, HP; Lawson, LD. Garlic: The science and therepeutic applications of *Allium sativum L.* and related species. In: Koch HP, Lawson LD (editors). 2nd ed. Maryland: Williams & Wilkins, 1996, 135–212.

Rosaline, H; Kandaswamy, D; Gogulnath, D; Rubin, M. Influence of various herbal irrigants as a final rinse on the adherence of Enterococcus faecalis by fluorescence confocal laser scanning microscope. *J Conserv Dent*, 2013, 16(4), 352-5.

Ruviére, DB; Machado, AC; Novais, RZ; Gaetti Jardim-Junior, E; Dezan Junior, E. Evaluation of the tissue response to inactivated microorganisms associated with aqueous and hydroalcoholic araça (Psidium cattleianum) solutions. *J Appl Oral Sci*, 2008, 432.

Sabir, A; Tabbu, CR; Agustiono, P; Sosroseno, W. Histological analysis of rat dental pulp tissue capped with propolis. *J Oral Sci*, 2005, 47, 135–8.

Sadr Lahijani, MS; Raoof Kateb, HR; Heady, R; Yazdani, D. The effect of German chamomile (Marticaria recutita L.) extract and tea tree (Melaleuca alternifolia L.) oil used as irrigants on removal of smear layer: a scanning electron microscopy study. *Int Endod J*, 2006, 39(3), 190-5.

Saha, S; Dhinsa, G; Ghoshal, U; Afzal Hussain, ANF; Nag, S; Garg, A. Influence of plant extracts mixed with endodontic sealers on the growth of oral pathogens in root canal: an *in vitro* study. *J Indian Soc Pedod Prev Dent*, 2019, 37(1), 39-45.

Sahebi, S; Khosravifar, N; SedighShamsi, M; Motamedifarc, M. Comparison of the Antibacterial Effect of Sodium Hypochlorite and Aloe Vera Solutions as Root Canal Irrigants in Human Extracted Teeth Contaminated with *Enterococcus Faecalis*. *J Dent (Shiraz)*, 2014, 15(1), 39–43.

Sangalli, J; Júnior, EGJ; Bueno, CRE; et al. Antimicrobial activity of *Psidium cattleianum* associated with calcium hydroxide against *Enterococcus faecalis* and *Candida albicans*: an in *vitro study*. *Clin Oral Investig*, 2018, 22(6), 2273–79.

Satti, P; Kakarla, P; Jogendra Avula, SS; Muppa, R; Kiran Rompicharla, SV; Biswas, S. Indigenous irrigants as potent antimicrobials in endodontic treatment: An *in vitro* study. *J Indian Soc Pedod Prev Dent*, 2019, 37, 275-81.

Seal, M; Rishi, R; Satish, G; Divya, KT; Talukdar, P; Maniyar, R. Herbal panacea: The need for today in dentistry. *J Int Soc Prev Community Dent*, 2016, 6(2), 105-9.

Sérvio, EML; Araujo, KS; Nascimento, LRS; Costa, CLS; Mendes, LMS; Filho, ALMM. Wound healing using *Chenopodium ambrosioides* (mastruz) extract and sterile secondary coverage in rats. *ConScientiae S*, 2011, 10, 441-8.

Siqueira, JF; Rôças, IN. Clinical implications and microbiology of bacterial persistence after treatment procedures. *J Endod*, 2008, 34(11), 1291-301.

Soares, CD; Carvalho, MG; Carvalho, RA; Trindade, SR; Rêgo, A C; Araújo-Filho, I; Marques, M. Chenopodium ambrosioides L. extract prevents bone loss. *Acta Cirur Bras*, 2015, 30, 812– 8.

Song, M; Yu, B; Kim, S; Hayashi, M; Smith, C; Sohn, S; Kim, E; Lim, J; Stevenson, RG; Kim, RH. Clinical and Molecular Perspectives of Reparative Dentin Formation: Lessons Learned from Pulp-Capping Materials and the Emerging Roles of Calcium. *Dent Clin North Am*, 2017, 61(1), 93-110.

Sousa, JNL. Effect of topical administration of mastic (Schinus terebinthifolius Raddi) and of the mastruço (*Chenopodium ambrosioides* L.) in the repair process of reimplanted rat teeth. (dissertation). *Natal: Universidade Potiguar*, 2010.

Sun, M; Zhou, Z; Dong, J; Zhang, J; Xia, Y; Shu, R. Antibacterial and antibioflm activities of docosahexaenoic acid (DHA) and eicosapentaenoic acid (EPA) against periodontopathic bacteria. *Microb Pathogen*, 2016, (99), 196–203.

Sunder, J; Jeyakumar, S; Kundu, A; Srivastava, RC; Kumar, A. Effect of Morinda citrifolia extracts on *in-vitro* growth of Ralstonia solanacearum. *Schol Res Libr*, 2011, 3(3), 394-402.

Tandon, S; Gupta, K; Rao, S; Malagi, KJ. Effect of Triphala mouthwash on caries status. *Int J Ayurveda Res*, 2010, 1, 93–9.

Tilburt, J; Kaptchuk, T. WHO | Herbal medicine research and global health: an ethical analysis. 2008. (online) Who.int. Available at: https://www.who.int/bulletin/volumes/86/8/07-042820/en/ (Accessed 28 Sep. 2019).

Torabinejad, M; Pitt Ford, TR; McKendry, DJ; Abedi, HR; Miller, DA; Kariyawasam, SP. Histologic assessment of mineral trioxide aggregate as a root-end filling in monkeys. *J Endod*, 1997, 23, 225–8.

Tronstad, L. Root resorption—etiology, terminology and clinical manifestations. *Endod Dent Traumatol*, 1988, 4(6), 241–52.

Tsai, YC; Wang, YH; Liou, CC; Lin, YC; Huang, H; Liu, YC. Induction of oxidative DNA damage by flavonoids of propolis: its mechanism and implication about antioxidant capacity. *Chem Res Toxicol*, 2012, 25(1), 191-6.

Valentim, D; Bueno, CRE; Marques, VAS; Vasques, AMV; Cury, MTS; Cintra, LTA; Dezan-Junior, E. Calcium hydroxide associated with a new vehicle: *Psidium cattleianum* leaf extracts. Tissue response evaluation. *Braz. Oral Res*, 2017, 31, 1-8.

Vinothkumar, TS; Rubin, MI; Balaji, L; Kandaswamy, D. *In vitro* evaluation of five different herbal extracts as an antimicrobial endodontic irrigant using real time quantitative polymerase chain reaction. *J Conserv Dent*, 2013, 16(2), 167-70.

Vishnuvardhini, S; Sivakumar, A; Vaiyapuri, R; Prasad, AS; Sivakumar, JS. Herbendodontics – Phytotherapy In Endodontics: A Review. *Biomed Pharmacol J*, 2018, 11(2), 1073-82.

Von Arx, T; Jensen, SS; Hänni, S. Clinical and radiographic assessment of various predictors for healing outcome 1 year after periapical surgery. *J Endod*, 2007, 33, 123-8.

Wang, Q; Xiong, SJ; Lin, XJ; et al. Scanning electron microscopic study on the use of traditional Chinese medical irrigant in ultrasonic root canal instrumentation. *Shanghai Kou Qiang Yi Xue*, 2006, 15(1), 77–80.

Yuanita, T; Kunarti, S; Zubaidah, N. East java extract propolis as potential intracanal medicament in experimentally induced chronic apical periodontitis. *Indian J Dent Res*, 2019, 30, 342-6.

Yuanita, T; Zubaidah, N; Kunarti, S. Expression of Osteoprotegrin and Osteoclast Level in Chronic Apical Periodontitis Induced with East Java Propolis Extract. *Iran Endod J*, 2018, 13(1), 42b–6.

In: Contemporary Use of Plant Extracts … ISBN: 978-1-53617-650-6
Editor: C. R. Emerenciano Bueno

Chapter 6

PHYTOTHERAPY IN PERIODONTICS

Ana Maria Veiga Vasques[1,*],
Henrique Rinaldi Matheus[2],
David Jonathan Rodrigues Gusman[2,3],
Marina Tolomei Sandoval Cury[1],
Alexandre Henrique dos Reis-Prado[4],
Juliana Quintino Trizzi[1]
and Carlos Roberto Emerenciano Bueno[1]

[1]Department of Endodontics, São Paulo State University (UNESP), Araçatuba School of Dentistry, Araçatuba, SP, Brazil
[2]Department of Surgery and Integrated Clinic, Division of Periodontics, São Paulo State University (UNESP), Araçatuba School of Dentistry, Araçatuba SP, Brazil
[3]Department of Periodontics, Presidente Prudente Dental School, University of Western São Paulo (UNOESTE), Presidente Prudente, SP, Brazil
[4]Department of Restorative Dentistry, Federal University of Minas Gerais (UFMG), School of Denstitry, Belo Horizonte, Minas Gerais, Brazil

---

* Corresponding Author's Email: anavvasques@hotmail.com.

ABSTRACT

Periodontal diseases continue to be the most commonly occurring oral diseases in modern times. Plaque-induced gingivitis and periodontitis are caused by the penetration of pathogens from the bacterial plaque into the connective tissue, resulting in an inflammatory condition. Gingivitis affects the connective tissue of the gingiva, while periodontitis affects the entire periodontal apparatus. Many adjuvant therapeutic modalities have been tested for the treatment of these conditions. Among them, herbal therapies have shown anti-inflammatory, antioxidant and antimicrobial properties. These phytotherapic are incorporated into mouth rinses, dentifrices, chewing gums, adhesives, and gels in order to prevent and even treat gingivitis.

With respect to periodontitis, gels, chips and extracts containing herbs have provided many benefits when used as adjuvants to scaling and root planning. In addition, its benefits are also observed in wound healing following periodontal surgery. Hence, this chapter will present aspects of phytotherapy in periodontics.

Keywords: herbal medicine, gingivitis, plant extracts, periodontics

1. THE USE OF PHYTOTHERAPY IN PERIODONTICS

In order to understand the effects of any medicine over a disease, it is essential to know not only its pathogenesis but also their pristine features. The periodontium (peri = around, odontos = tooth) comprises the gingiva, the periodontal ligament, the root cementum, and the alveolar bone. Gingiva is named the masticatory mucosa which covers the alveolar process and surrounds the cervical portion of the teeth. The gingiva is characterized by coral pink, firm consistency and dull surface. Between teeth, the gingiva receives a particular denomination, the interdental gingiva or the interdental papillae, which may occupy the entire area below contact points. The periodontal ligament is the soft, richly vascular and cellular connective tissue that joints the teeth (root cementum) to the alveolus (socket wall). Root cementum is a specialized mineralized tissue covering the root surface and, occasionally, small portions of the crowns. It has many features in common with bone tissue, however, with no blood, lymph vessels or innervation. The alveolar process is described as the bony parts of the mandible and maxillae that form and support the sockets of the teeth. (Attström et al. 1975, Ainamo 1977).

The diseases affecting periodontal tissues can be didactically divided in two big groups, the ones strictly affecting the gingiva (gingivitis), and the ones affecting the entire periodontal apparatus (periodontitis). Plaque-induced gingivitis is an inflammatory condition of the gingiva resulting from bacteria located at the gingival margin. The trigger of this inflammation is due to a disbiotic environment, in which periodontopathogens penetrate the connective tissues and release virulence factors (e.g., Lipopolysaccharides, Lipoteichoic acid, enzymes that degrade collagen fibers) that will initiate the hosts' inflammatory response. The common clinical findings of plaque-induced gingivitis include erythema, edema, bleeding, sensitivity, tenderness and enlargement (Löe *et al.* 1965, Suzuki 1988).

Important knowledge has been updated by the American Academy of Periodontology and the European Federation of Periodontology (Caton et al. 2018). Among them, was stated that plaque-induced gingivitis is reversible. This means that after treatment, the architecture of the gingiva is completely restored (Murakami et al. 2018). On the other hand, non-treated plaque-induced gingivitis is likely to lead to periodontitis, a site-specific condition characterized by permanent and irreversible loss of the connective attachment and bone (Kinane et al. 2008, Pappapanou et al. 2018).

Bacterial plaque, the main etiologic factor of plaque-induced periodontal diseases, presents a columnar arrangement of morphologically distinct microorganisms. After initial supragingival accumulation, its apical progression creates an environment frequently distinguished by a zone of gram negatives and/or species with high mobility, adjacent to the pocket epithelium. Rods and gram-positive cocci compose a layer of microorganisms strongly adhered to the enamel and root surface (Listgarten 1994).

Once the periodontal pocket is arranged, the features of subgingival bacterial deposits become significantly more complex. Subgingival biofilm takes advantage of the additional protection consequential from its localization, because the periodontal tissues provide a protective scenario to supragingival threats. In periodontitis, the more apical biofilm reaches, the more virulent bacteria of Socransky's et al. 1998 complex are found (e.g., *Porphyromonas gingivalis*, *Tannerella forsythia* e *Treponema denticule*). Recent researches suggest the inclusion of *Dialister pneumosintes* to the group of periodontal pathogens, due to its high prevalence in advanced periodontal lesions and low prevalence in children and young with gingivitis (Contreras et al. 2000, Doan et al. 2000).

The only two tools that could limit subgingival biofilm's growth are small area and hosts' immune response (Ximénez-Fyvie et al. 2000). When not removed by daily oral care, bacterial place is susceptible to be mineralized by the salivary ionic compounds calcium and phosphate. Once mineralized, the mineral content of the calculus reaches, in average, about 37%. This structure was not capable to result in inflammation when sterile (Allen & Kerr 1965), indicating that calculus may be considered a retentive factor to microorganisms, the triggers to periodontal breakdown.

For the treatment of periodontal diseases with strict plaque, not calculus, the mechanical control with toothbrushes and dental floss, and chemical control mouth rinses are sufficient to revert gingivitis to health. When are observed mineralized deposits, patient control is not sufficient, and, then professional care is needed. These deposits are not always confined to the gingival margin, and when associated with increased probing depth and attachment loss (periodontitis), the reversibility of this condition is more challenging than in gingivitis.

Even the gold standard for the treatment of periodontitis being the removal of plaque and calculus through scaling and root planning (SRP) (Dentino et al. 2013), not always this therapeutic modality reaches the best results for all patients (Genco & Borgnake 2013, Lyons & Darby 2017). This may occur due to different reasons, since periodontitis represents a collection of complex diseases involving iterative interactions between the host inflammatory and immune systems, subgingival microbiota and modifying environmental factors (Bartold & Van Dyke 2017). Hence, based on this limitation, periodontal therapy can be performed combining SRP to adjuvant therapies aiming to enhance its positive effects.

Over the past decades, pharmaceutical companies have increased their interest in investigating plants as therapy for many conditions. Herbal medicine has shown to present the properties of been antioxidant, anti-inflammatory, antimicrobial, antiseptic, and anticollagenase features (Moro et al. 2018). Once periodontal diseases include an interaction between pathogenic microorganisms and hosts' immune and inflammatory responses, herbal medicine is capable to interact with this complex environment in a positive and effective manner.

2. Phytotherapy in Periodontics

One of the groups of medicines most studied in dentistry is the antimicrobials. Interestingly, 73% of the new antimicrobials approved by the US Food and Drug Administration are phytotherapic agents (Freires & Rosalen 2016). Phytotherapics are prepared with active principles from plants that have therapeutic benefits. The benefits of antimicrobial, antioxidant, antiseptic anti-inflammatory and anticollagenase properties were already reported (Balunas & Kinghorn 2005). Additionally, aiming to avoid systemic toxicity and prevent problems with patient compliance, the local application of phytotherapics may be an alternative to maximize its effects at the specific sites (Kumar et al. 2009).

Independent on methods of administration (local or systemic), the use of herbal drugs has been reported since ancient times in the treatment of several diseases, including gingivitis and periodontitis (Cragg & Newman 2013).

2.1. Phytotherapics for the Treatment of Gingivitis

2.1.1. Mouth Rinses

2.1.1.1. *Lippia sidoides*

Lippia sidoides is an herb natural from Northeastern Brazil, historically used by Indians of that region. Its camphorous leaves are used as antiseptics for the skin and mucosal surfaces, and also for the treatment of throat infections. The essential oil obtained from this phytotherapic is mainly composed of thymol, carvacrol and other substances such as felandrene, caryophyllene, p-cymene and mircene. (Botelho et al. 2007a, Lemos et al. 1990). Previous studies indicated that these compounds exhibit potent antimicrobial activity against fungi and bacteria (Botelho et al. 2007a, Lacoste et al. 1996, Lemos et al. 1990), including *Streptococcus mutans* (Botelho et al. 2007a).

The mouth rinse containing *Lippia sidoides'* oil was evaluated by Botelho et al. (2007b) and was observed that it reduced the plaque accumulation and gingival inflammation, reaching similar results of 0.12% Chlorhexidine. Even chlorhexidine being considered effective for plaque reduction, its daily use during home care is limited due to side effects (Flotra et al. 1971).

2.1.1.2. *Triphala*

Triphala is the combination of three extracts obtained from medicinal plants: *Terminalia bellerica*, *Terminalia chebula* e *Emblica officinalis*. It has an Ayurvédic Indian origin and is traditionally used for reduction in cholesterol, indigestion, hypertension and ulcerative colitis (Mukherjee et al. 2006).

Triphala's extract is widely used as mouth rinse against bacterial plaque, gingivitis, and caries (Bajaj et al. 2011). These positive effects may be explained by its antimicrobial effect over gram-positive and gram-negative microorganisms (Mehta et al. 1993), besides being antioxidant, anti-inflammatory, with a potent healing property (Baliga et al. 2012).

Patients with periodontal abscesses reported relief of the symptoms after using a *Triphala*-based mouth rinse (Maurya et al. 1997). While used and adjuvant therapy to scaling and root planning, this phytotherapic seems to improve periodontal indices when compared to mechanical treatment alone (Desai et al. 2010). Based on its beneficial effects, *Triphala*-based mouth rinse can be used as an alternative to chlorhexidine (Narayan et al. 2012).

2.1.1.3. *Punica granatum*

Punica granatum belongs to *Punicaceae's* family, popularly known as pomegranate (Salgado et al. 2006). Almost all compounds of this herb can be explored. The pericarp (peel) contains pulicalagins and flavonoids that exhibit antifungal and anti-inflammatory activities. Pomegranate's leaves show excellent antioxidant activity by the presence of tannin, punicaline, and punicafolin (Viuda-Martos et al. 2010). The flowers contain ursolic and asiatic acids, which present antioxidant and liver-protecting actions, and, therefore, are used for the treatment of diabetes (Bhandari et al. 2012, Saxena et al. 2004).

Pomegranate is capable to suppress the initial stages of periodontal diseases. The protein levels in saliva are higher in periodontitis patients and correlated to bacterial plaque formation. Narhi et al. (1994) conducted a study in which patients were submitted to daily use of a pomegranate-based mouth rinse and confirmed its plausible antimicrobial activity based on the reduction in the salivary levels of proteins. *In* vitro assessments have already shown the antimicrobial effects of flavonoids over microorganisms related to gingivitis, such as *Streptococcus sanguis* and *Streptococcus sobrinus*, similarly to chlorhexidine (Badria et al. 2004, Pereira et al. 2001, Pereira et al. 2006). A plausible explanation for this antimicrobial property are the tannins, that are capable to increase bacteriolysis, interfering on the mechanisms of bacterial adhesion to tooth surfaces (Pereira et al. 2001).

Punica granatum used after scaling and root planing significantly improved probing depths and clinical attachment levels when compared with mechanical debridement alone. *Punica granatum's* extract may present a synergic action over collagen stabilization due to tannin's affinity to proteins. Hence, this feature could improve collagen adhesion to the root surface (Sastravaha et al. 2003).

A recent investigation showed that a pomegranate-based mouth rinse was effective to eliminate important periodontopathogens (e.g., *Aggregatibacter actinomicetemcomitans*, *Porphyromonas gingivalis* e *Prevotella intermedia*) (Bhadbhade et al. 2011). Other formulations containing pomegranate, such as toothpaste and gels also presented positive effects on the treatment of gingivitis. (Salgado et al. 2006, Somu et al. 2012, Mazumdar et al. 2013).

2.1.1.4. Punica granatum var. pleniflora

Punica granatum var. pleniflora is a Persian herbal, named Golnaar in its native language. This phytotherapic is a subspecies of pomegranate, known as its male plant, that has the blooms with no fruit generation (Aghili 2013). In the Persian culture, vinegar is a famous vehicle for many pharmacologic compounds in traditional medicine (Jorjani 2001, Mortenson et al. 2012).

The combination of punica granatum var. pleniflora and vinegar is known as Golnaar mouthwash, a formula used to control gingivitis (Jorjani 2001). Sedigh-Rahimabadi et al. (2017) compared this mouthwash with chlorhexidine and concluded that the Persian combination is a safe and effective modality in treatment of gingivitis in diabetic patients and may be considered as a good alternative.

2.1.2. Dentifrice

2.1.2.1. *Scutellaria baicalensis*

Scutellaria baicalensis is a plant widely used in Chinese conventional medicines and is a part of the diet in China, Pajan, Korea, Russia and United States. Its roots are composed of innumerous chemical-bioactive substances. Among them, the flavanoids baicalein, baicalin, wogonin and acteoside have been reported with antimicrobial, anti-inflammatory, anti-allergic and diuretic activities (Bensky et al. 1986, Guo et al. 2009).

More recent findings showed some benefits of *S. baicalensis* as adjuvant therapy in prostate cancer, (Bemis et al. 2004, 2005), hepoatocellular carcinoma (Ye et al. 2009) and on the prevention of oral cancer (Yang et al. 2005).

Due to its promising features, the extract of *Scutellaria baicalensis* was incorporated to toothpastes in order to prevent and to treat gingivitis, with positive effects of reduction of plaque formation and gingival bleeding. When compared with conventional fluoride toothpaste, the plant-based dentifrice may be an efficient option for the treatment of gingivitis (Arweiler et al. 2011).

2.1.2.2. *Aloe vera*

Aloe vera is a succulent plant that belongs to the family *Aloeaceae* (subfamily *Asphodelaceae*) (Eggli et al. 2001). There are over 400 different species of *Aloe*, however, the *Aloe vera* is the most accepted specie for medical use (Grindlay et al. 1986). Its basic properties are anti-inflammatory (Kornman et al. 1993, Cobb et al. 1996), anti-ulcerative (McNabb et al. 1992, Hellstrom et al. 1996), and the capacity to improve wound healing (Yates et al. 1993, Nogueira-Filho et al. 2000, Lee et al. 2004).

The antimicrobial effect of the dentifrice containing *Aloe vera* was shown by and *in vitro* experiment in which this phytotherapic agent inhibited the growth of de *Streptococcus mutans*, *Streptococcus sanguis*, *Actinomyces viscosus* and *Candida albicans* (Lee et al. 2004).

Pradeep et al. (2012a) compared the dentifrice containing *Aloe vera* with a conventional triclosan-based dentifrice, observing that bot presented reduction of the gingival bleeding index and reduction on the overall number of microorganisms. De Oliveira et al. (2008) concluded that the *Aloe vera*-toothpaste and the conventional fluoride toothpaste significantly reduced the bacterial plaque and gingivitis.

Based on the literature on this topic, the preparations of herbal-based products remain popular, and the *Aloe vera* dentifrice may be useful to improve the periodontal status.

2.1.3. Chewing Gum

2.1.3.1. *Salvadora Persica*

Salvadora Persica is a plant commonly used in Middle East (Eid et al. 1994), known as Miswak (World Health Organization 1987). The World Health Organization recommends the chewing of stick of *Persica* (Miswak) to improve oral hygiene.

The chewing gum can be used as a vehicle for release of *Persica* extract and is related to benefits for gingival health, since this gum reduces the plaque accumulation (Simons et al. 1997, Smith et al. 1996). Also, *Persica's* extract contains substances with antimicrobial and prophylactic activities over bascteria related to caries and periodontal diseases (e.g., *Streptococcus mutans, Streptococcus salivarius, Staphylococcus aureus* and *anaerobia strepcococci*) (Eid et al. 1994, Al lafi et al. 1995, Khalessi et al. 2004, Almas et al. 2005, Sofrata et al. 2007).

The *Percica*-based gum has a slightly bitter, but not unpalatable, flavour (Lewis et al. 1980), which can increase the salivary flow and express an anti-plaque effect. A research conducted by Amoian et al. (2010) reported that the gum with *Persica* in its composition reduces the gingival bleeding and can be indicated for the treatment of mild gingivitis.

2.1.3.2. *Magnólia officinalis*

The extract obtained from the peel of *Magnólia* has been used in Chinese medicine for 2000 years for the treatment of acute pain, cough and urinary issues (Watanabe et al. 1983). The main compounds of the peel of this plant are *magnolol* and *honokiol*, known because of their anti-inflammatory effect (Wang et al. 1995), antimicrobial activity (Clark et al. 1981), antioxidant and eliminator of free radicals (Lo et al. 1994).

In vitro studies demonstrated that *magnolol* and *honokiol* inhibit the growth of *Streptococcus mutans*, *Streptococcus sobrinus*, *Porphyromonas gingivalis*, *Fusobacterium nucleatum*, *Aggregatibacter actinomycetemcomitans, Capnocytophaga gingivalis* and *Veillonella disper* (Chang et al. 1998, Ho et al. 2001, Li et al. 2004, Greenberg et al. 2007).

The incorporation of Magnólia officinalis's extract to the chewing gum was performed by Campus et al. (2011), who reported a reduction on the bleeding on probing in this study. The main reason to explain this improvement is the extract's inhibitory effect over the growth of oral bacteria, leading to reduction on plaque (Chang et al. 1998, Ho et al. 2001).

2.1.3.3. *Mastique*

Mastique is obtained from the leaves of *Pistacia lentiscus* and was considered a traditional medicine in Greece and other areas of the Mediterranean region for many centuries. Clinically, *Mastique* has been shown to be effective for the treatment of benign gastric and duodenal ulcers (Al-Habbal et al. 1984), and capable to inhibit the activity of *Helicobacter pylori* (Huwez et al. 1998).

Th inhibitory effect of *Mastique*-based chewing gum was tested and the resulted showed a significantly decreased bacterial growth in samples of saliva when compared to the placebo group of the study (Greenstein et al. 1986). The salivary plaque corresponds to the oral microbial load, which can result in plaque accumulation on the surface of the teeth, and, therefore, based on its positive effects, the gum containing *Mastique* can be considered an adjuvant to daily practices of oral hygiene (Takahashi et al. 2003).

2.1.3.4. *Eucalyptus globulus*

Eucalyptus globulus is an Australia's native representant of the species *Eucalipto*. Its leaves are used for medical purposes and in the diet. The extract of *E. globulus* displays antimicrobial activity over cariogenic (e.g., *Streptococcus mutans* and *Streptococcus sobrinus*) (Deans et al. 1987, Osawa et al. 1995, 1996, Nagata et al. 2006) and periodontopathogenic (*Porphyromonas gingivalis* e *Prevotella intermedia*) bacteria (Nagata et al. 2006).

The antimicrobial property of the extract of *E. globulus* is resultant from some of its compounds, the macrocarpals A, B and C (Osawa et al. 1996, Nagata et al. 2006). Among the bacteria directly involved with periodontal diseases, the growth of *Porphyromonas gingivalis* was substantially reduced by the extract of *E. globulus*, even in low concentrations (Saito et al. 2003).

The chewing gum containing *E. globulus* was tested in patients with gingivitis (Nagata et al. 2008). At the end of the experiment, was observed statistically significant improvements in the periodontal indices of plaque accumulation, gingival index, bleeding on probing and probing depths (Nagata et al. 2008). These results sustain that the chewing gum containing eucalyptus extract may be beneficial to revert a scenario of gingivitis back to a healthy periodontium.

2.1.4. Adhesive

2.1.4.1. ***Centella asiatica (gotu kola), Echinacea purpurea e Sambucus nigra***

The transmucosal herbal periodontal patch (THPP) was elaborated to treat specific sites with gingivitis (Grbic et al. 2011). THPP encompasses extracts obtained from the herbs *Centella asiatica (gotu kola), Echinacea purpurea* and *Sambucus nigra*. These plants' extract exhibits antioxidant and immunomodulatory properties capable to suppress the inflammatory response (Harokopakis et al. 2006, Mishima et al. 2004, Punturee et al. 2005, Sastravaha et al. 2005, Woelkart et al. 2006).

This system of transmucosal adhesives covers the inflamed gingiva and allows the intimate contact of the extracts with the gingiva. The results published by Grbic et al. (2001) shows that this adhesive reduces the scores of gingival index within the first 24 yours of use. The side effects that could be associated to the use of THPP, such as changes in taste and mucosal reactions, were tolerated by the patients.

Centella asiatica is known due to its healing properties, mainly regarding wound healing and microangiopathy (Cesarone et al. 2001, Kimura et al. 2008). Its inner anti-inflammatory properties reduce the levels of ß-glucuronidase, an enzyme found in high concentration in inflamed tissues, including gingiva (Noguchi et al. 2007).

Echinacea purpurea is one of the most used medicinal herbs. Its compounds exhibit immunomodulatory effects related to the pro-inflammatory interleukins interferon-γ and tumor necrosis factor 1-α (Mishima et al. 2004, Woelkart et al. 2006, Matthias et al. 2007). Additionally, *Sambucus nigra* suppresses the pro-inflammatory potential of bacteria involved with periodontal diseases (Harokopakis et al. 2006).

The local specific therapy consists an important adjuvant to the standard treatment of gingivitis, since conventional forms of treating this condition can result in refractory inflammation of gingival sites.

2.1.5. Gel

2.1.5.1. *Acácia arábica*

Acacia arabica's gum has been commercialized for thousands of years. The tree from where this gum is extracted was reported during the reign of Ramsés III, in ancient Egypt, as the "Egyptiac gum" (Tyler et al. 1977). In some African and Asian countries, *Acacia*-based products are used to treat stomach disturbs, to cover inflamed surfaces and over burn injuries. Also, the compounds extracted from the peels of *Acacia* are used for the treatment of stomatitis and gingival bleeding (Kirtikar et al. 1984).

The gum of *Acacia arabica* is basically composed by *arabica*, a complex mixture of calciumn, magnesium and potassium from the arabic acid. Adiotionally, it contains cyanogenic glycosides and many other enzymes, such as oxidases, peroxidases and pectinases with antimicrobial properties (Tyler et al. 1977, Kirtikar et al. 1984).

A study evaluating the efficacy of a gel containing *Acacia* reported a reduction of plaque and gingival indices, as well as significant decrease on the counting of microbial species, very similar to the effects found for chlorhexidine gel (Pradeep et al. 2012b).

The positive clinical and microbiological effects of *Acacia's* gel may be assigned to the distinct effects of its compounds, and was pointed to be a herbal formulation efficient to chemical control in gingivitis patients.

2.2. Phytotherapics for the Treatment of Periodontitis

2.2.1. Gel

2.2.1.1. *Garcinia mangostana*

Garcinia mangostana, popularly known as mangosteen is composed, among other substances, by chrysantemin, garcinone A, B and C, sesquiterpene, gartanin, fructose, sucrose, tannins, xanthones and their derivatives (Fansworth et al. 1992).

Mangostana can inhibit the vines of *Staphylococcus aureus* resistant to penicillin (Phongpaichit et al. 1994), suppress the growth of *Helicobacter pyroli* (Hasegawa et al. 1996), and also to potentially inhibit the expression of prostaglandin E_2 (Nakatani et al. 2002). Besides the antimicrobial activity, *mangostana*, *1-isomangostana* and *mangostana* triacetate are inti-inflammatory (Shankaranarayan et al. 1979).

A study performed by Rassameemasmaung et al. (2008) showed that the gel of *Garcinia mangostana* applied adjuvant to scaling and root planning in periodontitis patients reduced the probing depths and the gingival bleeding when compared with the control group, treated with mechanical debridement alone.

2.2.1.2. *Lippia sidoides*

Lippia sidoides is a constituent of the family *Verbenacea,* that has many species spread all over Brazil, mainly in its Northeast (Veras et al. 2011, Bitu et al. 2014). The essential oil obtained from this plant in rich in *thymol, carvacrol* and phenolic compounds with anti-inflammatory and antimicrobial properties (Veras et al. 2014, Botelho et al. 2007a, 2007b, 2007c).

The thymol-based nanogel was tested in induced acute periodontitis in rats, and the results tended to confirm reduced inflammatory response due to the observation of neutrophil influx (Botelho et al. 2016). In addition, another study (Botelho et al. 2008) observed a reduction in the number of *Streptococcus mutans* in saliva and gingivitis status, indicating that *thymol* can be used for treatment and prevention or periodontal injuries (Botelho et al. 2007c).

2.2.1.3. *Cranberry*

The medicinal use of *Cranberry* is dated from the 17th century, for the treatment of gastric diseases and scurvy. *Cranberry* (*Vaccinium macrocarpon*) is a North America's native fruit, commercialized in India as fresh fruits, juices and jams. This phytotherapic consists of a rich source of bioactive flavonoids, such as flavanols, anthocyanins and proanthocyanins, that provide substantial therapeutic potential.

In vitro assessments reported that *Cranberry's* compounds inhibited the activity of *Streptococcus sorbinus* and *Streptococcus mutans* (Steinberg et al. 2004, Duarte et al. 2006, Koo et al. 2010, Babu et al. 2012), hindering the formation of the bacterial plaque (Yamanaka et al. 2007, La et al. 2010, Polak et al. 2013) and the activity of some periodontopathogens such as *Porphyromonas gingivalis* and *Fusubacterium nucleatum* (Weiss et al. 2004, Yamanaka et al. 2004, Labrecque et al. 2006, Feldman et al. 2012, Polak et al. 2013).

A gel for the treatment of periodontal diseases was manufactured from the concentrated juice of Cranberry (CJC). The thermosensitive gel, when compared to commercial 0.12% chlorhexidine, displayed very similar results regarding antimicrobial activity over microorganisms related to periodontal infections (Howell 2007). Another point that might explain its efficacy is the anti-adhesive feature of the epicatechins, another bioactive molecule of the CJC (Howell 2007).

Even scaling and root planning to be the first step for periodontitis treatment, this modality is not always completely effective, and, therefore, adjuvant therapies are necessary to maximize its benefits (Mombelli et al. 2000). An important characteristic of adjuvant therapies would be the absence of side effects, which can be pointed as one of the phytotherapics such as *Cranberry*.

2.2.1.4. *Carvacrol*

Carvacrol is a phenolic product of the *Lippia sidoides*. Phenolic compounds have been widely used for the treatment of experimental periodontitis, mainly ruled by their anti-inflammatory and antimicrobial properties (Botelho et al. 2007c, 2008).

The *Carvacrol* gel showed to be an efficient inhibitor of periodontal pathogens (Tomasi & Wennström 2004), capable to reduce the activity of myeloperoxidase (MPO), an enzyme responsible to catalyze oxidative species that contribute to tissues' breakdown during inflammation (Botelho et al. 2008). This gel has a constitutive effect on the progression of periodontitis (Stoltze 1992). More than reducing the total number of neutrophils infiltrated in the gingival tissue, *Carvacrol* suppresses the mediators of chronic inflammatory processes, interleukin-1β and tumor necrosis factor-α. (Botelho et al. 2007c, 2008), strengthening its protective effects over periodontal tissues.

An experimental model was used to evaluate the effects of *Carvacrol* gel over induced periodontal disease (Botelho et al. 2009). The authors reported significant reduction on the alveolar bone loss in tested group when compared with the control (Botelho et al. 2009). This finding is supported by many characteristics of this phytotherapic, including its direct effect over periodontal pathogens (Botelho et al. 2008).

Also, the systemic administration of antibiotics adjuvant to scaling and root planning is related to gastrointestinal side effects (Gencosmanoglu et al. 2004). Therefore, this side effect can be suppressed by the use of *Carvacrol* instead of traditional medicine.

2.2.2. Chip

2.2.2.1. *Azadirachta indica (neem)*

Azadirachta indica (neem) is native from India, known as "holy tree" (Sharma et al. 2011) and declared the "Tree of the XXI century" by the United Nations. Its leaves, roots, bark and fruit are used for the treatment of inflammations, infections.

Some compounds such as *nimbin, nimbidin, ninbidol and sodium nimbinate* have been reported as the responsible for its anti-microbial, anti-inflammatory and analgesic properties (Biswas et al. 2002, Girish et al. 2008).

Periodontitis may be considered a multifactorial disease with microorganisms present in subgingival plaque being the main local ethiologic fator. *Porphyromonas gingivalis* and *Aggregatibacter actinomycetemcomitans* are two of the main bacteria related with periodontitis (Slots et al. 1999). A study evaluated the capacity of *Azadirachta indica's (neem)* extract to inhibit subgingival microbiota, through the placement of a *chip* inside the periodontal pocket. In this study, in group test was observed complete absence of *Porphyromonas gingivalis* when compared with control group (Vennila et al. 2016).

While evaluated in the formulation of a tooth paste, *Azadirachta indica's (neem)* extract also showed to be effective for reduction on the amount of bacterial plaque, maybe due to its inhibitory effect over gran-negative bacteria when compared with conventional formulations of tooth paste (Rao et al. 1986).

2.2.3. Extracts

2.2.3.1. Grape Seed

Over the past years, the literature has reported the benefits of the consumption of dried fruit, green tea and red wine, which were mainly explained by the high concentration of proanthocyanidins in these aliments (Hertog et al. 1993, Santos-Buelga et al. 2000). The proanthocyanidins are among the more concentrated phenols in grape seeds (*Vitis vinífera*) and is related to the protective effect of red wine over cardiovascular diseases (Pace-Asciak et al. 1995, Hayek et al. 1997) and reduction on the risk of developing cancer (Singh et al. 1998, Hong et al. 1997).

The plausible mechanisms in which the protective features of proanthocyanidins are based on are antioxidant properties, elimination of oxygen and nitrogen reactive species (Hayek et al. 1997, Belguendouz et al. 1997, Plumb et al. 1998), inhibitory effects on arachidonic acid cascade and modulation of the expression and synthesis of inducible nitric oxide synthase (iNOS) (Kim et al. 1999, Tsai et al. 1999).

The stimulation of hosts' immune response by pathogenic bacteria results on the production of oxygen and nitrogen reactive species (Sheikhi et al. 2000, Knight et al. 2000, Katsuragi et al. 2003). The excess of free radicals can lead to damages on the gingiva, periodontal ligament and alveolar bone.

Researches have shown the efficacy of the extract obtained from grape seeds against oxidative stress (Ariga, 2004, Bagchi et al. 2003) due its capacity of elimination of oxygen reactive species. An *in vitro* experiment confirmed that the proanthocyanidins strongly inhibit the release of nitrogen by the macrophages (Houde et al. 2006). The proanthocyanidins are a valuable natural resource for the development of medicines for the treatment of inflammatory illness, including periodontitis.

2.2.3.1. Green-Tea

Green tea extract (GTE) manufactured using dried leaves of *Camellia sinensis* has been proposed for the treatment of inflammatory illness (Afzal, Safer, & Menon 2015). The catechins found in this phytotherapic play their protective role in the periodontium by different paths. They are capable to inhibit expression of COX-2 (Tominari et al. 2015), reduces osteoclastic activity (Yun et al. 2004) and displays antimicrobial effects (Yun et al. 2004). Also, GTE induces the expression of human beta-defensin, enhancing the barrier function of epithelial cells against bacterial threads in the periodontium (Lagha et al. 2018).

A pre-clinical model of ligature-induced periodontitis in rats was used to access the effects of the green tea extract used as local adjuvant therapy to scaling and root planning (de Almeida et al. 2019). de Almeida et al. (2019) reported higher amount of bone in the furcation in animals treated with mechanical debridement combined with adjuvant GTE when compared with rats treated with debridement alone. This was assumed as the primary outcome variable, that was supported by the other analysis. The authors (de Almeida et al. 2019) found a lower inflammatory process in the periodontium, as well as decreased expression of pro-inflammatory cytokines and increased expression of interleukin-10, an anti-inflammatory biomarker. The less intense and less persistent inflammatory response may be the explanation for reduction on the expression of active osteoclasts, also described by the authors, and an important factor to support the higher amount of bone in group tested with green tea.

2.3. Phytotherapics for the Treatment of Surgical Areas

2.3.1. *Curcuma Longa*, *Ghee*

The *Curcuma Longa* (turmeric) has been used for a long time in asiatic medical practice as stomacal tonic, blood "purifier" and for wound healing. It has been widely investigated by the pharmaceutical industry due to its anti-inflammatory, antimicrobial and antioxidant properties. *Curcumin* is the active component of the *Curcuma*, obtained from its rhizomes.

Previous studies showed favorable results of the use of *curcumin* for the repair of surgical wounds, usually explained by the increased cellular component and revascularization of the area. Also, *curcumin* seems to induce the endogenous expression of the transforming growth factor-1, improving wound healing (Sidhu et al. 1998, Mani et al. 2002).

Ghee (refined animal fat) also displays therapeutically effects on the repair process of wounds (Sharma 1981). Its components, such as saturate fatty acids polyunsaturated fatty acids are capable to stimulate the proliferation of epithelial cells (Calder 2001).

Habiboallah et al. 2008 studied a novel formulation of sheep's' *Ghee* combined with *curcumin*. The results indicated that the wounds treated with this combination showed reduced inflammatory process, presence of higher amount of collagens fibers and epithelialization of the wound, suggestive of complete repair at 7 days postoperatively, indicating a possible used in periodontal therapy, both surgically and nonsurgically.

References

Afzal M, Safer AM & Menon M. Green tea polyphenols and their potential role in health and disease. *Inflammopharmacology* 2015;23(4):151–161.

Aghili MH. Makhzan-Al-Advieh (The Store of Drugs) [in Persian], 5th ed. Tehran, Iran: Sabzarang; 2013. Jorjani SE. *Zakhireye Kharazmshahi* [in Persian]. Vol. 1, Part 1, Section 3. Tehran, Iran: *Academy of Medical Sciences*; 2001:379-381.

Ainamo A. Optimal reference line for determination of the location of the maxillary mucogingival junction in the orthopantomogram. *Proc Finn Dent* 1977;73(2):70-75.

Al lafi T, Ababneh H. The effect of the extract of the miswak (chewing sticks) used in Jordan and the Middle East on oral bacteria. *Int Dent J* 1995;45(3):218–22.

Al-Habbal MJ, Al-Habbal Z, Huwez FU. A double-blind controlled clinical trial of mastic and placebo in the treatment of duodenal ulcer. *Clin Exp Pharmacol Physiol* 1984;11(5):541-544.

Allen DL, Kerr DA. Tissue response in the guinea pig to sterile and non-sterile calculus. *J Periodontol* 1965; 36:121–126.

Almas K, Skaug N, Ahmad I. An in vitro antimicrobial comparison of miswak extract with commercially available non-alcohol mouthrinses. *Int J Dent Hyg* 2005;3(1):18–24.

Amoian B, Moghadamnia AA, Barzi S, Sheykholeslami S, Rangiani A. Salvadora Persica extract chewing gum and gingival health: improvement of gingival and probe-bleeding index. *Complement Ther Clin Pract* 2010;16(3):121-123.

Ariga T. The antioxidative function, preventive action on disease and utilization of proanthocyanidins. *Biofactors* 2004;21(1-4):197-201.

Arweiler NB, Pergola G, Kuenz J, Hellwig E, Sculean A, Auschill TM. Clinical and antibacterial effect of an anti-inflammatory toothpaste formulation with Scutellaria baicalensis extract on experimental gingivitis. *Clin Oral Investig* 2011;15(6):909-13.

Attström R, Graf-De Beer M, Schroeder HE. Clinical and Histologic Characteristics of Normal Gingiva in Dogs. *J Periodontal Res* 1975;10(3):115-127.

Babu J, Blair C, Jacob S, Itzhak O. Inhibition of *Streptococcus gordonii* metabolic activity in biofilm by cranberry juice high-molecular-weight componente. *J Biomed Biotechnol* 2012:590384.

Badria FA, Zidan OA. Natural products for dental caries prevention. *J Med Food* 2004;7(3):381-4.

Bagchi D, Sen CK, Ray SD et al. Molecular mechanisms of cardioprotection by a novel grape seed proanthocyanidin extract. *Mutat Res* 2003;523-524:87-97.

Bajaj N, Tandon S. The effect of triphala and chlorhexidine mouthwash on dental plaque, gingival inflammation, and microbial growth. *Int J Ayurveda Res* 2011;2(1):29–36.

Baliga MS, Meera S, Mathai B, Rai MP, Pawar V, Palatty PL. Scientific validation of the ethnomedicinal properties of the ayurvedic drug triphala: a review. *Chin J Integr Med* 2012;18(12):946–54.

Balunas MJ, Kinghorn AD. Drug discovery from medicinal plants. *Life Sci*. 2005;78(5):431-441.

Bartold PM, Van Dyke TE. Host modulation: controlling the inflammation to control the infection. *Periodontol 2000* 2017;75(1):317-329.

Belguendouz L, Fremont L, Linard A. Resveratrol inhibits metal ion-dependent and independent peroxidation of porcine low-density lipoproteins. *Biochem Pharmacol* 1997;53(9):1347-1355.

Bemis DL, Capodice JL, Anastasiadis AG, Katz AE, Buttyan R. Zyflamend, a unique herbal preparation with nonselective COX inhibitory activity, induces apoptosis of prostate cancer cells that lack COX-2 expression. *Nutr Cancer* 2005;52(2):202–212.

Bemis DL, Capodice JL, Desai M, Buttyan R, Katz AE. A concentrated aglycone isoflavone preparation (GCP) that demonstrates potent anti-prostate cancer activity in vitro and in vivo. *Clin Cancer Res* 2004;10(15):5282–5292.

Bensky D, Gamble A, Kaptchuk T. *Chinese herbal medicine*. Materia Medica: Eastland Press, Seattle, 1986;107–9.

Bhadbhade SJ, Acharya AB, Rodrigues SV, Thakur SL. The antiplaque efficacy of pomegranate mouthrinse. *Quintessence Int.* 2011;42(1): 29-36.

Bhandari PR. Pomegranate (*Punica granatum* L). Ancient seeds for modern cure? Review of potential therapeutic applications. *Int J Nutr Pharmacol Neurol Dis* 2012;2(3):171-84.

Biswas K, Chattopadhyay I, Banerjee RK, Bandyopadhyay U. Biological activities and medicinal properties of neem (*Azadirachta indica*). *Curr Sci* 2002;82(11):1336-45.

Bitu VC, Fecundo HD, da Costa JG et al. Chemical composition of the essential oil of Lippia gracilis Schauer leaves and its potential as modulator of bacterial resistance. *Nat Prod Res* 2014;28(6):399-402.

Botelho MA, Barros G, Queiroz DB, Carvalho CF, Gouvea J, Patrus L, Bannet M, Patrus D, Rego A, Silva I, Campus G, Araújo-Filho I. Nanotechnology in Phytotherapy: Antiinflammatory Effect of a Nanostructured Thymol Gel from Lippia sidoides in Acute Periodontitis in Rats. *Phytother Res* 2016;30(1):152-9.

Botelho MA, Bezerra Filho JG, Correa LL et al. Effect of a novel essential oil mouthrinse without alcohol on gingivitis: a double-blinded randomized controlled trial. *J Appl Oral Sci* 2007a;15(3):175–180.

Botelho MA, Nogueira NA, Bastos GM et al. Antimicrobial activity of the essential oil from Lippia sidoides, carvacrol and thymol against oral pathogens. *Braz J Med Biol Res* 2007b;40(3):349–356.

Botelho MA, Rao VS, Carvalho CB et al. Lippia sidoides and Myracrodruon urundeuva gel prevents alveolar bone resorption in experimental periodontitis in rats. *J Ethnopharmacol* 2007c;113(3): 471–478.

Botelho MA, Rao VS, Montenegro D et al. Effects of a herbal gel containing carvacrol and chalcones on alveolar boné resorption in rats on experimental periodontitis. *Phytother Res* 2008;22(4):442–449.

Botelho MA, Martins JG, Ruela RS, I R, Santos JA, Soares JB, França MC, Montenegro D, Ruela WS, Barros LP, Queiroz DB, Araujo RS, Sampio FC. Protective effect of locally applied carvacrol gel on ligature-induced periodontitis in rats: a tapping mode AFM study. *Phytother Res* 2009;23(10):1439-48.

Calder PC. 1. *n*-3 polyunsaturated fatty acid, inflammation and immunity: pouring oil on trouble waters or another fishy tales. *Nutr Res* 2001;21(1):309–341.

Campus G, Cagetti MG, Cocco F, Sale S, Sacco G, Strohmenger L, Lingström P. Effect of a sugar-free chewing gum containing magnolia bark extract on different variables related to caries and gingivitis: a randomized controlled intervention trial. *Caries Res* 2011;45(4):393-9.

Caton JG, Armitage G, Berglundh T, Chapple ILC, Jepsen S, Kornman KS et al. A new classification scheme for periodontal and peri-implant diseases and conditions – introduction and key changes from the 1999 classification. *J Periodontol* 2018;89(1):1-8.

Cesarone MR, Incandela L, De Sanctis MT, et al. Evaluation of treatment of diabetic microangiopathy with total triterpenic fraction of *Centella asiatica:* a clinical prospective randomized trial with a microcirculatory model. *Angiology* 2001;52(suppl 2): S49-S54.

Chang B, Lee Y, Ku Y, Bae K, Chung C. Antimicrobial activity of magnolol and honokiol against periodontopathic microorganisms. Planta Med 1998;64(4):367–369.

Clark AM, Elferaly FS, Li WS. Antimicrobial activity of phenolic constituents of *Magnolia grandiflora*. *J Pharm Sci* 1981;70(8):951–952.

Cobb CM. Non-surgical pocket therapy: Mechanical. *Ann Periodontol* 1996;1(1):443-490.

Contreras A, Doan N, Chen C, Rusitanonta T, Flynn Mj, Slots J. Importance of dialister pneumosintes in human periodontitis. *Oral Microbiol Immunol* 2000;15(4):269-272.

Cragg GM, Newman DJ. Natural products: a continuing source of novel drug leads. *Biochem Biophys Acta* 2013;1830(6):3670-3695.

de Almeida JM, Marques BM, Novaes VCN, de Oliveira FLP, Matheus HR, Fiorin LG, Ervolino E. Influence of adjuvant therapy with green tea extract in the treatment of experimental periodontitis. *Arch Oral Biol* 2019;102:65-73.

de Oliveira SM, Torres TC, Pereira SL, Mota OM, Carlos MX. Effect of a dentifrice containing Aloe vera on plaque and gingivitis control. A double-blind clinical study in humans. *J Appl Oral Sci* 2008;16(4): 293-296.

Deans SG, Ritchie G. Antibacterial properties of plant essential oils. *Int J Food Microbiol* 1987;5(2):165-180.

Dentino A, Lee S, Mailhot J, Hefti AF. Principles of periodontology. *Periodontol 2000* 2013;61(1):16-53.

Desai A, Anil M, Debnath S. A clinical trial to evaluate the effects of triphala as a mouthwash in comparison with chlorhexidine in chronic generalized periodontitis patients. *Indian J Dent Adv* 2010; 2:243-7.

Doan N, Contreras A, Flynn J, Slots J, Chen C. Molecular identification of Dialister pneumosintes in subgingival plaque of humans. *J Clin Microbiol* 2000;38(8):3043-3047.

Duarte S, Gregoire S, Singh AP, Vorsa N, Schaich K, Bowen WH, Koo H. Inhibitory effects of cranberry polyphenols on formation and acidogenicity of *Streptococcus mutans* biofilms. *FEMS Microbiol Lett* 2006;257(1):50-56.

Eggli U. Illustrated Handbook of Succulent Plants: Monocotyledons. Berlin: Springer-Verlag; 2001:102-186.

Eid MA, Selim HA. A retrospective study on the relationship between miswak chewing stick and periodontal health. *Egypt Dent J* 1994;40(1):589–92.

Fansworth NR, Bunyapraphatsara N. Thai medicinial plants recommended for primary health care system. Bangkok: Prachachon; 1992: 402 p.

Feldman M, D. Grenier. Cranberry proanthocyanidins act in synergy with licochalcone a to reduce *Porphyromonas gingivalis* growth and virulence properties, and to suppress cytokine secretion by macrophages. *J Appl Microbiol* 2012;113(2):438-447.

Flotra L, Gjermo P, Rolla G, Waerhaug J. Side effects of chlorhexidine mouth washes. *Scand J Dent Res* 1971;79(2):119-25.

Freires IA, Rosalen PL. How natural product research has contrib- uted to oral care product development? A critical view. *Pharm Res* 2016;33(6):1311-1317.

Genco RJ, Borgnakke WS. Risk factors for periodontal disease. *Periodontol 2000* 2013;62(1):59-94.

Gencosmanoglu R, Kurtkaya-Yapicier O, Tiftikci A, Avsar E, Tozun N, Oran ES. Mid-esophageal ulceration and candidiasis-associated distal esophagitis as two distinct clinical patterns of tetracycline or doxycycline-induced esophageal injury. *J Clin Gastroenterol* 2004;38(6):484–489.

Girish K, Bhat SS. Neem - A green treasure. *Electron J Biol* 2008;4(3):102-11.

Grbic J, Wexler I, Celenti R, Altman J, Saffer A. A phase II trial of a transmucosal herbal patch for the treatment of gingivitis. *J Am Dent Assoc* 2011;142(10):1168-75.

Greenberg M, Urnezis P, Tian M: Compressed mints and chewing gum containing magnólia bark extract are effective against bactéria responsible for oral malodor. *J Agric Food Chem* 2007;55(23):9465–9469.

Greenstein G, Berman C, Jaffin R. Chlorhexidine. Na adjunct to periodontal therapy. *J Periodontol* 1986;57(6):370-377.

Grindlay D, Reynolds T. The Aloe vera phenomenon: A review of the properties and modern uses of the leaf parenchyma gel. *J Ethnopharmacol* 1986;16(2-3):117-151.

Guo HX, Liu DH, Ma Y, Liu JF, Wang Y, Du ZY, Wang X, Shen JK, Peng HL. Long-term baicalin administration ameliorates metabolic disorders and hepatic steatosis in rats given a highfat diet. *Acta Pharmacol Sin* 2009;30(11):1505–1512.

Habiboallah G, Nasroallah S, Mahdi Z, Nasser MS, Massoud Z, Ehsan BN, Mina ZJ, Heidar P. Histological evaluation of Curcuma longa-ghee formulation and hyaluronic acid on gingival healing in dog. *J Ethnopharmacol* 2008;120(3):335-41.

Harokopakis E, Albzreh MH, Haase EM, Scannapieco FA, Hajishengallis G. Inhibition of proinflammatory activities of major periodontal pathogens by aqueous extracts from elder flower (*Sambucus nigra). J Periodontol* 2006;77(2):271-279.

Hasegawa H, Sakai S, Aimi N, Takayama H, Koyano T. Helicobacter pylori inhibitors containing xanthones from Garcinia mangostana. Patent: Jpn Kokai Tokkyo Koho JP 08, 231, 396 (96,231,396) (1996): 5 p.

Hayek T, Fuhrman B, Vaya J, et al. Reduced progression of atherosclerosis in apolipoprotein E-deficient mice following consumption of red wine, or its polyphenols quercetin or catechin, is associated with reduced susceptibility of LDL to oxidation and aggregation. *Arterioscler Thromb Vasc Biol* 1997;17(11):2744-2752.

Hellstrom MK, Ramberg P, Krok L, Lindhe J. The effect of supragingival plaque control on the subgingival microflora in human periodontitis. *J Clin Periodontol* 1996;23(10):934-940.

Hertog MG, Hollman PC, Katan MB, Kromhout D. Intake of potentially anticarcinogenic flavonoids and their determinants in adults in The Netherlands. *Nutr Cancer* 1993;20(1):21-29.

Ho KY, Tsai CC, Chen CP, Huang JS, Lin CC. Antimicrobial activity of honokiol and magnolol isolated from *Magnolia officinalis*. *Phytother Res* 2001;15(2):139–141.

Hong W, Sporn M. Recent advances in chemoprevention of cancer. *Science* 1997;278(5340):1073-1077.

Houde V, Grenier D, Chandad F. Protective effects of grape seed proanthocyanidins against oxidative stress induced by lipopolysaccharides of periodontopathogens. *J Periodontol* 2006;77 (8):1371-9.

Howell AB. Bioactive compounds in cranberries and their role in prevention of urinary tract infections. *Mol Nutr Food Res* 2007;51: 732–7.

Huwez FU, Thirlwell D, Cockayne A, Ala'Aldeen DA. Mastic gum kills *Helicobacter pylori. N Engl J Med* 1998;24(26):339-1946.

Jorjani SE. Zakhireye Kharazmshahi [in Persian]. Vol. 1, Part 1, Section 3. Tehran, Iran: *Academy of Medical Sciences*; 2001: 379-381.

Katsuragi H, Ohtake M, Kurasawa I, Saito K. Intracellular production and extracellular release of oxygen radicals by PMNs and oxidative stress on PMNs during phagocytosis of periodontopathic bacteria. *Odontology* 2003;91(1):13-18.

Khalessi AM, Pack AR, Thomson WM, Tompkins GR. An in vivo study of the plaque control efficacy of Persica: a commercially available herbal mouthwash containing extracts of *Salvadora persica*. *Int Dent J* 2004;54(5):279–83.

Kim HP, Lee JY, Jeong JK, et al. Nongenomic stimulation of nitric oxide release by estrogen is mediated by estrogen receptor alpha localized in caveolae. *Biochem Biophys Res Commun* 1999;263(1):257-262.

Kimura Y, Sumiyoshi M, Samukawa K, Satake N, Sakanaka M. Facilitating action of asiaticoside at low doses on burn wound repair and its mechanism. *Eur J Pharmacol* 2008;584(2-3):415-423.

Kinane DF, Lindhe J, Trombelli L. Chronic periodontitis. In: Lindhe J, Thorklid K, Lang NP(eds). Clinical periodontology and implantology. 5th ed. Oxford: Munksgaard; 2008:420-27.

Kirtikar KR, Basu BD. Indian medicinal plants. 2nd edn. Allahabad. Lalit Mohan Basu, 1984;2: 919–93.

Knight JA. Review: Free radicals, antioxidants, and the immune system. *Ann Clin Lab Sci* 2000;30(2):145-158.

Koo H, Duarte S, Murata RM, Scott-Anne K, Gregoire S, Watson GE, Singh AP, Vorsa N. Influence of cranberry proanthocyanidins on formation of biofilms by *Streptococcus mutans* on saliva-coated apatitic surface and on dental caries development in vivo. *Caries Res* 2010;44:116-126.

Kornman KS, Loe H. The role of local factors in the etiology of periodontal diseases. *Periodontol 2000* 1993;2:83-97.

Kumar P, Ansari SH, Ali J. Herbal remedies for the treatment of periodontal disease—a patent review. *Recent Pat Drug Delivery Formul* 2009;3(3):221-228.

La VD, Holwee AB, Grenier D. Anti-*Porphyromonas gingivalis* and anti-inflammatory activities of A-type cranberry proanthocyanidins. *Antimicrob Agents Chemother* 2010, 54(5):1778-1784.

Labrecque J, Ch. Bodet, F. Chandad, D. Grenier. Effects of a high-molecular-weight cranberry fraction on growth, biofilm formation and adherence of *Porphyromonas gingivalis*. *J Antimicrob Chemother* 2006;58(2):439-443.

Lacoste E, Chaumont JP, Mandin D, Plumel MM, Matos FJ. Antisseptic properties of essential oil of Lippia sidoides Cham: application to the cutaneous microflora. *Ann Pharm Fr* 1996;54(3):228-30.

Lagha AB, Groeger S, Meyle J, & Grenier D. Green tea polyphenols enhance gingival keratinocyte integrity and protect against invasion by Porphyromonas gingivalis. *Pathog Dis* 2018;76(4).

Lee SS, Zhang W, Li Y. The antimicrobial potential of 14 natural herbal dentifrices: Results of an in vitro diffusion method study. *J Am Dent Assoc* 2004;135(8):1133-1141.

Lemos TL, Craveiro AA, Alencar JW, Matos FJ, Clarck AM, Mac-Chesney JD. Antimicrobial activity of essential oil of Brazilian plants. *Phytother Res* 1990;4(3):82-4.

Lewis ME. Plants and dental health. *J Prevent Dent* 1980; 6:75–80.

Li J, Lu YY, Xu XH. Cariostatic activity of gargle with compounded herb medicine in rat. *ZJU Med* 2004; 26: 187–189.

Listgarten M A. The structure of dental plaque. *Periodontol 2000* 1994;5:52-65.

Lo YC, Teng CM, Chen CF, Chen CC, Hong CY: Magnolol and honokiol isolated from *Magnolia officinalis* protect rat heart mitochondria against lipid peroxidation. *Biochem Pharmacol* 1994;47(3):549–553.

Löe H, Theilade E, Jensen SB. Experimental Gingivitis In Man. *J Periodontol* 1965;36:177-87.

Lyons KM, Darby I. Interdisciplinary periodontics: the multidisciplinary approach to the planning and treatment of complex cases. *Periodontol 2000* 2017;74(1):7-10.

Mani H, Sidhu GS, Kumari R, Gaddipati JP, Seth P, Maheshwari RK. Curcumin differentially regulates TGF-_1, its receptors and nitric oxide synthesis during impaired wound healing. *Biofactors* 2002;16(1-2):29–43.

Matthias A, Banbury L, Stevenson LM, Bone KM, Leach DN, Lehmann RP. Alkylamides from echinacea modulate induced imune responses in macrophages. *Immunol Invest* 2007;36(2):117-130.

Maurya DK, Mittal N, Sharma KR, Nath G. Role of triphala in the management of periodontal disease. *Anc Sci Life*. 1997;17(2):120-7.

Mazumdar M, Chatterjee A, Majumdar S, Chandrika M, Patki PS. Evaluation of the safety and efficacy of complete care herbal toothpaste in controlling dental plaque, gingival bleeding and periodontal diseases. *J Homeop Ayurv Med* 2013;2:124.

McNabb H, Mombelli A, Lang NP. Supragingival cleaning 3 times a week. The microbiological effects in moderately deep pockets. *J Clin Periodontol* 1992; 19(5):348-356.

Mehta BK, Shitut S, Wankhada H. In vitro antimicrobial efficacy of triphala. *Fitoterapia* 1993; 64:371–2.

Mishima S, Saito K, Maruyama H, et al. Antioxidant and immuno-enhancing effects of *Echinacea purpurea. Biol Pharm Bull* 2004;27(7):1004-1009.

Mombelli A, B Schmid, A Rutar, NP Lang. Persistence patterns of Porphyromonas gingivalis, Prevotella intermedia/nigrescens, and Actinobacillus actinomycetemcomitans after mechanical therapy of periodontal disease. *J. Periodontol* 2000;71(1):14–21.

Moro MG, Silveira Souto ML, Franco GCN, Holzhausen M, Pannuti CM. Efficacy of local phytotherapy in the nonsurgical treatment of periodontal disease: A systematic review. *J Periodontal Res* 2018;53(3):288-97.

Mortenson D, Sadilek M, Flake NM, et al. The effect of using an alternative irrigant between sodium hypochlorite and chlorhexi- dine to prevent the formation of para-chloroaniline within the root canal system. *Int Endod J* 2012;45(9):878-882.

Mukherjee PK, Sujay R, Sauvik B et al. Clinical study of 'triphala'- a well known phytomedicine from India. *Iranian J Pharmacol Therapeut* 2006;5(1):51–4.

Murakami S, Mealey BL, Mariotti A, Chapple ILC. Dental plaque-induced gingival conditions. *J Periodontol* 2018;89(1):S17- S27.

Nagata H, Inagaki Y, Yamamoto Y, et al. Inhibitory effects of macrocarpals on the biological activity of Porphyromonas gingivalis and other periodontopathic bacteria. *Oral Microbiol Immunol* 2006;21(3):159-163.

Nagata H, Inagaki Y, Tanaka M, Ojima M, Kataoka K, Kuboniwa M, Nishida N, Shimizu K, Osawa K, Shizukuishi S. Effect of eucalyptus extract chewing gum on periodontal health: a double-masked, randomized trial. *J Periodontol* 2008;79(8):1378-85.

Nakatani K, Nakahata N, Arakawa T, Yasuda H, Ohizumi Y. Inhibition of cyclooxygenase and prostaglandin E2 synthesis by gamma-mangostin, a xanthone derivative in mangosteen, in C6 rat glioma cells. *Biochem Pharmacol* 2002;63(1):73-9.

Narayan A, Mendon C. Comparing the effect of different mouth rinses on de novo plaque formation. *J Contemp Dent Pract* 2012;13(4):460–3.

Narhi TO, Tenovuo J, Ainamo A, Vilja P. Antimicrobial factors, sialic acid, and protein concentration in whole saliva of the elderly. *Scan J Den Res* 1994;102(2):120-5.

Noguchi K, Ishikawa I. The roles of cyclooxygenase-2 and prostaglandin E2 in periodontal disease. *Periodontol 2000* 2007; 43:85-101.

Nogueira-Filho GR, Toledo S, Cury JA. Effect of 3 dentifrices containing triclosan and various additives. An experimental gingivitis study. *J Clin Periodontol* 2000;27(7):494-498.

Osawa K, Yasuda H, Morita H, Takeya K, Itokawa H. Eucalyptone from Eucalyptus globulus. *Phytochemistry* 1995;40(1):183-184.

Osawa K, Yasuda H, Morita H, Takeya K, Itokawa H. Macrocarpals H, I, and J from the leaves of Eucalyptus globulus. *J Nat Prod* 1996;59(9):823-827.

Pace-Asciak CR, Hahn S, Diamandis EP, Soleas G, Goldberg DM. The red wine phenolics trans-resveratrol and quercetin block human platelet aggregation and eicosanoid synthesis: Implications for protection against coronary heart disease. *Clin Chim Acta* 1995;235(2):207-219.

Papapanou PN, Sanz M, Buduneli N, Dietrich T, Feres M, Fine DH et al. Periodontitis: Consensus report of workgroup 2 of the 2017 World Workshop on the Classification of Periodontal and Peri-Implant Diseases and Conditions. *J Periodontol* 2018;89(1):S173-S182.

Pereira JV, Pereira MSV, Sampo FC, Sampio MCC, Alves PM, Araujo CRF, et al. *In vitro* antibacterial and adherence effect of the extract of *Punica granatum* Linn. upon dental biofilm microorganisms. *J Braz Pharmacogn* 2006;16(1):88-93.

Pereira JV, Silva SC, Filho LS, Higino JS. Antimicrobial activity of hyroalcoholic extract of *Punica granatum* Linn. on plaque forming microorganisms. *Periodontics Ver* 2001;12:57-64.

Phongpaichit S, Ongsakul M, Nilrat L, Tharavichitkul P, Bunchoo S, Chuaprapaisilp T. Antibacterial activities of extracts from *Garcinia mangostana* pericarps on methicillin-resistant *Staphylococcus aureus* and *Enterococcus* species. *Songklanakarin J Sci Technol* 1994;16:399-405.

Plumb GW, De Pascual-Teresa S, Santos-Buelga C, Cheynier V, Williamson G. Antioxidant properties of catechins and proanthocyanidins: Effect of polymerisation, galloylation and glycosylation. *Free Radic Res* 1998;29(4):351-358.

Polak D, Naddaf R, Shapira L, Weiss El, Houri-Haddad Y. Protective potential of non-dialyzable material fraction of cranberry juice on the virulence of *P. gingivalis* and *F. nucleatum* mixed infection. *J Periodontol* 2013;84(7):1019-1025.

Pradeep AR, Agarwal E, Bajaj P, Naik SB, Shanbhag N, Uma SR. Clinical and microbiologic effects of commercially available gel and powder containing Acacia arabica on gingivitis. *Aust Dent J* 2012b;57(3):312-8.

Pradeep AR, Agarwal E, Naik SB. Clinical and microbiologic effects of commercially available dentifrice containing aloe vera: a randomized controlled clinical trial. *J Periodontol* 2012a;83(6):797-804.

Punturee K, Wild CP, Kasinrerk W, Vinitketkumnuen U. Immunomodulatory activities of *Centella asiatica* and *Rhinacanthus nasutus* extracts. *Asian Pac J Cancer Prev* 2005;6(3):396-400.

Rao DV, Singh I, Chopra P, Chhabra PC, Ramanujalu G. *In vitro* antibacterial activity of neem oil. *Indian J Med Res* 1986;84:314-6.

Rassameemasmaung S, Sirikulsathean A, Amornchat C, Maungmingsook P, Rojanapanthu P, Gritsanaphan W. Topical application of Garcinia mangostana L. pericarp gel as an adjunct to periodontal treatment. *Complement Ther Med* 2008;16(5):262-7.

Saito MV, Nagata H, Maeda K, et al. Antibacterial activity of extracts from eucalyptus leaves on periodontopathic bacteria. *J Dent Health* (Tokyo) 2003;53:585-591.

Salgado AD, Maia JL, Pereira SL, de Lemos TL, Mota OM. Antiplaque and antigingivitis effects of a gel containing *Punica granatum linn* extract. A double-blind clinical study in humans. *J Appl Oral Sci* 2006;14(3):162-166.

Santos-Buelga C, Scalbert A. Proanthocyanidins and tannin-like compounds in human nutrition. *J Food Sci Agric* 2000;80(7):1094-1117.

Sastravaha G, Gassmann G, Sangtherapitikul P, Grimm WD. Adjunctive periodontal treatment with *Centella asiatica* and *Punica granatum* extracts in supportive periodontal therapy. *J Int Acad Periodontol* 2005;7(3):70-79.

Sastravaha G, Yotnuengnit P, Booncong P, Sangtherapitikul P. Adjunctive periodontal treatment with *Centella asiatica* and *Punica granatum* extracts. A preliminary study. *J Int Acad Periodontol* 2003;5(4): 106-15.

Saxena A, Vikram NK. Role of selected Indian plants in management of type 2 diabetes: A review. *J Altern Complement Med* 2004;10(2): 369-78.

Sedigh-Rahimabadi M, Fani M, Rostami-Chijan M, Zarshenas MM, Shams M. A Traditional Mouthwash (Punica granatum var pleniflora) for Controlling Gingivitis of Diabetic Patients: A Double-Blind Randomized Controlled Clinical Trial. *J Evid Based Complementary Altern Med* 2017;22(1):59-67.

Shankaranarayan D, Gopalakrishnan C, Kameswaran L. Pharmacological profile of mangostin and its derivatives. *Arch Int Pharmacodyn Ther* 1979;239(2):257-69.

Sharma P, Tomar L, Bachwani M, Bansal VM. Review of neem (Azadirachta indica): Thousand problems one solution. *Int Res Pharm* 2011;2(12):97-102.

Sharma RS. Ghee: a resume of recent research. *J food Sci Technol* 1981;18:70–75.

Sheikhi M, Gustafsson A, Jarstrand C. Cytokine, elastase and oxygen radical release by Fusobacterium nucleatum-activated leukocytes: A possible pathogenic factor in periodontitis. *J Clin Periodontol* 2000;27(10):758-762.

Sidhu GS, Singh AK, Thaloor D, Banaudha KK, Patnaik GK, Srimal RC, Maheshwari RK. Enhancement ofwound healing by curcumin in animals. *Wound Repair Regen* 1998;6(2):167–177.

Simons D, Kidd EA, Beighton D, Jones B. The effect of chlorhexidine/xylitol chewing-gum on cariogenic salivary microflora: a clinical trial in elderly patients. *Caries Res* 1997;31(2):91–6.

Singh D, Lippman S. Cancer chemoprevention part 2: Hormones, nonclassic antioxidant natural agents, NSAIDs, and other agents. *Oncology* 1998;12(12):1787-1800.

Slots J, Ting M. *Actinobacillus actinomycetemcomitans* and *Porphyromonas gingivalis* in human periodontal disease: Occurrence and treatment. *Periodontol 2000* 1999; 20:82-121.

Smith AJ, Moran J, Dangler LV, Leight RS, Addy M. The efficacy of an antigingivitis chewing gum. *J Clin Periodontol* 1996;23(1):19–23.

Socransky SS, Haffajee AD, Cugini MA, Smith C, Kent RL Jr. Microbial Complexes in Subgingival Plaque. *J Clin Periodontol* 1998;25(2):134-144.

Sofrata A, Lingstrom P, Baljoon M, Gustafsson A. The effect of miswak extract on plaque pH. An in vivo study. *Caries Res* 2007;41(6):451–4.

Somu CA, Ravindra S, Ajith S, Ahmed MG. Efficacy of a herbal extract gel in the treatment of gingivitis: A clinical study. *J Ayurveda Integr Med* 2012;3(2):85-90.

Steinberg D, Feldman M, Ofek I, Weiss EI. Effect of a high-molecular-weight component of cranberry on constituents of dental biofilm. *J Antimicrob Chemother* 2004;54(1):86-89.

Stoltze K. Concentration of metronidazole in periodontal pockets after application of a metronidazole 25% dental gel. *J Clin Periodontol* 1992; 19:698–701.

Suzuki JB. Diagnosis and classification of the periodontal diseases. *Dent Clin North Am* 1988;32(2):195-216.

Takahashi K, Fukazawa M, Motohira H, Ochiai K, Nishikawa H, Miyata T. A pilot study on antiplaque effects of mastic chewing gum in the oral cavity. *J Periodontol* 2003;74(4):501-5.

Tomasi C, Wennström JL. Locally delivered doxycycline improves the healing following non-surgical periodontal therapy in smokers. *J Clin Periodontol* 2004;31(8): 589–595.

Tominari T, Matsumoto C, Watanabe K, Hirata M, Grundler FM, Miyaura C, et al. Epigallocatechin gallate (EGCG) suppresses lipopolysaccharide-induced in- flammatory bone resorption, and protects against alveolar bone loss in mice. *FEBS Open Bio* 2015;5:522–527.

Tsai SH, Lin-Shiau SY, Lin JK. Suppression of nitric oxide synthase and the down-regulation of the activation of NFkB in macrophages by resveratrol. *Br J Pharmacol* 1999;126(3):673-680.

Tyler V, Brady L, Robbers J. *Pharmacognosy*. 7th ed. Philadelphia: Lea & Febiger, 1977:64-8.

Vennila K, Elanchezhiyan S, Ilavarasu S. Efficacy of 10% whole Azadirachta indica (neem) chip as an adjunct to scaling and root planning in chronic periodontitis: A clinical and microbiological study. *Indian J Dent Res* 2016;27(1):15-21.

Veras HN, Campos AR, Rodrigues FF, et al. Enhancement of the antibiotic activity of erythromycin by volatile compounds of Lippia alba Mill. NE. Brown against Staphylococcus aureus. *Pharmacogn Mag* 2011;7(28):334–337.

Veras HN, Rodrigues FF, Botelho MA, Menezes IR, Coutinho HD, da Costa JG. Antimicrobial effect of Lippia sidoides and thymol on Enterococcus faecalis biofilm of the bacterium isolated from root canals. *Scie World J* 2014; 6:471580.

Viuda-Martos M, Fernández-López J, Pérez-Álvarez JA. Pomegranate and its many functional components as related to human health: A review. *Compr Rev Food Sci Food Saf* 2010;9(6):635-54.

Wang JP, Ho TF, Chang L, Chen CC. Anti-inflammatory effect of magnolol, isolated from *Magnolia officinalis*, on A23187 induced pleurisyinmice. *J Pharm Pharmacol* 1995; 47(10):857–860.

Watanabe K, Watanabe H, Goto Y, Yamaguchi M, Yamamoto N, Hagino K. Pharmacological properties of magnolol and honokiol extracted from *Magnolia officinalis*: central depressant effects. *Planta Med* 1983;49(2):103–108.

Weiss EI, A. Kozlovsky, D. Steinberg, R. Lev-Dor, R.B.N. Greenstein, M. Feldman, *et al.* A high molecular mass cranberry constituent reduces mutans streptococci level in saliva and inhibits in vitro adhesion to hydroxyapatite. *FEMS Microbiol Lett* 2004; 232:82-92.

Woelkart K, Marth E, Suter A et al. Bioavailability and pharmacokinetics of *Echinacea purpurea* preparations and their interaction with the immune system. *Int J Clin Pharmacol Ther* 2006;44(9):401-408.

World Health Organization. Prevention of oral diseases. Geneva: WHO; 1987.

Ximénez-Fyvie LA, Haffajee AD, Socransky SS. Microbial composition of supra- and subgingival plaque in subjects with adult periodontitis. *J Clin Periodontol* 2000;27(10):722-732.

Yamanaka A, Kimizuka R, Kato T, Okuda K. Inhibitory effects of cranberry juice on attachment of oral streptococci and biofilm formation. *Oral Microbiol Immunol* 2004;19(3):150-154.

Yamanaka A, Kouchi T, Kasai K, Kato T, Ishihara K, Okuda K. Inhibitory effect of cranberry polyphenol on biofilm formation and cysteine proteases of *Porphyromonas gingivalis. J Periodontal Res* 2007;42(6):589-592.

Yang X, Chen MW, Terry S, Vacherot F, Chopin DK, Bemis DL, Kitajewski J, Benson MC, Guo Y, Buttyan R. A human and male-specific protocadherin that acts through the wnt signaling pathway to induce neuroendocrine transdifferentiation of prostate cancer cells. *Cancer Res* 2005;65(12):5263–5271.

Yates R, Jenkins S, Newcombe RG, Wade WG, Moran J, Addy M. A 6-month home usage trial of a 1% chlorhexidine toothpaste (1). Effects on plaque, gingivitis, calculus and toothstaining. *J Clin Periodontol* 1993;20(2):130-138.

Ye F, Che Y, McMillen E, Gorski J, Brodman D, Saw D, Jiang B, Zhang DY. The effect of Scutellaria baicalensis on the signaling network in hepatocellular carcinoma cells. *Nutr Cancer* 2009;61(4):530–537.

Yun JH, Pang EK, Kim CS, Yoo YJ, Cho KS, Chai JK, et al. Inhibitory effects of green tea polyphenol (-)-epigallocatechin gallate on the expression of matrix metalloproteinase-9 and on the formation of osteoclasts. *J Periodontal Res* 2004;39(5):300–307.

In: Contemporary Use of Plant Extracts … ISBN: 978-1-53617-650-6
Editor: C. R. Emerenciano Bueno

Chapter 7

OTHER APPLICATIONS OF PLANT EXTRACTS IN DENTISTRY

Christine Men Martins[1,*], Juliana Quintino Trizzi[2], Victor Eduardo de Souza Batista[3,4], Bruno Piazza[1], Henrique Rinaldi Matheus[5], Eloi Dezan Junior[2] and Carlos Roberto Emerenciano Bueno[2]

[1]Department of Endodontics,
University of Western Sao Paulo (UNOESTE), Presidente Prudente,
Sao Paulo, Brazil
[2]Department of Endodontics, São Paulo State University (UNESP),
Araçatuba School of Dentistry, Araçatuba, SP, Brazil
[3]Department of Dentistry, Presidente Prudente Dental School,
University of Western São Paulo (UNOESTE),
Presidente Prudente, SP, Brazil
[4]Department of Dental Materials and Prosthodontics,
São Paulo State University (UNESP), Araçatuba School of Dentistry,
Araçatuba, SP, Brazil
[5]Department of Surgery and Integrated Clinic, Division of Periodontics,
São Paulo State University (UNESP), Araçatuba School of Dentistry,
Araçatuba SP, Brazil

[*] Corresponding Author's Email: christinemen@hotmail.com.

ABSTRACT

Alternative treatments or coadjutants should be studied and proposed, especially considering the global trend and boosting the world health organization towards natural substances and medicinal plants, regarding their advantages as a function of its diversity, flexibility, accessibility, availability and wide acceptance. In this context, current researches have evaluated the effectiveness of natural substances, medicinal plants, phytoterapy and homeopathics: (1) as storage media for avulsed teeth or root surface treatment before teeth replantation; (2) as coadjutant to improve osteointegration and reduce peri-implantitis in dental implants; (3) as an alternative for anesthetic agents; (4) within treatment for bone remodeling during orthodontic movement or rapid maxillary expansion; (5) as hemostatic agents; and (6) as dental plaque disclosing agents. This chapter will discuss several studies regarding to all these related topics.

Keywords: dental implants, hemostatic agents, phytotherapy, plant extracts, tooth avulsion

THE USE OF PLANT EXTRACTS AND PHYTOTHERAPY IN DENTISTRY

The World Health Organization stated that medicinal plants are the best and largest source of drugs for humanity and researches should be performed to generate evidence-based indications of their use. This chapter outlines the use of several herbal alternatives or coadjutants in tooth avulsion, dental implants, anesthetic agents, bone remodeling in orthodontic treatment, hemostatic agents and dental plaque disclosing agents.

1. PHYTOTHERAPY IN TOOTH AVULSION

One of the most severe forms of dental trauma is tooth avulsion, which is referred to as the complete displacement of a tooth from the alveolar socket (Andersson et al. 2012, Andersson 2013). Faced with this injury, the ideal treatment is the immediate replantation of the tooth into the socket (Andersson et al. 2012, Andersson 2013, Poi et al. 2013). However, this rarely occurs (Poi et al. 2013, Resende et al. 2019, Osmanivic et al. 2018), leading to late dental replantation (Andersson et al. 2012, Andersson 2013, Poi et al. 2013). Its success is related to extra alveolar time, non-manipulation of root portion, endodontic therapy, administration of systemic antibiotics, minimal bacterial contamination and storage medium for avulsed teeth (Poi et al. 2013).

Characteristics of an ideal storage media are physiologic osmolality and pH, temperature, grow factors, nutrients for fibroblasts and be easily accessible and inexpensive (Andersson et al. 2012, Andersson 2013, Poi et al. 2013, Resende et al. 2019, Osmanivic et al. 2018). All of these characteristics are important to minimize the damage on PDL cells because, when the blood supply is interrupted, the stored metabolites become depleted and cells begin to die. If the major quantity of cells die after tooth replantation, a huge inflammatory response can begin, which leads to inflammatory root resorption. On the other hand, if the inflammatory process is controlled, abnormal attachment can occur after healing, which might be in the form of ankylosis (Hiremath & Kidiyoor 2011).

Various types of wet storage media have been investigated, from tissue culture solutions, medical/hospital products, contact lens solutions and rehydrating solutions to natural products (Osmanovic et al. 2018, Resende et al. 2019, Hiremath & Kidiyoor 2011, Poi et al. 2013, Adnan et al. 2018).

Natural products have been investigated as an alternative or complementary source of drugs and in the last years many researchers were performed. Also, it has been studied the use of natural products as storage media for avulsed teeth (Resende et al. 2019). Even though the use of natural substances and medicinal plants is encouraged due to their diversity, flexibility, accessibility, availability and wide acceptance, the World Health Organization stated that medicinal plants are the best and largest source of drugs for humanity (Resende et al. 2019, Poi et al. 2013).

To evaluate the efficacy of storage media for avulsed teeth, many protocols have been written in the literature. Primary PDL cell culture from extracted premolars and molars, fibroblast cell culture and PDL cell directly from extracted teeth were examples of cells types used under trypan blue and MTT assays (Martins et al. 2016). Trypan blue assay is an easy and cheap method to evaluate cell viability related to the maintenance of cellular membrane integrity; however, it cannot be evaluated the cell metabolism activity, which gap is suppressed using the MTT or MTS assays (Martins et al. 2016, Hwang et al. 2011). Also, different cell types from peripheral blood mononuclear cells can be stimulated to the process of osteoclastogenesis and evaluate parameters which will suggest resorption activity (Wimolsantirungsri et al. 2018). Furthermore, histological and histomorphometric analysis can be performed using an animal model that simulates tooth avulsion and tooth replantation (Mori et al. 2010, Poi et al. 2018).

1.1. Propolis

Propolis is a resinous hive substance produced by honeybees from collected plant products. The precise chemical composition of propolis is not stable, being variable according to the plant source, the climate, season, year and location (Al-Haj Ali et al. 2013) but, regardless, it has good properties.

In general, propolis is composed of 50% resin and vegetable balsam, 30% wax, 10% essential and aromatic oils, 5% pollen and 5% various other substances. The principal characteristics of propolis are antifungal, antibacterial and anti-inflammatory resinous material (Ahangari et al. 2013).

Propolis have been introduced in medicine and dentistry treatments as coadjutant and mainly therapies as we can observe in previously chapters. This natural product has been widely studied in tooth avulsion and tooth replantation also.

Ozan et al. (2007) evaluated viability of primary PDL cell culture from extracted premolars and molars thru trypan blue assay along 24 h (1, 3, 6, 12 and 24 h). It was observed that 20% propolis presented a great result on maintaining cell viability. As a complementary analysis, an evaluation of cell metabolism activity was performed under same cells but thru MTT. Al-Haj Ali et al. (2013) subjected the cells during 0, 30, 45, 60, 90 and 120 minutes dry storage times then incubated with Jordanian propolis for 45 minutes at room temperature. It was observed that when PDL cells are left dry and treated with propolis, negative effects of PDL cell viability can be observed. However, they hypothesized that soaking in propolis should be extended more than 45 minutes to be beneficial. Awawdeh et al. (2018) evaluated different concentrations of propolis in Dulbecco's Modified Eagles Medium (DMEM) for 1 h, 2 h, 6 h, 24 h, 48 h, 72 h, and 168 h. It was observed that propolis at 6.25 mg/mL in DMEM resulted in 138% viable PDL and it was able to preserve PDL cells for up to 168 hours.

Studies have observed PDL cell viability directly from extracted teeth and analyzed by trypan blue assay. Martin et al. (2004) used extracted teeth dried for 30 min to stock in 50 and 100% propolis during 45 min. It was observed both concentrations of propolis lead to better PDL cell viability than HBSS, milk and saline. Ahangari et al. (2013) obtained same result in their research changing only the stocked time to 1 h and 3 h. Prueksakorn et al. (2016) used different concentrations of Thai propolis during 3 hours and a non-toxic dose of 2.5 mg/ml-1 of propolis extract yielded the greatest percentage of cell viability, similar to HBSS and higher than milk. However, they also observed that 2.5 mg/ml-1 of the extract did not induce PDL cell proliferation. Likewise, Babaji et al. (2017) selected extracted teeth and immersed in 50% propolis for 45 min and cell viability were assessed by trypan blue and great results were observed.

Casaroto et al. (2010) evaluated the efficacy of propolis extract in maintaining the viability of human periodontal ligament (PDL) cells, and to radiographically analyze tooth replantation and the adjacent periodontium in dogs after storage in this extract. The result showed great performance thru MTT assay, with optical density over than 0.8 along all experimental time (1, 3, 6, 12 and 24h), but did not prevent root resorption of avulsed and replanted teeth in dogs. Gjertsen et al. (2011) evaluated not only PDL cell viability, but also PDL cell apoptosis and mitochondrial enzymatic activity and as result they have observed that cells maintained in propolis increased cell viability, increased mitochondrial enzymatic activity and decreased apoptotic levels of PDL cells.

Complementary analysis was performed by Yuan et al. (2018) comparing osteogenic differentiation potential PDL using alkaline phosphatase (ALP) staining, ALP activity, osteogenic marker gene expression and protein production. The results showed that cells stored in propolis presented no significant difference in ALP activity, ALP expression, and protein levels compared with control group, which suggested that Propolis maintained the original early osteogenic differentiation character of PDL. Furthermore, expression of RUNX2 was similar among the different groups, which reflect that RUNX2 was not affected by Propolis. To examine the late stage osteogenic differentiation potential, Alizarin Red S staining and real-time PCR of OCN and OSX showed that Propolis and HBSS exhibited similar effects. To complete, it was analyzed anti-inflammatory effect of Propolis. PDL were stimulated with LPS to increase the expression of inflammatory cytokines and, after treatment with Propolis, the expression levels of inflammatory cytokines were significantly downregulated. So, they concluded propolis could be used as an alternative storage medium to preserve the viability and osteogenic potential of PDL. It also has a superior effect in downregulating the expression of pro-inflammatory cytokines in hPDLCs when used as a storage medium.

An *in vitro* induction of osteoclastogenesis affected by propolis were evaluated in Wimolsantirungsri et al. (2018) research. They used peripheral blood mononuclear cells cultured in the presence or absence of various non-toxic concentrations of propolis extract, as determined by the alamar Blue® assay. Osteoclast formation was examined by tartrate-resistant acid phosphatase staining, actin ring formation, and real-time polymerase chain reaction. The resorption pit assay was performed to determine osteoclast function. They have observed that non-toxic concentrations of propolis extract suppressed osteoclast formation by significantly decreasing the percentages of tartrate-resistant acid phosphatase-positive multinuclear cells and the ratios of cells with F-actin ring formation in a dose-dependent fashion. Expression of several osteoclast-specific genes was significantly downregulated by propolis in a dose-dependent manner. The percentages of resorption areas on dentin slices were significantly decreased by propolis. So, Thai propolis can inhibit human osteoclast formation and function, which may be beneficial for prevention of root resorption following replantation of avulsed teeth.

Some histomorphometric analisys were performed in mice model of tooth avulsion followed by tooth replantation. Gulinelli et al. (2008) extracted the teeth, kept teeth dried for 60 min and then used 15% propolis as surface treatment comparing with 2% sodium fluoride solution. After 60 days of replantation, it was observed that 15% propolis yield similar external root resorption in teeth with delayed tooth replantation to 2% sodium fluoride, which had almost 50% of the area with root resorption. Similarly, Mori et al. (2010) simulated an avulsion in a murine tooth, the teeth were maintained in 20% propolis during 60 min and 6 h and then replantation was performed. After 15 and 60 days was observed low incidence of inflammatory and replacement resorption and preservation of both the cementum layer and root surface after 6 h storing teeth. However, in 60 min it could be observed the reduction of the cementum presence on the root and the lack of periodontal repair after tooth reimplantation in this group. This demonstrated that the maintenance of the avulsed tooth in propolis for 6 h was more effective. It has been believed that there would be the best action and the highest incorporation of the active principles of propolis which have been responsible for the antimicrobial, anti-inflammatory and healing actions when the tooth has been kept in propolis for 6 h.

de Souza et al. (2017) kept PDL cells at 5°C and 20°C, in Propolis, for 3, 6, 24, 48, 72, 96, and 120 h, through the analysis of MTT assay. They have observed that cell maintained in propolis were not influenced by temperature and is a suitable medium to be used up to 3 hours.

Propolis is widely studied and, in general, results indicate that it can be used as interim storage media for avulsed teeth.

1.2. Coconut Water

Coconut water is a natural product and has been widely used as a blood plasma substitute because of its sterility and biocompatibility (Bharath et al. 2015). Its consumption is related to replace fluids, electrolytes (potassium, calcium and magnesium), and sugars lost from the body. Coconut`s water characteristic is biologically pure, sterile and rich in amino acids, proteins, vitamins and minerals (Moreira-Neto et al. 2009).

A bunch of studies have suggested coconut water as a storage media for avulsed teeth, but the results are conflicting.

A classical method to evaluate periodontal ligament (PDL) cell viability is using human primary PDL cell culture from extracted premolars and molars thru MTT assay was performed. Bharath et al. (2015) tested tender coconut water and observed no statistically difference between HBSS (cell culture media) within 15 min, 30 min, 60 min and 90 min. Similarly, Al-Haj Ali et al. (2013) evaluated at 0 min, 30 min, 45 min, 60 min, 90 min and 120 min dry storage times then incubated with 100% mature coconut water for 45 minutes at room temperature; it was observed that when PDL cells are left dry for over than 45 minutes may benefit from soaking for 45 minutes in mature coconut water; on the other hand, PDL cells left dry less than 45 min, the best scenario should be immediate replantation. Kokkali et al. (2017) storage PDL primary culture cells for 75 min and they have observed medians results for coconut water, whereas milk presented the best performance.

Same MTT method were performed in fibroblast cell cultured. Awawdeh et al. (2018) tested immature, half mature, and mature coconut water incubated for 1 h, 2 h, 6 h, 24 h, 48 h, 72 h, and 168 h. It was observed that coconut water showed significantly higher viability of cells than DMEM and water at 6 hours with half mature coconut water being superior. de Souza et al. (2017) kept PDL cells at 5°C and 20°C, in natural coconut water for 3, 6, 24, 48, 72, 96, and 120 h, through the analysis of MTT assay. They have observed that cell maintained in natural coconut water were not influenced by temperature and is a suitable medium to be used up to 3 hours.

Another method to evaluate cell viability is thru trypan blue assay. Thomas et al. (2008) tested coconut water in fibroblast cell culture at 15, 30, 45, 60 and 120 min thru trypan blue assay. As result, they observed that coconut water is as effective as HBSS during all experimental time. Gopikrishna et al. (2008) extracted teeth and maintained dry for 30 min and, later on, the teeth were maintained in coconut storage media for 45 min. Trypan blue assay have demonstrated highest number of viable PDL cells followed in rank order by HBSS and milk.

Although above studies presented promising results to the use of coconut water as storage media for avulsed teeth, Moreira-Neto et al. (2009) evaluated the effectiveness of coconut water in maintaining PDL cell viability at 1 h, 2 h and 4 h, by the analysis of cell metabolism using the neutral red assay. It was observed that the performance of coconut water was similar to mineral water, which is not adequate. The explanation can be because of its pH acid around 4.1, which is deleterious to cell metabolism. This explanation is supported to the fact of the group to added sodium bicarbonate to coconut water and it was more effective as storage medium than coconut alone.

Corroborating with this theory, De Paula Reis et al. (2014) extracted dogs' teeth and maintained in coconut water with pH adjusted during 50 min. All teeth were replanted in the socket with finger pressure and splinted with semirigid contention for 14 days. After 28 days, the dogs were euthanized and it was performed microCT and histomorphometric analysis. Coconut water showed a performance similar to whole milk group, being a promising storage media. Also, Moura et al. (2014) performed a research of PDL cell viability from extracted dog's teeth thru trypan blue assay after stored 50 min and 24 hours. They observed pH-adjusted coconut water had similar performance after 50 min significantly higher cell viability at 24 h period than long shelf-life skim milk, long shelf-life whole milk, and HBSS. Also, pH-adjusted coconut water resulted in cell viability similar to the level obtained immediately after tooth avulsion.

Due to great properties presented by coconut water and the researches performed cited above, it can be a potential storage media for avulsed teeth, but the best result can be observed when pH is adjusted.

1.3. Green Tea

Green tea was chosen as a test solution because the increased consumption nowadays and maybe will be an easily available alternative in the event of an accident (Bharath et al. 2015). In the dental field, green tea extract was known to protect alveolar bone resorption from periodontal disease because it inhibited the expression of matrix metalloproteinase-9 (MMP) in osteoblasts and the formation of osteoclasts (Bharath et al. 2015). Furthermore, its anti-bacterial, anti-oxidative, and anti-inflammatory effects raised the interest in its use as a storage media for avulsed teeth (Ghasempour et al. 2015).

It is produced from leaves of *Camellia sinensis* plant, which is considered a major source of polyphenols, like catechin, epicatechin, epigallocatechin, epigallocatechin-3-gallate, epicatechingallate, and quercetin glycosides (Ghasempour et al. 2015). This medium also contains critical elements for cell growth such as calcium, magnesium, selenium, zinc, iron, and fluoride as well as some carbohydrates such as glucose, fructose, sucrose, and vitamins B, C, and E (Ghasempour et al. 2015).

Although its potential to have good results, Bharath et al. (2015) tested a commercial green tea as storage media and observed after 90 min an inferior viability compared to HBSS and Ringer's lactate using cultured PDL cells from extracted premolars thru MTT assay. The result was clarified due the very low osmolality, which might lead to cell death. On the other hand, Ghasempour et al. (2015) also tested a commercial green tea, but along 1 h, 3 h and 15 hall medium were kept at 4o C. By this way, the viability of PDL cells directly from extract teeth were like those kept in HBSS and higher than those kept in distilled water.

Interestingly, Hwang et al. (2011) performed a research using primary culture of PDL cell in a commercial green tea and in a green tea extract.

The have examined cell characteristics under optical microscope and cell viability thru nucleocounter and MTS assay. Microscopic analysis showed that the PDL cells stored in the HBSS and green tea extract kept almost the spindle-like morphology as time passed, differently from commercial green tea and water. Corroborating to the microscope examination, nucleocounter method and MTS assay showed higher viabilities to green tea extract and HBSS, over than 90% to nucleocounter and on the verge of 0.4 optical density to MTS assay.

Still, few studies were performed. It can be suggested to better evaluate green tea and specially compare the extract with commercial available green tea.

1.4. Aloe Vera

Aloe Vera is a member of *Liliaceae* family and is a medicinal plant composed by 96% water and 75 active properties such as vitamins, enzymes, minerals, sugars, salicylic acids, and amino acids. It has been reported that Aloe Vera has significant anti-inflammatory, antioxidant, antibacterial, antifungal, anticarcinogenic activities and leads to a great wound healing effect (Badakhsh et al. 2014).

Aloe Vera has been studied due to its potential to be a storage media for avulsed teeth. Badakhsh et al. (2014) tested different concentrations of Aloe Vera as storage media on viability thru MTT assay of PDL cells directly from extract teeth and observed that after 1 h, 3 h, 6 h and 9 h 10, 30 and 50% concentration of Aloe Vera had the greatest ability to preserve the cell viability at least for up to 9 hours and 100% Aloe Vera were significantly the worst experimental media within the first hour. It is important to explain that dilutions were made with DMEM, which is a cell culture media. Also 100% Aloe Vera concentration is highly viscous, at the time of experiment it entirely covered the surface of the experimented cells and may have possibly prevented the accessibility of oxygen to them.

On the other hand, same method was performed by Babaji et al. (2017), which immersed selected extracted teeth were immersed in Aloe

Vera gel obtained directly from the leaves for 45 min. Regarding to the result, Aloe vera was considered a suitable storage media. Moazzami et al. (2017) kept teeth 30 min dry followed by a 45 min immersion in 50% aloe vera extract and they observed thru trypan blue assay high percentages of cell viability, being similar to HBSS. Corroborating those results, Fulzele et al. (2016) concluded in their research that, highest viable cells found in HBSS followed by Aloe vera over a period of 120 min. Sharma et al. (2015) found highest viable cells with A. vera when compared to egg white and milk.

1.5. Soymilk

Studies have proposed soymilk as an alternative storage medium because of the increased consumption of soy products in many countries and the fact that soymilk is a good source of minerals, carbohydrates, sugars, proteins, fats, calcium and vitamins A, C, D, and E. Also, it presents a physiological pH (de Paula Reis et al. 2014, Moura et al. 2014).

Moazzami et al. (2017) used a dog model for dental trauma such as tooth avulsion and replantation. Teeth were maintained dry for 30 min followed by a 45-min immersion in soymilk and viable cells were counted via trypan blue assay. High percentages of cell viability were seen in soymilk group, being similar to HBSS. Moura et al. (2014) performed a similar research but using PDL cell viability from dog's teeth and did not maintained dry but stored for 50 min and 24 hours. They observed soymilk had similar performance after 50 min and significantly higher cell viability at 24 h period than long shelf-life skim milk, long shelf-life whole milk, and HBSS. Also, soymilk resulted in cell viability similar to the level obtained immediately after tooth avulsion.

On the other hand, de Paula Reis et al. (2014) extracted dogs' teeth and maintained in soymilk during 50 min. All teeth were replanted in the socket with finger pressure and splinted with semirigid contention for 14 days. After 28 days, the dogs were euthanized and it was performed microCT and histomorphometric analysis. Although the soymilk properties its used caused higher ankylosis than the control group (immediate replantation).

1.6. Natural Products Little Studied in Tooth Avulsion and Replantation

Pomegranate is the fruit of *Punica granatum* (*Punicaceae*) that has been extensively used in the folk medicine of many cultures to treat acidosis, dysentery, microbial infections, diarrhea, hemorrhage, respiratory pathologies, and hypertension. Besides, pomegranate is a rich source of polyphenolic flavonoids; which possess direct antioxidant properties. Pomegranate flavonoids also have anti-inflammatory and antibacterial properties, besides stimulating osteoblasts proliferation and differentiation.

Tavassoli-Hojjati et al. (2014) used primary culture of human PDL cells in contact with pomegranate juice during 1, 3, 6 and 24 ha and cell viability was assessed by neutral red assay and also it was analyzed cell morphology under phase contrast microscope. The more concentrated the juice solution, the better the performance in maintaining cell viability. Concentration of 5 and 7,5% presented better results than HBSS and preserved spindle-like cell morphology even after 24 hours. An interesting result is pomegranate increased cell proliferation. It can be explained because of the numerous antioxidants and flavonoids. In the same way, Babaji et al. (2017) observed good performance of pomegranate juice on maintained viable PDL cells from selected extracted teeth and assessed by trypan blue.

Dragon`s blood sap (*Chroton lechleri*) presents significant chemical and pharmacological properties, such as anti-inflammatory, healing, anticancer, antimycotic, antiviral, antifungal and antibacterial, and antioxidant activities. In addition, this sap demonstrated potential to enhance osteogenesis, mineralization and bone formation (Martins et al. 2016). Martins et al. (2016) performed a research to verify the viability of human peripheral blood mononuclear and cultured periodontal ligament cells thru Trypan Blue and MTT assay after 1, 3, 6, 10 and 24 h of incubation. For trypan blue test, the dragon's blood sap was similar to milk and both presented the highest viability values. For MTT, the dragon's blood sap showed better results than all storage media, even better than milk. This result suggested not only maintenance of cell integrity, but also cell metabolism activity.

Capparis spinosa is one of the most commonly found aromatics in the Mediterranean kitchen. It is used in medicine for its diuretic, constipant and tonic properties. Different parts of this plant, including the flower buds, fruits, seeds, shoots, and bark of roots, were traditionally used as folk medicines in the treatment of disorders, such as rheumatism, stomach problems, headache, and toothache. These properties can be related to the presence of alkaloids, lipids, flavonoids, polyprenols, and aliphatic glucosinolates (Ozan et al. 2015). Ozan et al. (2015) performed a research using primary culture of PDL cells and analyzed by the xCELLigence - which measures the impedance changes due to electrode surface occupation by (proliferated/migrated/invaded) cells during the course of time. They have observed that the cell index values of the light milk and HBSS were significantly lower compared with the DMEM and *C. spinosa* groups, suggesting that *C. spinosa* have a proliferative effect with time.

Morus rubra is another plant that the juice has been tested as an alternative storage media. Due its oxygen radicals and oxygen tension, it has been reported that *Morus rubra* modulates osteoblast and osteoclast activities, as far as presents antioxidant and antioxidative properties (Ozan et al. 2008). Ozan et al. (2008) evaluated primary culture of PDL cell viability assessed by trypan blue exclusion at 37°C for 1, 3, 6, 12, or 24 hours maintained in *Morus rubra* juice in different concentrations. They observed that at 3, 6, and 12 hours was found to be significantly better than HBSS. At 24 hours, 4% *M. rubra* was found to be similar to HBSS, but 2.5% *M. rubra* was found to be significantly worse than HBSS. The results showed that juice of the fruit sample of *Morus rubra* studied at a concentration of 4% was a more effective storage medium than other groups.

Resveratrol (trans-3 5 4′-trihydroxystilbene) is a natural polyphenolic substance found in plants (blackberries), peanuts, nuts, vegetables and red grape peels, which is why certain red wines have high concentrations of it. Its properties are related to strong antioxidant, anti-inflammatory, antiplaque and antiproliferative. In dentistry, Resveratrol has also been proven to decrease periodontal damage induced in rats and increase type I collagen synthesis and the microcondrial respiration in fibroblasts of human gingival tissue under oxidative stress induced by hydrogen peroxide (Poi et al. 2018). Despite, Poi et al. (2018) performed a research simulating teeth avulsion in mices and evaluated histomorphometric after teeth were stored in resveratrol diluted in DMSO. They have observed thru acute inflammatory process in the epithelial insertion, the organization of the periodontal ligament, chronic inflammatory infiltrate and the depth and extent of resorption that teeth storage in resveratrol diluted in DMSO solution did not inhibit root resorption after delayed replantation in rat teeth.

Castor oil is a colorless to very-pale-yellow liquid with a distinct taste, obtained from the seeds of castor oil plant (*Ricinus communis*). Castor oil as a vegetable oil has several advantages such as antimicrobial and antioxidant properties, low toxicity, and glutathione preservation capability, low cost, and high availability. It also has the capacity to repair bone defects. Although great propertied demonstrated, Nabavizadeh et al. (2018) used extracted human teeth stored dry for 30 min, immersed for 45 min in castor oil and the number of viable PDL cells were counted by trypan blue. It was observed that castor oil was significantly lower than HBSS and milk, so it appears that castor oil cannot be served as an ideal medium for storage of avulsed tooth.

2. Phytotherapy in Dental Implants

The use of dental implants has become an alternative in the rehabilitation of edentulous patients, with a success rate of approximately 96%. The causes of the failures may be related to patient's general health and oral hygiene habits, which can trigger peri-implantitis. Peri-implantitis is defined as an inflammation of the mucosa with the presence of suppuration, bleeding, and continuous bone loss around the implants, generally caused by accumulation of biofilm.

Treatment for that is mechanically and chemically remove the infection. Chlorhexidine is widely used in this context, but new agents have been proposed in order to minimize unwanted reactions presented by users with the use of antimicrobials, such as increased resistance by microorganisms, unpleasant taste, taste changes, pigmentation of teeth, and oral desquamation.

Among the substances obtained from plants, the essential oils stand out as natural, complex compounds characterized by strong odor and volatility. Trindade et al. (2015) investigated the biological activity of the essential oil from *Cymbopogon nardus* and of the phytoconstituent citronellal on *Candida spp* strains as to the inhibition of adherence to dental implants and cover screws. The essential oil significantly inhibited the adherence of *Candida albicans* to the dental implants and cover screws. Citronellal inhibited yeast adherence only to the dental implants, and no significant results were found for the cover screws compared to the growth control. As conclusion, the essential oil and citronellal have proven antifungal activity and are able to inhibit the *in vitro* adherence of *C. albicans.*

Also, a successful dental implant treatment requires stability of the implant fixture with the living bone, which could be achieved through the process of osseointegration. Titanium is widely used as dental implant materials owing to its low density, good biocompatibility, high corrosion resistance and appropriate mechanical properties. Nevertheless, its bioinert nature warrants more time to achieve complete osseointegration. To overcome this limitation, various physical, chemical, and biochemical treatments are explored to modify the surface of the titanium implant (de Oliveira et al. 2014; Somsanith et al. 2018). Another attempt to improve osseointegration is use natural extracts as drugs or homeopathy (Sakakura et al. 2008, Spin-Neto et al. 2010).

Anodic oxidation (anodizing) is a simple, versatile and cost-effective surface treatment process to generate nanostructures on titanium and its alloys, called TNT. Propolis is a resinous natural product, which contains a mixture of different plant exudates collected by the honeybees from the buds and leaves of various types of trees and plants and the honeybee's salivary enzymes. It presents anti-microbial and antiprotozoal, anti-inflammatory, and immunomodulatory activities. The use of propolis is also explored in dental treatment which includes aphthous ulcers, candidiasis, gingivitis, periodontitis, pulpitis and tooth avulsion/ replantation. Somsanith et al. (2018) performed an *in vitro* and *in vivo* study. For *in vitro* studies the TNT were prepared on titanium plates whereas for *in vivo* studies using a rat model, the TNT were prepared on a titanium dental implant. Both were loaded with propolis to study the effect of propolis on osseointegration. In a cytotoxicity test using osteoblast, PL-TNT-Ti group exhibited an increased cell proliferation and differentiation. A Sprague Dawley rat mandibular model was used to evaluate the osseointegration and bone bonding of TNT or PL-TNT-Ti. From the μ-CT and hematoxylin and eosin (HE) histological results after implantation at 1 and 4 weeks to rat mandibular, an increase in the extent of new bone formation and mineral density around the PL-TNT-Ti implant was confirmed. The Masson's trichrome staining showed the expression of well-formed collagenous for bone formation on the PL-TNT-Ti. Immunohistochemistry staining indicate that bone morphogenetic proteins (BMP-2 and BMP-7) around the PL-TNT-Ti increased the expression of collagen fibers and of osteogenic differentiation whereas the expression of inflammatory cytokine such as interleukin-1 beta (IL-1ß) and tumor necrosis factor-alpha (TNF-α) is decreased.

Avocado and soybean unsaponifiables extract is produced from the fruits and seeds of avocados and soybeans in a ratio 1:2, respectively, and is indicated as a supplement of rheumatoid arthritis and osteoarthritis thru controlling the action of several pro-inflammatory mediators such as IL-1β, IL-6, IL-8, TNFα, prostaglandins PGE2, inducible nitric oxide synthase iNOS, metalloproteinase MMP-2 and MMP-3, and bone morphogenetic protein BMP-2. De Oliveira et al. (2014) performed a surgery to consolidate titanium implant in tibia`s mice and they have systemically administrated avocado and soybean unsaponifiables extract thru gavage since the day of the surgery or before 7 days until 60 days postoperatively. Implant osseointegration and bone maturation were assessed by biomechanical and radiographic bone density analysis; descriptive histology; immunohistochemistry for bone morphogenetic protein 2 (BMP-2), transforming growth factor beta 1 (TGF-β1), and osteocalcin; and histomorphometric evaluation of bone-to-implant contact and mineralized bone area fraction within the threads of the implant. As results, they observed that the systemic administration of avocados and soybeans unsaponifiables showed three times higher expression of BMP-2 and nine times higher expression of TGF-β1 compared with without administration. Histomorphometric analysis, however, showed that both ASU1 and ASU2 groups presented significantly higher bone-to-implant contact values only in the cortical bone compartment. By this way, the administration of these extracts seems to exert only a subtle effect on implant osseointegration. De Paula et al. (2018) performed a similar research however using mices with experimental arthritis and they have observed that systemically administrated avocado and soybean unsaponifiables extract improved the osseointegration, particularly in animals with induced arthritis.

Resveratrol is a natural component found in black grape skin, has become important in light of various findings of pharmacological and clinical studies. Beyond the protective effect of resveratrol against several tumour and pathological mechanisms, its inhibitory effect on osteoclast differentiation and its potential to induce bone formation have also been studied. Casarin et al. (2014) investigated the effect of systemic resveratrol on bone healing and its influence on the gene expression of osteogenic markers through calvaria defects and screw-shaped titanium implant was inserted in the tibia. Histomorphometric analysis revealed higher remaining defect in the calvaria defects of the control group than the resveratrol; also this natural compound increased the counter-torque values of implant removal, up-regulate the gene expression of important osteogenic markers (BMP-2, BMP-7 and OPN). Ribeiro et al. (2019) investigated the effect of resveratrol on peri-implant repair, and its influence on bone-related markers in rats submitted to cigarette smoking inhalation and they concluded that resveratrol reverses the negative effects of smoking in the peri-implant repair, benefiting the modulation of bone-related markers.

Symphytum officinale (Comfrey) is a common garden plant that has been used in herbal medicine for a long time. The homeopathic preparation *Symphytum* 6CH is reported to improve bone healing after trauma or fractures (Spin-Neto et al. 2010, Mazzocchi & Montanaro 2012). Sakakura et al. (2008) and Spin-Neto et al. (2010) observed that systemic consumption of *Symphytum officinale* in homeopathic potency (comfrey) resulted in increased implant removal torque values and peri-implant radiographic bone density compared with placebo treatment thru mice model of implants placed in tibiae. Interestingly, Mazzocchi & Montanaro (2012) also reported that adding *Symphytum* 5CH to conventional analgesia may reduce pain and swelling after minor surgery in patients subjected to titanium dental implant.

Pectins are plant-specific polysaccharides that provide mechanical strength for the cell walls of higher plants in addition to playing an important role in various cellular processes. In medicine, it has been demonstrated capacity to improve cell adhesion and behavior, stimulated osteoblastogenesis, and anti-inflammatory property. Kokkonen et al. (2008) investigated how titanium coated with modified pectins supports osteoblast differentiation; the data indicate that modified pectin nanocoatings may enhance the biocompatibility of bone and dental implants.

The leaves of the tea plant (*Camellia Sinensis*) are rich in extractable polyphenols which make up around 10–15% of the weight and are responsible for anti-inflammatory, antioxidant, anticancer, and antibacterial effects, as well as effects on bone health by improving osteoblast mineralization and differentiation. Cazzola et al. (2018) evaluated a chemically-treated titanium alloy surface functionalized with a polyphenolic extract from green tea. The cells and titanium surfaces were characterized for monitoring cell viability and hydroxyapatite production. A higher production of extracellular matrix was highlighted on the functionalized samples and the fluorescence images showed higher viability of cells and greater presence of osteocalcin in these samples, indicating the ability of polyphenols to improve cell differentiation and to stimulate biological mineralization.

3. Anesthetic Agents of Plant Origin

Pain is one of the most common symptom in dentistry practice nowadays, despite it is an undesired experience caused by pathologic conditions, injury, surgery or procedures during various dentistry treatments (Rios et al. 2007, Rita et al. 2012, Andrade et al. 2013, Nomura et al. 2013, Santana de Freitas-Blanco et al. 2016). It can prostrate and/or psychologically traumatize the patient (Andrade et al. 2013). By the way, controlling pain has always been a major concern for health professionals (Tsuchiya et al. 2017). The process of nociception involves the transduction, transmission, modulation and perception being afferent nociceptors (αdelta and c-fibers) the responsible for initiate that (Rios et al. 2007). To abolish or interrupt these nociceptive procedure, two types of medications are widely used, analgesics and anesthetics. Local and topical application of local anesthetics on oral mucosa generally produces superficial anesthesia; benzocaine and lidocaine are commonly used for this purpose. However, medicinal plants and herbs have been used since ancient times for relieving pain and herbal can be alternative due its low cost, easy access and good properties (Rios et al. 2007, Rita et al. 2012, Andrade et al. 2013, Nomura et al. 2013, Santana de Freitas-Blanco et al. 2016, Tsuchiya et al. 2017).

Acmella oleracea is a flowering herb species popularly known as "jambu", its leaves and yellow flowers cause a mild tingling and numbness of the tongue (Andrade et al. 2013, Nomura et al. 2013, Santana de Freitas-Blanco et al. 2016, Rondanelli et al. 2019). Current literature is revealing pharmacological properties such as its efficiency as a topical anesthetic.

Santana de Freitas-Blanco et al. (2016) evaluated the permeation of spilanthol and topical anesthetic efficacy in mice of ethanolic extracts from aerial parts of jambu in mucoadhesive films. They have concluded that mucoadhesive film containing crude extract of jambu treated with activated carbon is a potential alternative for oral, topical use, encouraging future clinical studies. In this line, Andrade et al. (2013) applied 15% or 30% of *Acmella oleracea* ointment in one side of the mouth, in the mucobuccal fold above the maxillary canine eminence. Each volunteer served as his/her own control, whereas on the other side were applied benzocaine. Next, a twenty-seven-gauge short needle was inserted into the mucosa just past the bevel and then immediately removed and pain measurement was performed thru visual analogue scale. As result it was observed that no statistically significant differences between the medicinal plant and benzocaine; so *Acmella oleracea* ointment was effective and safe in reducing the pain.

Another line of research, Nomura et al. (2013) administrated systemically an ethanolic extract obtained from the flowers of *Acmella oleracea* in mice model and observed reduction of neurogenic and inflammatory phases of the formalin- and also capsaicin- and cinnamaldehyde-induced orofacial nociception. The extract also reversed capsaicin-induced heat hyperalgesia, reduced mechanical allodynia caused by partial sciatic nerve ligation for 3h and did not alter the locomotion of animals. They concluded that ethanolic extract of *Acmella oleracea* produces prevalent antinociceptive effects and does not cause adverse effects.

Recently, Rondanelli et al. (2019) performed a literature review about the anti-inflammatory, anti-oxidant and painkiller properties of *Acmella oleracea*. They explained that all of these properties are attributed to phytosterols and phenolic compounds, especially N-alkylamides, the spilanthol, responsible for primarily anesthetic. Different process for antinociceptive effect has been demonstrated, related to inhibition of prostaglandin synthesis, activation of opioidergic, serotoninergic and GABAergic systems. Anesthetic activity was related to the blockage of voltage-gated Na Channels.

Others medicinal herbs also have been related to analgesic activity. *Heliopsis longipes* is a Mexican plant that presented fungistatic and bacteriostatic activity, as well as analgesic activity. Rios et al. (2007) evaluated gama amino butyric acid (GABA) concentration in a region of the cerebral cortex, because increasing this concentration, it is produced lasting analgesia by enhancing the descending inhibition of spinal nociceptive neurons. They have observed that affinin (an active compound) evoked the GABA release and suggested its possible analgesic activity.

Sterculia tragacantha presented anti-inflammatory and anti-oxidant properties related to neutrophil-derived free radicals, reactive oxygen species, nitric oxide, prostaglandins and cytokines. Rita et al. (2012) injected intra-dermally the extracts and fractions of *Sterculia tragacantha* in guinea pig and sensitivity test were performed every 5 min for a period of 30 min. It was observed that both the extract and fractions of *Sterculia tragacantha* were able to inhibit nerve impulse conduction in the skin of Guinea pigs and the alkaloids and saponins contained may be responsible for this activity.

4. Phytotherapy in Bone Remodeling during Orthodontic Treatment

Orthodontic tooth movement is achieved by the process of repeated alveolar bone resorption on the pressure side and new bone formation on the tension side (Wang et al. 2012). The idea of corroborating chemical and mechanical acting might lead to faster orthodontic tooth movement than with mechanical orthodontic force alone (Wang et al. 2012). Therefore, some medical plants were studied.

Dipsacus asper Wall (*Dipsacaceae*), commonly known as gusuibu, has been used in Chinese traditional medicine to treat bone fractures, especially because it improves circulation, has a tonic effect, an analgesic and anti-inflammatory properties (Wang et al. 2012). *Salvia miltiorrhiza* (Salvia), commonly known as danshen, is traditionally used for treating inflammatory and cardiovascular diseases due to organ protective, anti-inflammatory and anti-oxidative effects. Also this herbal inhibits platelet aggregation and promotes fibrinolysis (Wang et al. 2012). *Drynaria fortunei* (Drynaria), commonly known as Gusuibu, is frequently used for the prevention or treatment of bone-related diseases (Wang et al. 2012). Wang et al. (2012) used a mice model simulating orthodontic tooth movement and they had administrated intragastrical administration the cited plants extract every day until 28 days. They have seen that new bone formation in periodontal tissue were significantly higher in the herbal groups compared with the control group, as well the quantity of osteoclastic cells.

Another aspect that deserves respect during orthodontic treatment is related to bone formation after rapid maxillary expansion. This a common orthodontic procedure used to correct the narrowness of the upper jaw. After the procedure, it is important the velocity and the quality of new bone formed is an important factor to avoid post-expansion relapse (Kara et al. 2012, Erdogan et al. 2015, Halicioglu et al. 2015, Irgin et al. 2016). A mice model simulating orthopedic expansion force to maxillary incisors in rats is widely used to evaluate important parameters, and some researches were developed to evaluate different types of medicinal plants (Kara et al. 2012, Erdogan et al. 2015, Halicioglu et al. 2015, Irgin et al. 2016), and interestingly that all of them presented great results, indicating the use of these extracts as stimulator of bone formations after rapid maxillary expansion.

Capparis spinosa presents antihypertensive, anti-inflammatory, antiviral, diuretics, astringents, tonics and antioxidant properties which may play a crucial act in the hastening of bone regeneration and decreasing the consolidation duration. Erdogan et al. (2015) administrated *Caparis spinosa* orogastrically and observed higher quantity of new bone area, new bone volume, connective tissue space, and connective tissue volume for *Capparis spinosa* groups after 7 days; however, after 14 days, same performance was observed for both control group and herbal group. They concluded that systemic administration of *Capparis spinosa* accelerated fastened osteoblastic activity in the early period.

Urtica dioica (Urticaceae family), also known as Stinging nettle (SN) or Common nettle, is among the common green plants widely used to treat rheumatoid arthritis, osteoarthritis, urinary tract infections, coronary heart disease and high blood pressure, diabetes, cancer, inflammation, viral and parasitic diseases, and psychotic disorders because of its components (Irgin et al. 2016). Irgin et al. (2016) administrated Stinging nettle and the response was accelerating new bone formation and reducing inflammation in the maxillary expansion procedure.

Ginkgo biloba (Maidenhair tree) leaf extract is used in medicine as coadjutant treatment for memory impairment and dementia as well as Alzheimer's disease; it presents antioxidant, antiplatelet, antihypoxic, antiedemic, hemorheologic, and microcirculatory properties and can improve athletic ability and promote recovery (Kara et al. 2012). Kara et al. (2012) observed new bone formation, number of capillaries, and the ratio of inflammatory cells in maxillary sutures were higher in the *Ginkgo biloba* group than in the control, as well the quantity of osteoblasts and osteoclasts.

St John's wort (*Hypericum perforatum*) has been traditionally used for the treatment of excitability, neuralgia, fibrositis, sciatica, menopausal neurosis, anxiety, and depression, as well as a nerve tonic, and in topical preparations for the treatment of wounds (Halicioglu et al. 2015). Halicioglu et al. (2015) have observed higher number of osteoclasts, capillaries, inflammatory cells infiltration and bone formation using St John's wort.

5. Hemostatic Agents

Hemostatic is characterized by a complex physiological process related to endothelial wall, platelets and plasma factors (Saville & Brow 2008). It can be divided in two parts: primary and secondary hemostatic. Primary hemostatic involves vasoconstriction and platelet adhesion to vascular endothelium. Secondary hemostatic interferes the coagulant formation, during coagulation cascade (Arthus & Pagès 1890, Davie & Ratnoff 1964).

Hemostatic is important for surgical procedures and is related to proper operative technique and anesthetic procedure. However, situations can promote bleeding which can be controlled thru surgical maneuvers and/or hemostatic solutions (Torre et al. 2007).

As in other areas of dentistry and medicine, hemostatic can also be achieved through herbal medicines (Achneck et al. 2010). However, this topic is still little studied. This subchapter comes to elucidate the use of some herbal extracts and their hemostatic action.

5.1. Ankaferd Blood Stopper ABS: Thymus Vulgaris, Glycyrrhiza Glabra, Vitis Vinifera, Alpinia Officinarum e Urtica Dioica

This herbal compound is a potent hemostatic agent of Turkish origin. Its use is applied for management and control of external bleeding and during dental surgeries. Its action occurs through encapsulated protein scaffold formation that allows at focal points the aggregation of erythrocytes. Induced protein formation in erythroid vital aggregation encompasses the entire physiological hemostatic process. Elements such as RBCs (such as spectrin and ankrin surface receptors in addition to the internal ferrocellatase enzyme), related transcription factors (such as GATA-1), and RBC-related proteins (such as urotensin II) are the main objectives of ABS. These proteins, in addition to adenosine triphosphate bioenergy, are also targets during the coagulation process by the product (Kurt et al. 2010).

Cipil et al. (2009) verified the efficacy of this drug on controlling the bleed in rats previously treated with warfarin. The efficacy was assessed by the duration of bleeding and the amount of bleeding occurred. As result they have observed marked decrease in both bleeding duration and amount of blood lost in groups treated topically with ABS. Corroborating this result, Sogut et al. (2015) performed a similar research, however compared with heparin and they concluded that ABS acts more effectively than irrigation using saline in the treatment for hemostasis after tail tip amputation in rats, with or without pretreatment heparin, and the use of compressive dressings.

Complementing these scientific findings, İşler et al. (2010) reported that ABS, besides promoting hemostasis, presents a decrease in inflammatory process and necrosis in bone tissue repair after tibiae defects in rats. Also, no foreign body reactions were found in the ABS groups. Beyond animal researches, Kazancıoğlu et al. (2012) performed a controlled clinical study and have demonstrated the efficacy of ABS during dental extractions performed on hemophiliac patients. By this way, ABS can be a good alternative for hemostatic agents.

5.2. Regenerated Oxidized Cellulose (ROC)

Regenerated oxidized cellulose has been in use since the 1960s, when the first trademark emerged called Surgicel (Sundaram & Keenan 2010). It is classified as vegetal origin because its regeneration of pure cellulose in interlaced and subsequently oxidized cotton fabric. The mainly active ingredient of this hemostatic is anhydroglucuronic acid, which promotes decrease in local pH. Lower pH promotes hemolysis by releasing hemoglobin which will react forming acid hematin (Achneck et al. 2010); however, it can promote significant increase in the inflammatory process and delayed healing process (Tomizawa 2005).

Kim et al. (2016) demonstrate the efficiency of the product in the elimination of bleeding in abdominal surgeries in swine and the results showed no difference in blood loss; however small amounts of fibrosis, foreign bodies and hemorrhages were verified.

The use of ROC may also be indicated for dental patients during dental extractions. Salam et al. (2007) observed that ROC provides excellent hemostasis, even in patients previously treated with warfarin; they concluded that the association of ROC and local suture allows satisfactory hemostasis even for patients using blood thinners. This result was confirmed by Karslı et al. in 2011. In order to evaluated histologically, Gabrielli et al. (2008) extracted rabbit's teeth and applied ROC as hemostatic agents. They saw lower inflammatory infiltrate, as consequence do not interfere during the repair process.

6. Dental Plaque Disclosing Agents

The use of dental plaque disclosing agents is well stablished in scientific literature, as a paramount motivator for oral hygiene, since its use demonstrates the presence and local accumulation of biofilm on dental surface, facilitating visualization and removal (personal or professional), to reduce incidence of caries and periodontal disease (Duarte et al. 1990, Larsen & Fiehn 2017). The dental plaque can be evidenced with special dyes, as fuchsin, iodine, gentian violet, fast green, fluorescein, among others, mainly in the form of tablets, solutions or mouth rinses (Dipayan et al. 2017), whereas the intensity of the color is directly correlated with plaque thickness (Zoya et al. 2015). Interestingly, the presence of dental plaque in specific areas of the oral cavity seems to be influenced by factors such as age, socioeconomic level, body mass index and oral health (Fasoulas et al. 2019). Unusually, an allergenic case caused by synthetic plaque disclosing agent was previously reported (Sania et al. 2016).

6.1. Euterpe Oleracea and Bixa Orellana

In the search for herbal medicines and other natural substances as a substitute of synthetic components, Ribeiro de Nazaré et al. (2007) proposed the formulation of a dental plaque disclosing agent from two natural plants from the Amazonian biodiversity. The extract from açaí berry (*Euterpe oleracea*) and annatto/urucum (*Bixa orellana*) generate dyes entitled anthocyanins (from açaí) and bixin and norbixin (from annatto), which can be used to replace the synthetic dyes available in the dentistry market.

An *in vivo* study was conducted by Ribeiro de Nazaré et al. (2007) to compare the natural with the synthetic disclosing agents, regarding effectiveness in staining dental plaque. The groups consisted in natural dying agents from *Euterpe oleracea* and *Bixa orellana* and commercial dying agents Replak® (Dentsply) and Plakstesim® (Probem), applied in 42 undergraduate students from Pará Federal University (UFPA-Brazil) dentistry course, with intervals of 7 days each. Comparison analysis was performed using a visible plaque index before the application of the disclosing agent and a dye plaque index after the application of the dye substance. Statistical tests of t-Student and ANOVA showed that the disclosing agents based on natural source were more efficient, evidencing about 62% more plaque under naked eye visual perception.

Based on the observed results, the use of dental plaque disclosing agents from *Euterpe oleracea* and *Bixa orellana* extracts are viable alternatives to synthetic agents. In Brazil, patented were required under No. PI 0202465-9 and registered in the United States of America under patent US 7182935B2 (Ribeiro de Nazaré et al. 2007).

References

Achneck, HE; Sileshi, B; Jamiolkowski, RM; Albala, DM et al. A comprehensive review of topical hemostatic agents: efficacy and recommendations for use. *Ann Surg*, 2010, 251, 217-228.

Adnan, S; Lone, MM; Khan, FR; Hussain, SM; Nagi, SE. Which is the most recommended medium for the storage and transport of avulsed teeth? A systematic review. *Dent Traumatol*, 2018, 34(2), 59-70.

Ahangari, Z; Alborzi, S; Yadegari, Z; Dehghani, F; Ahangari, L; Naseri, M. The effect of propolis as a biological storage media on periodontal ligament cell survival in an avulsed tooth: an *in vitro* study. *Cell J*, 2013 Fall, 15(3), 244-9.

Al-Haj, Ali SN; Al-Jundi, S; Mhaidat, N. Comparison of Coconut Water and Jordanian Propolis on Survival of Bench-dried Periodontal Ligament Cells: An *in vitro* Cell Culture Study. *Int J Clin Pediatr Dent*, 2013, 6(3), 161-5.

Andersson, L; Andreasen, JO; Day, P; Heithersay, G; Trope, M; DiAngelis, AJ; et al. International Association of Dental Traumatology guidelines for the management of traumatic dental injuries: 2. Avulsion of permanent teeth. *Dent Traumatol*, 2012, 28(2), 88–96.

Andersson, L. Epidemiology of traumatic dental injuries. *Pediatr Dent*, 2013, 35, 102-5.

Andrade, LC; Rotta, IW; Chaves, SR; Uchida, DT; Gazim, ZC; Ferreira, FBP; Jacomassi, E; Boleta-Ceranto, DCF. Effectiveness of Acmella oleracea for topical anesthesia on buccal mucosa. *Rev Odonto Cienc*, 2013, 28(3), 61-5.

Arthus, M; Pagès, C. Nouvelle theorie chimique de la coagulation du sang. *Arch Physiol Norm Pathol*, 1890, 5, 739-46.

Awawdeh, L; Haimour, RN; Al-Jundi, SH; Al-Qaoud, K. Human periodontal fibroblasts viability stored in Custodiol®; coconut water, and propolis. An *ex vivo* study. *Dent Traumatol*, 2018, 34(4), 264-70.

Babaji, P; Melkundi, M; Devanna, RSSB; Chaurasia, VR5; VGP. *In vitro* comparative evaluation of different storage media (hank's balanced salt solution, propolis, Aloe vera, and pomegranate juice) for preservation of avulsed tooth. *Eur J Dent*, 2017, 11(1), 71-5.

Badakhsh, S; Eskandarian, T; Esmaeilpour, T. The use of aloe vera extract as a novel storage media for the avulsed tooth. *Iran J Med Sci*, 2014, 39(4), 327-32.

Bharath, MJ; Sahadev, CK; Ramachandra, PK; Rudranaik, S; George, J; Thomas, A. Comparative evaluation of four transport media for maintaining cell viability in transportation of an avulsed tooth - An *in vitro* study. *J Int Soc Prev Community Dent*, 2015, 5(1), 69-73.

Casarin, RC; Casati, MZ; Pimentel, SP; Cirano, FR; Algayer, M; Pires, PR; Ghiraldini, B; Duarte, PM; Ribeiro, FV. Resveratrol improves bone repair by modulation of bone morphogenetic proteins and osteopontin gene expression in rats. *Int J Oral Maxillofac Surg*, 2014, 43(7), 900-6.

Casaroto, AR; Hidalgo, MM; Sell, AM; Franco, SL; Cuman, RK; Moreschi, E; Victorino, FR; Steffens, VA; Bersani-Amado, CA. Study of the effectiveness of propolis extract as a storage medium for avulsed teeth. *Dent Traumatol*, 2010, 26(4), 323-31.

Cazzola, M; Ferraris, S; Boschetto, F; Rondinella, A; Marin, E; Zhu, W; Pezzotti, G; Vernè, E1; Spriano, S. Green Tea Polyphenols Coupled with a Bioactive Titanium Alloy Surface: *In Vitro* Characterization of Osteoinductive Behavior through a KUSA A1 Cell Study. *Int J Mol Sci*, 2018, 19(8), 2255.

Cipil, HS; Kosar, A; Kaya, A; Uz, B; et al. *In vivo* hemostatic effect of the medicinal plant extract Ankaferd Blood Stopper in rats pretreated with warfarin. *Clin Appl Thromb Hemost*, 2009, 15, 270-6.

Davie, EW; Ratnoff, OD. Waterfall sequence for intrinsic blood clotting. *Science*, 1964, 1310-12.

de Oliveira, GJ; de Paula, LG; Spin-Neto, R; Stavropoulos, A; Spolidório, LC; Marcantonio, E; Jr. Marcantonio, RA. Effect of avocado/soybean unsaponifiables on osseointegration: a proof-of-principle preclinical *in vivo* study. *Int J Oral Maxillofac Implants*, 2014, 29(4), 949-57.

de Paula, LGF; Lopes de Oliveira, GJP; Pinotti, FE; Grecchi, BB; de Aquino, SG; Chiérici Marcantonio, RA. Effect of Avocado/Soybean Unsaponifiables (ASU) on Osseointegration in Rats with Experimental Arthritis. *Int J Oral Maxillofac Implants*, 2018, 33(3), 603-612.

de Paula Reis, MV; Moura, CC; Soares, PB; Leoni, GB; Souza-Neto, MD; Barbosa, DZ; Soares, CJ. Histologic and micro-computed tomographic analyses of replanted teeth stored in different kind of media. *J Endod*, 2014, 40(5), 665-9.

de Souza, BD; Bortoluzzi, EA; Reyes-Carmona, J; Dos Santos, LG; Simões, CM; Felippe, WT; Felippe, MC. Effect of temperature and seven storage media on human periodontal ligament fibroblast viability. *Dent Traumatol*, 2017, 33(2), 100-5.

Dipayan, D; Ramesh Kumar, SG; Aswath Narayanan, MB; Leena Selvamary, A. Sujatha. Disclosing solutions used in dentistry. *World J Pharmaceut Res*, 2017, 6(6), 1648-56.

Duarte, CA; Lascala, NT; Muench, A. Influence of bacterial plaque disclosing agents on patient oral hygiene motivation under direct supervision and direction. *Rev Odontol Univ Sao Paulo*, 1990, 4, 278-283.

Erdogan, MS; Babacan, H; Kara, MI; Gurler, B; Akgul, H; Soyler, DA. Effect of Capparis spinosa extract on sutural ossification: A stereological study. *Arch Oral Biol*, 2015, 60(8), 1146-52.

Fasoulas, A; Pavlidou, E; Petridis, D; Mantzorou, M; Seroglou, K; Giaginis, C. Detection of dental plaque with disclosing agents in the context of preventive oral hygiene training programs. *Heliyon*, 2019, 5(7), e02064.

Fulzele, P; Baliga, S; Thosar, N; Pradhan, D. Evaluation of Aloe vera Gel as a Storage Medium in Maintaining the Viability of Periodontal Ligament Cells - An *in Vitro* Study. *J Clin Pediatr Dent*, 2016, 40(1), 49-52.

Gabrielli, MAC; Hochuli-Vieira, E; Paleari, AG; Cerri, OS et al. Histologic Evaluation of Hemostatic Agents in the Rabbit Mandible. *Rev Cir Traumatol. Buco-Maxilo-fac*, 2019, 9, 97-106.

Ghasempour, M; Moghadamnia, AA; Abedian, Z; Amir, MP; Feizi, F; Gharekhani, S. *In vitro* viability of human periodontal ligament cells in green tea extract. *J Conserv Dent*, 2015, 18(1), 47-50.

Gjertsen, AW; Stothz, KA; Neiva, KG; Pileggi, R. Effect of propolis on proliferation and apoptosis of periodontal ligament fibroblasts. *Oral Surg Oral Med Oral Pathol Oral Radiol Endod*, 2011, 112(6), 843-8.

Gopikrishna, V; Thomas, T; Kandaswamy, D. A quantitative analysis of coconut water: a new storage media for avulsed teeth. *Oral Surg Oral Med Oral Pathol Oral Radiol Endod*, 2008, 105(2), e61-5.

Gulinelli, JL; Panzarini, SR; Fattah, CM; Poi, WR; Sonoda, CK; Negri, MR; Saito, CT. Effect of root surface treatment with propolis and fluoride in delayed tooth replantation in rats. *Dent Traumatol*, 2008, 24(6), 651-7.

Halicioglu, K; Çörekçi, B; Akkaş, İ; Irgin, C; Özan, F; Yilmaz, F; Türker, A. Effect of St John's wort on bone formation in the orthopaedically expanded premaxillary suture in rats: a histological study. *Eur J Orthod*, 2015, 37(2), 164-9.

Hiremath, G; Kidiyoor, KH. Avulsion and storage media. *J Investig Clin Dent*, 2011, 2(2), 89-94.

Hwang, JY; Choi, SC; Park, JH; Kang, SW. The use of green tea extract as a storage medium for the avulsed tooth. *J Endod*, 2011, 37(7), 962-7.

Irgin, C; Çörekçi, B; Ozan, F; Halicioğlu, K; Toptaş, O; Birinci Yildirim, A; Türker, A; Yilmaz, F. Does stinging nettle (*Urtica dioica*) have an effect on bone formation in the expanded inter-premaxillary suture? *Arch Oral Biol*, 2016, 69, 13-8.

İşler, SC; Demircan, S; Cakarer, S; Cebi, Z; et al. Effects of folk medicinal plant extract Ankaferd Blood Stopper on early bone healing. *J Appl Oral Sci*, 2010, 18, 409-14.

Kara, MI; Altan, AB; Sezer, U; Erdoğan, MŞ; Inan, S; Ozkut, M; Nalcacı, R. Effects of *Ginkgo biloba* on experimental rapid maxillary expansion model: a histomorphometric study. *Oral Surg Oral Med Oral Pathol Oral Radiol*, 2012, 114(6), 712-8.

Karslı, ED.; Erdogan, Ö; Esen, E; Acartürk, E. Comparison of the Effects of Warfarin and Heparin on Bleeding Caused by Dental Extraction: A Clinical Study. *J Oral Maxillofac Surg*, 2011, 69, 2500–2507.

Kazancıoğlu, HO; Cakır, O; Ak, G; Zülfikar, B. The Effectiveness of a New Hemostatic Agent (Ankaferd Blood Stopper) for the Control of Bleeding following Tooth Extraction in Hemophilia: A Controlled Clinical Trial. *Turk J Haematol*, 2013, 30, 19-24.

Kim, SH; Kim, SH; Yoon, HS; Kim, HK; et al. Efficacy of Oxidized Regenerated Cellulose, SurgiGuard®, in Porcine Surgery. *Yonsei Med J*, 2017, 58, 195-205.

Kokkali, VV; Bendgude, V; Sharangpani, G. Comparative evaluation of post-traumatic periodontal ligament cell viability using three storage media. *Eur Arch Paediatr Dent*, 2017, 18(3), 209-214.

Kokkonen, H; Cassinelli, C; Verhoef, R; Morra, M; Schols, HA; Tuukkanen, J. Differentiation of osteoblasts on pectin-coated titanium. *Biomacromolecules*, 2008, 9(9), 2369-76.

Kurt, M; Kekilli, M; Goker, H; Haznedaroglu, IC. Evaluation of hemostatic effects of Ankaferd as an alternative medicine. *Altern Med Rev*, 2010, 15, 329-336.

Larsen, T; Fiehn, NE. Dental biofilm infections - an update. *APMIS*, 2017, 125(4), 376–84.

Martin, MP; Pileggi, R. A quantitative analysis of Propolis: a promising new storage media following avulsion. *Dent Traumatol*, 2004, 20(2), 85-9.

Martins, CM; Hamanaka, EF; Hoshida, TY; Sell, AM; Hidalgo, MM; Silveira, CS; Poi, WR. Dragon's Blood Sap (*Croton Lechleri*) As Storage Medium for Avulsed Teeth: *In Vitro* Study of Cell Viability. *Braz Dent J*, 2016, 27(6), 751-6.

Mazzocchi, A; Montanaro, F. Observational study of the use of Symphytum 5CH in the management of pain and swelling after dental implant surgery. *Homeopathy*, 2012, 101(4), 211-6.

Moazzami, F; Asheghi, B; Sahebi, S. Effect of Four Different Media on Periodontal Ligament Cells Viability of Dry- Stored Dog Teeth. *J Dent (Shiraz)*, 2017, 18(1), 24-29.

Moreira-Neto, JJ; Gondim, JO; Raddi, MS; Pansani, CA. Viability of human fibroblasts in coconut water as a storage medium. *Int Endod J* 2009, 42(9), 827-30.

Mori, GG; Nunes, DC; Castilho, LR; de Moraes, IG; Poi, WR. Propolis as storage media for avulsed teeth: microscopic and morphometric analysis in rats. *Dent Traumatol*, 2010, 26(1), 80-5.

Moura, CC; Soares, PB; de Paula Reis, MV; Fernandes Neto, AJ; Zanetta Barbosa, D; Soares, CJ. Potential of coconut water and soy milk for use as storage media to preserve the viability of periodontal ligament cells: an *in vitro* study. *Dent Traumatol*, 2014, 30(1), 22-6.

Nabavizadeh, M; Abbaszadegan, A; Khodabakhsi, A; Ahzan, S; Mehrabani, D. Efficiency of Castor Oil as a Storage Medium for Avulsed Teeth in Maintaining the Viability of Periodontal Ligament Cells. *J Dent (Shiraz)*, 2018, 19(1), 28-33.

Nomura, EC; Rodrigues, MR; da Silva, CF; Hamm, LA; Nascimento, AM; de Souza, LM; Cipriani, TR; Baggio, CH; Werner, MF. Antinociceptive effects of ethanolic extract from the flowers of *Acmella oleracea* (L.) R. K. Jansen in mice. *J Ethnopharmacol*, 2013, 150(2), 583-9.

Osmanovic, A; Halilovic, S; Kurtovic-Kozaric, A; Hadziabdic, N. Evaluation of periodontal ligament cell viability in different storage media based on human PDL cell culture experiments-A systematic review. *Dent Traumatol*, 2018, 34(6), 384-393.

Ozan, F; Özan, Ü; Oktay, EA; Toptas, O; Özdemir, H; KürÞat, E. Dynamic assessment of Capparis spinosa buds on survival of periodontal ligament cells using a real-time cell analysis method. *Niger J Clin Pract*, 2015, 18(3), 395-9.

Ozan, F; Polat, ZA; Er, K; Ozan, U; Değer, O. Effect of propolis on survival of periodontal ligament cells: new storage media for avulsed teeth. *J Endod*, 2007, 33(5), 570-3.

Ozan, F; Tepe, B; Polat, ZA; Er, K. Evaluation of *in vitro* effect of Morus rubra (red mulberry) on survival of periodontal ligament cells. *Oral Surg Oral Med Oral Pathol Oral Radiol Endod*, 2008, 105(2), e66-9.

Poi, WR; Sonoda, CK; Amaral, MF; Queiroz, AF; França, AB; Brandini, DA. Histological evaluation of the repair process of replanted rat teeth after storage in resveratrol dissolved in dimethyl sulphoxide. *Dent Traumatol*, 2018, 34(4), 254-63.

Poi, WR; Sonoda, CK; Martins, CM; Melo, ME; Pellizzer, EP; de Mendonça, MR; Panzarini, SR. Storage media for avulsed teeth: a literature review. *Braz Dent J*, 2013, 24(5), 437-45.

Prueksakorn, A; Puasiri, S; Ruangsri, S; Makeudom, A; Sastraruji, T; Krisanaprakornkit, S; Chailertvanitkul, P. The preservative effect of Thai propolis extract on the viability of human periodontal ligament cells. *Dent Traumatol*, 2016, 32(6), 495-501.

Resende, KKM; Faria, GP; Longo, DL; Martins, LJO; Costa, CRR. *In vitro* evaluation of plants as storage media for avulsed teeth: A systematic review. *Dent Traumatol*, 2019, 00, 1-16.

Ribeiro de Nazaré, RF; Emmi, DT; Barroso, RFF; da Rocha, PO. Bacterial plaque evidencing composition based on natural colorants. *United States Patent* US 7182935B2 Feb 2007.

Ribeiro, FV; Pimentel, SP; Corrêa, MG; Bortoli, JP; Messora, MR; Casati, MZ. Resveratrol reverses the negative effect of smoking on peri-implant repair in the tibia of rats. *Clin Oral Implants Res*, 2019, 30(1), 1-10.

Rios, MY; Aguilar-Guadarrama, AB; Gutiérrez, Mdel C. Analgesic activity of affinin, an alkamide from *Heliopsis longipes* (Compositae). *J Ethnopharmacol*, 2007, 110(2), 364-7.

Rita, I. Udegbunam; Uzoma, I. Asuzu; Raphael, OC. Kene; Sunday, O. Udegbunam; Chinaka, O. Nwaehujor. Local Anesthetic and Tissue Effects of the Leaf Extract and Fractions of *Sterculia tragacantha Lindl*. *J Pharmacol Toxicol*, 2012, 7(4), 192-8.

Rondanelli, M; Fossari, F; Vecchio, V; Braschi, V; Riva, A; Allegrini, P; Petrangolini, G; Iannello, G; Faliva, MA; Peroni, G; Nichetti, M; Gasparri, C; Spadaccini, D; Infantino, V; Mustafa, S; Alalwan, T;

Perna, S. *Acmella oleracea* for pain management. *Fitoterapia*, 2019, 140, 104419.

Sakakura, CE; Neto, RS; Bellucci, M; Wenzel, A; Scaf, G; Marcantonio, E. Jr. Influence of homeopathic treatment with comfrey on bone density around titanium implants: a digital subtraction radiography study in rats. *Clin Oral Implants Res*, 2008, 19(6), 624-8.

Salam, S; Yusuf, H; Milosevic, A. Bleeding after dental extractions in patients taking warfarin. *Br J Oral Maxillofac Surg*, 2007, 45, 463-6.

Sania, Mohanty S; Aggarwal, MC; Chaubey, KK. An Overaction to Plaque disclosing agent: An Unsual case. *J Periodontal Med Clin Pract*, 2016, 03, 51-5.

Santana de Freitas-Blanco, V; Franz-Montan, M; Groppo, FC; de Carvalho, JE; Figueira, GM; Serpe, L; Oliveira Sousa, IM; Guilherme Damasio, VA; Yamane, LT; de Paula, E; Ferreira Rodrigues, RA. Development and Evaluation of a Novel Mucoadhesive Film Containing *Acmella oleracea* Extract for Oral Mucosa Topical Anesthesia. *PLoS One*, 2016, 11(9), e0162850.

Saville, M; Brown, V. Clinical aspects of coagulation. *Intensive Care Med*, 2007, 8(6), 234-8.

Sharma, M; Sharma, S; Reddy, YG; Mittal, R; Agarwal, V; Singh, C; Singh, A. Evaluation of Periodontal Ligament Cell Viability in Three Different Storage Media: An *in Vitro* Study. *J Dent (Tehran)*, 2015, 12(7), 524-31.

Sogut, O; Erdogan, MO; Kose, R; Boleken, ME; et al. Hemostatic efficacy of a traditional medicinal plant extract (Ankaferd Blood Stopper) in bleeding control. *Clin Appl Thromb Hemost*, 2015, 21, 348-53.

Somsanith, N; Kim, YK; Jang, YS; Lee, YH; Yi, HK; Jang, JH; Kim, KA; Bae, TS; Lee, MH. Enhancing of Osseointegration with Propolis-Loaded TiO_2 Nanotubes in Rat Mandible for Dental Implants. *Materials (Basel)*, 2018, 11(61), 14 p.

Spin-Neto, R; Belluci, MM; Sakakura, CE; Scaf, G; Pepato, MT; Marcantonio, E. Jr. Homeopathic *Symphytum officinale* increases removal torque and radiographic bone density around titanium implants in rats. *Homeopathy*, 2010, 99(4), 249-54.

Sundaram, CP; Keenan, AC. Evolution of hemostatic agents in surgical practice. *Indian J Urol*, 2010, 26, 374-8.

Tavassoli-Hojjati, S; Aliasghar, E; Babaki, FA; Emadi, F; Parsa, M; Tavajohi, S; Ahmadyar, M; Ostad, SN. Pomegranate juice (*Punica granatum*): a new storage medium for avulsed teeth. *J Dent (Tehran)*, 2014, 11(2), 225-32.

Thomas, T; Gopikrishna, V; Kandaswamy, D. Comparative evaluation of maintenance of cell viability of an experimental transport media "coconut water" with Hank's balanced salt solution and milk; for transportation of an avulsed tooth: An *in vitro* cell culture study. *J Conserv Dent*, 2008, 11(1), 22-9.

Tomizawa, Y. Clinical benefits and risk analysis of topical hemostats: a review. *J Artif Organs*, 2005, 8, 137-142.

Torre, RA; Bachman, SL; Wheeler, AA; Bartow, KN; et al. Hemostasis and hemostatic agents in minimally invasive surgery. *Surgery*, 2007, 142, 39-45.

Trindade, LA; de Araújo Oliveira, J; de Castro, RD; de Oliveira Lima, E. Inhibition of adherence of *C. albicans* to dental implants and cover screws by *Cymbopogon nardus* essential oil and citronellal. *Clin Oral Investig*, 2015, 19(9), 2223-31.

Tsuchiya, H. Anesthetic Agents of Plant Origin: A Review of Phytochemicals with Anesthetic Activity. *Molecules*, 2017, 22(8), pii: E1369.

Wang, Y; Wang, XX; Zhang, LN; Jin, SM; Zhang, J. Effects of traditional Chinese medicine on bone remodeling during orthodontic tooth movement. *J Ethnopharmacol*, 2012, 141(2), 642-6.

Wimolsantirungsri, N; Makeudom, A; Louwakul, P; Sastraruji, T; Chailertvanitkul, P; Supanchart, C; Krisanaprakornkit, S. Inhibitory effect of Thai propolis on human osteoclastogenesis. *Dent Traumatol*, 2018, 34(4), 237-44.

Yuan, XJ; Wang, YY; Shi, BQ; Zhao, YM. Effect of propolis on preserving human periodontal ligament cells and regulating pro-inflammatory cytokines. *Dent Traumatol*, 2018, 34(4), 245-53.

Zoya, C; Ranjana, M; Vandana, S; Rohit, R; Aruna, D. Disclosing agents in periodontics, an update. *J Dent Coll Azamgarh*, 2015, 1(1), 103–110.

About the Editor

Carlos Roberto Emerenciano Bueno

Professor, Post-Graduate Dental Science, Department of Endodontics, São Paulo State University (UNESP), Araçatuba School of Dentistry, Araçatuba, São Paulo, Brazil;

Department of Endodontics, São Paulo State University (UNESP), Araçatuba School of Dentistry, Araçatuba, São Paulo, Brazil

Email: dentistabueno@gmail.com

Professor Carlos Roberto Emerenciano Bueno studied dentistry at Federal University of Amazonas (UFAM), in Manaus city. After graduation, joined the Brazilian Army as a dentist, working in the frontier between Brazil and Colombia. There, in the free time, Dr. Carlos Bueno studied the beauty of Endodontics with his favorites books and after doing his time in the army, he specialized in Endodontics in Bauru dental school. After the course completion, he continued studying at the post-graduation program of Araçatuba School of Dentistry, in São Paulo State University (FOA/UNESP), obtaining the Master of Science (MSc) and Philosophy Doctor (PhD) degrees in endodontics, publishing several papers regarding biological response to endodontic materials and plant extracts, besides the publication of several chapters in different fields of dentistry.

INDEX

B

C

D

E

F

G

H

I

K

L

M

N

O

P

V

W

X

Z